Essentials of Aerosol Therapy in Critically ill Patients

Mohamed E. A. Abdelrahim
Haitham Saeed • Hadeer S. Harb
Yasmin M. Madney

Essentials of Aerosol Therapy in Critically ill Patients

Springer

Mohamed E. A. Abdelrahim
Department of Clinical Pharmacy
Beni-Suef University
Beni-Suef
Egypt

Haitham Saeed
Department of Clinical Pharmacy
Beni-Suef University
Beni-Suef
Egypt

Hadeer S. Harb
Department of Clinical Pharmacy
Beni-Suef University
Beni-Suef
Egypt

Yasmin M. Madney
Department of Clinical Pharmacy
Beni-Suef University
Beni-Suef
Egypt

ISBN 978-3-030-85025-8 ISBN 978-3-030-85026-5 (eBook)
https://doi.org/10.1007/978-3-030-85026-5

This Springer imprint is published by the registered company Springer Nature Switzerland AG
The registered company address is: Gewerbestrasse 11, 6330 Cham, Switzerland

Preface

Aerosol therapy is applied for the treatment of several pulmonary diseases in addition to some promising applications intended for systemic absorption. Nowadays, aerosol delivery to clinically stable patients in outpatient settings is done easily with a lot of focus on patient counseling and enhancement of lung deposition. A lot of guidelines are available for several diseases, and it could offer adequate guidance to the therapists concerning escalation or de-escalation of therapy to enhance treatment efficiency and safety. However, in critically ill patients, aerosol delivery is mostly done by the choice of the respiratory therapist only according to his or her knowledge.

This book describes the type of patients requiring aerosol therapy, different aerosol generators available for the treatment of critically ill patients, mechanisms of aerosol lung deposition, and factors affecting aerosol deposition. It also discusses the special needs of neonates and infants, transitioning of aerosol from hospital to home, and methods of aerosol delivery to different patients, e.g., nasal delivery patients and ventilated patients. Moreover, it reviews methods of detecting such aerosol delivery to the lung. At the end, it discusses the suggested monitoring plans and weaning protocols to ensure high efficacy and safety of the ventilatory support in such patients. We hope that this book could serve as guidelines or specific recommendations to maximize clinical benefits of medicated aerosols in critically ill patients.

The Editors.

Beni-Suef, Egypt Mohamed E. A. Abdelrahim
Beni-Suef, Egypt Haitham Saeed
Beni-Suef, Egypt Hadeer S. Harb
Beni-Suef, Egypt Yasmin M. Madney

Contents

Abbreviations

ACT	Asthma control test
AAD	Adaptive aerosol delivery
ABG	Arterial blood gases
ACQ	Asthma control questionnaire
AIM	Aerosol Inhalation Monitor
ATAQ	The Asthma Therapy Assessment Questionnaire
AC	Assist control
ACPE	Acute cardiogenic pulmonary edema
AHI	Apnea-hypopnea index
ARDS	Acute respiratory distress syndrome
AutoPEEP	Unintended positive end-expiratory pressure
BA-pMDIs	Breath-actuated pMDIs
BC-pMDIs	Breath-coordinated pMDIs
BDP	Beclometasone dipropionate
BP	Blood pressure
BTS/RCP	British Thoracic Society/Royal College of Physicians
BiPAP	Bilevel positive airway pressure
CAT	COPD assessment test
CCQ	Clinical COPD questionnaire
CF	Cystic fibrosis
CFC	Chlorofluorocarbons
CNS	Central nervous system
COPD	Chronic obstructive pulmonary disease
CFD	Computational fluid dynamic
C-ACT	Childhood asthma control test
CMD	Count median diameter
CPAP	Continuous positive air pressure
CV	Coefficient of variation
CMV	Continuous mandatory ventilation
CWD	Chest wall disease
CSV	Continuous spontaneous ventilation

DPI	Dry powder inhaler
DDAVP	1-Desamino-8-d-arginine vasopressin
DLCO	Carbon monoxide diffusing capacity
ECMO	Extracorporeal membrane oxygenation
ED	Emergency department
Hi-VNI	High-velocity nasal insufflation Vapotherm system
ECD	Effective cutoff diameter
EAdi	Electrical activity of the diaphragm
ECG	Electrocardiogram
EMG	Electromyography
EPAP	Expiratory positive airway pressure
EPO	Erythropoietin
ETCO2	End-tidal carbon dioxide
ETT	Endotracheal tube
EUCAST	European Committee on Antimicrobial Susceptibility Testing
F	Flow through the inhaler
FiO_2	Fractional inspired concentration of oxygen
FPD	Fine particle dose
FPF	Fine particle fraction
FVC	Forced vital capacity
FEV1	Forced expiratory volume in one second
GIT	Gastrointestinal tract
GINA	Global Initiative for Asthma
GOLD	Global Initiative for Chronic Obstructive Lung Disease
GSD	Geometric standard deviation
GSD	Geometric standard deviation
Hb A1C	Glycated hemoglobin
Heliox	Helium and oxygen
HFA	Hydrofluoroalkane
HFNC	High-flow nasal cannula
hGH	Human growth hormone
HME	Heat and moisture exchanger
HPLC	High-performance liquid chromatography
HFCs	Hydrofluorocarbons
HRQol	Health-related quality of life
HR	Heart rate
IM	Inhalation manager
IFR	Inspiratory flow rate
ICS	Inhaled corticosteroids
ICU	Intensive care unit
IMV	Invasive mechanical ventilation
INFα 2b	Interferon alpha-2b
IPAP	Inspiratory positive airway pressure
iPEEP	Intrinsic positive end-expiratory pressure
IV	Intravenous

IgE	Immunoglobulin E
JN	Jet nebulizer
LABA	Long-acting β_2-agonists
LAMA	Long-acting muscarinic antagonist
LFNC	Low-flow nasal cannula
LV	Low air volume
LTOT	Long-term oxygen therapy
MDR	Multidrug resistant
mMRC	Modified Medical Research Council score
MMAD	Mass median aerodynamic diameter
MAP	Mean airway pressure
MIC	Minimum inhibitory concentration
MIP	Maximal inspiratory pressure
MMI	Marple-Miller Cascade Impactor
MMD	Mass median diameter
MSLI	Multistage liquid impinger
MV	Mechanical ventilation
NAEPP	The National Asthma Education and Prevention Program
NFA	Near-fatal asthma
NIPPV	Noninvasive positive-pressure ventilation
MVV	Maximal voluntary ventilation
NGI	Next-generation impactor
NAVA	Neurally adjusted ventilatory assist
NIV	Noninvasive ventilation
NMD	Neuromuscular disease
OR	Operating room
OSA	Obstructive sleep apnea
OPCs	Optical particle counters
pMDI	Pressurized metered-dose inhaler
PET	Positron-emission tomography
SPECT	Single-photon emission computed tomography
SPE	Solid-phase extraction
O_2COB	Oxygen cost of breathing
OI	Oxygenation index
P0.1	Airway occlusion pressure (airway pressure generated in the first 100 ms of inspiration against an expiratory occlusion)
Pa_{O2}/FI_{O2}	Partial pressure of arterial oxygen/fractional inspired concentration of oxygen
PAO_2	Partial pressure of alveolar oxygen
*P*aw	Positive airway pressure
PC	Pressure-controlled
PaO_2	Partial pressure of oxygen
pCO_2	Partial pressure of carbon dioxide
*P*cw	Chest wall elastic recoil
PD	Pharmacodynamics

PAV	Proportional assist
*P*di	Transdiaphragmatic pressure
PEEP	Positive end-expiratory pressure
PEF	Peak expiratory flow
*P*es	Esophageal pressure
*P*ga	Gastric pressure
PIFR	Peak inspiratory flow rate
PIP	Peak inspiratory pressure
PK	Pharmacokinetics
*P*L	Transpulmonary pressure
*P*mus	Inspiratory muscle pressure
*P*pl	Pleural pressure
*P*plat	Plateau pressure
PS	Pressure support
P-SILI	Patient self-inflicted lung injury
PSV	Pressure-support ventilation
PTP	Pressure-time product
PVD	Patient-ventilator dyssynchrony
PC	Pressure-controlled
PC-CMV	Pressure-controlled continuous mandatory ventilation
PC-CSV	Pressure-controlled continuous spontaneous ventilation
PC-IMV	Pressure-controlled intermittent mandatory ventilation
PDE4	Phosphodiesterase-4
PEFR	Peak expiratory flow rate
PIFR	Peak inspiratory flow rate
PRVC	Pressure-regulated volume control
PSV	Pressure support ventilation
R	Resistance in the inhaler device
rhDNase	Recombinant human deoxyribonuclease
RR	Respiratory rate
SABA	Short-acting β_2-agonists
SAMA	Short-acting muscarinic antagonist
SaO_2	Oxygen saturation
SBT	Spontaneous breathing trial
sGaw	Specific airway conductance
SABA	Short-acting B2-agonist
SaO_2	Oxygen saturation
SIMV	Synchronized intermittent mandatory ventilation
SMI	Soft mist inhaler
SRT	Surfactant replacement therapy
TRACK	Test of respiratory and asthma control in kids
t1/2	Half-life
$TcpCO_2$	Transcutaneous partial pressure of carbon dioxide
Te	Expiratory time
TED	Total emitted dose

TFdi	Thickening fraction of diaphragm
Ti	Inspiratory time
TV	Tidal volume
TST	Tracheostomy tube
USN	Ultrasonic nebulizer
VMD	Volume median diameter
V50	50% of vital capacity
VAP	Ventilator-associated pneumonia
VC	Vital capacity
VC	Volume-controlled
VE	Exhaled volume/breath
VILI	Ventilator-induced lung injury
VMN	Vibrating mesh nebulizer
Vt	Tidal volume
VHC	Valved holding chamber
VAEs	Ventilator-associated events
VAP	Ventilator-associated pneumonia
VC-CMV	Volume-controlled continuous mandatory ventilation
VC-IMV	Volume-controlled intermittent mandatory ventilation
VTV	Volume-targeted ventilation
WOB	Work of breathing
β_2	Beta 2
ΔP	Driving pressure
ΔPL	Dynamic swing in the transpulmonary pressure
ΔPocc	Airway pressure swing during the occlusion
18FDG	18-Fluorodeoxyglucose

Chapter 1
The Type of Patients Requiring Aerosol Therapy (to Treat What and Where?)

Contents

Abbreviations

ABG	Arterial blood gases
CAT	COPD assessment test
COPD	Chronic obstructive pulmonary disease
ED	Emergency department
FEV_1	Forced expiratory volume in one second
FVC	Forced vital capacity
GINA	Global initiative for asthma
GOLD	Global initiative for chronic obstructive lung disease
ICs	Inhaled corticosteroids
ICU	Intensive care unit

M. E. A. Abdelrahim et al., *Essentials of Aerosol Therapy in Critically ill Patients*,
https://doi.org/10.1007/978-3-030-85026-5_1

IgE	Immunoglobulin E
LABA	Long-acting B2-agonists
LAMA	Long-acting muscarinic antagonists
mMRC	Modified Medical Research Council score
NAEPP	The National Asthma Education and Prevention program
NFA	Near-fatal asthma
NIV	Noninvasive ventilation
PDE4	Phosphodiesterase-4
PEFR	Peak expiratory flow rate
pMDIs	Pressurized metered-dose inhalers
SABA	Short-acting B2-agonist

1.1 Introduction

Aerosol therapy simply describes the delivery of drug molecules loaded on inhaled gases to the patient which represents the mainstay of treating respiratory diseases e.g. asthma, chronic obstructive pulmonary disease (COPD), and cystic fibrosis. Its use is mainly indicated to produce bronchodilator and anti-inflammatory activities and also inhaled antibiotics can be used to treat infections as in cystic fibrosis [1, 2]. The inhaled drugs are not limited to treat pulmonary diseases only but also have a role in the management of non-pulmonary disorders. This route of drug administration exhibits many advantages supporting its use such as the need for lower drug doses when compared with traditional routes e.g. oral and intravenous, rapid onset of action, and produced local effect with minimal systemic adverse effects [3]. Targeting a certain drug to specific diseased areas in the lung is a major purpose of using aerosolized medicines. There are two approaches to target a drug to the lung: passive and active targeting. Passive targeting mainly depends on enhancing aerosol deposition in the peripheral airways and the alveolar region by adjusting many factors such as particle size, aerosol dosage, gas density, breathing pattern, duration of breath-hold, and others. The modification of these factors also decreases the oropharyngeal deposition of the delivered drug which lowers the local and systemic side effects of the swallowed fraction. On the other hand, active targeting aims at localizing the deposition of the drug in the pulmonary diseased area through using biological or molecular recognition [3]. Aerosol therapy is largely prescribed for various patient populations e.g. neonates, pediatrics, and adults either at home for stable conditions or during hospitalization when dealing with critical situations. Of note, pediatrics show different anatomical, physiological, and behavioral characteristics than adults which in turn can affect aerosol delivery [4]. Inhalation therapy is largely given in pulmonary critical care. Patients in intensive care units (ICUs are typically ventilator-dependent but treatment in critical care units can be also provided for non-invasively ventilated patients and those with artificial airways [5].

1.2 Differences Between Pediatrics and Adults Influencing Aerosol Delivery

Aerosol therapy is affected by airway size, lung volume, inspiratory flow, inhalation route, and breathing pattern which are completely different in pediatrics when compared with adults. So, effective inhalation therapy will be determined at any development stage based on these factors. Children have slower inspiratory flow and smaller lung volume than adults. During aerosol inhalation, slow inspiratory flow results in lower aerosol loss due to inertial impaction in the oronasopharyngeal region [6]. The increase in age results in a subsequent elevation in both lung volume and inspiratory flow but with a more regular breathing pattern and slower respiratory rate. Stabilization of respiratory variables is reached by the age of 12 years where these variables are approximately the same as adults. Additionally, children are obligate nose breathers and exhibit smaller airways which largely attribute to higher aerosol deposition in upper airways and lower deposition in the lower respiratory tract than adults. Children also show differences in the rate of drug clearance and elimination half-life over adults as they are more rapid drug metabolizers exhibiting a smaller drug half-life [6].

1.3 Diseases Treated by Aerosol Therapy

1.3.1 Asthma

Asthma is a condition accompanied by airflow obstruction that markedly differs spontaneously or with treatment. Asthmatic patients exhibit a particular form of airway inflammation that makes them more susceptible to various stimuli than non-asthmatics which results in excessive airway narrowing with a subsequent airflow reduction and breathlessness. This existing airway narrowing is reversible in most cases but chronic asthmatic patients can exhibit irreversible airflow obstruction. At any age, asthma can occur at the age of 3 years which can be considered the peak age for its occurrence. Additionally, asthma affects women twice as men but this ratio is equalized by puberty. Symptoms of asthma usually disappear during adolescence but may return in adulthood in those with severe disease and persistent symptoms [7, 8]. Asthma etiology is multifactorial where the inflammation of airways developed in a genetically susceptible person with atopy on exposure to certain environmental stimuli. Atopy refers to the tendency of an individual when exposed to small quantities of an antigen to produce large amounts of immunoglobulin E (IgE). The incidence of other diseases like urticaria, allergic rhinitis, and eczema is also elevated in atopic individuals. Asthma triggers may be seasonal (outdoor) or perennial (indoor). Recognizing the trigger factors which induce the respiratory attack or crisis plays a great role in determining the treatment of asthma [9]. Outdoor allergens include pollen from weeds, grass, or trees, detected throughout the year at different times while indoor allergens include exposures to dust traces, cockroaches, mice, molds, and dander from pets. Other asthma triggers include cigarette smoke, passive smoking, occupational exposures, strong odors, extreme changes in temperature, and exercise [10, 11].

1.3.1.1 Asthma Diagnosis

To have a confident asthma diagnosis, patients should undergo pulmonary function testing with reporting existing symptoms. Of note, asthma symptoms are always nonspecific and mimic several diseases so the exclusion of these diseases is critical especially in elderly patients [10]. The clinical presentation of asthma includes many allergic symptoms like breathlessness, tachycardia, wheezing, and coughs, where up to 27% of asthmatic patients have daily symptoms. There is an extreme variation in the clinical presentation between each asthma attack not only in different individuals but also in a single patient [8]. Additionally, a strong relationship is found between asthma development and genetic predisposition so the family history regarding asthma or allergies, in general, is so important to rule out asthma. Asthma can be diagnosed and classified into mild, moderately severe, severe, and imminent respiratory failure based on frequency and duration of symptoms, exacerbation intensity, and frequency of administering a reliever medication. The most important tests used for asthma diagnosis are spirometry, x-ray findings, and methacholine challenge test besides the presence of asthma risk factors as allergies, pollution, smoking, and poverty [9, 12]. Global Initiative for Asthma (GINA) considers spirometry as the preferred diagnostic tool for asthma where airflow limitation measurement, reversibility, or methacholine challenge test can also aid the diagnosis. The interpretation of the findings by a specialist can maximize the benefits from these diagnostic tools [12–14]. Table 1.1 illustrates findings of physical examination based on the classification of an asthma attack. If asthma is the likely diagnosis based on the history of the patient and physical examination findings, the following step is to conduct spirometry testing pre and post-bronchodilator inhalation to determine the two main characters fundamental to accurately diagnose the disease: airflow limitation reversibility and expiratory airflow obstruction. Of note, spirometry

Table 1.1 Risk factors for asthma-related mortality [15]

Comorbidities as heart diseases or another chronic pulmonary disease
Unauthorized drug use
Low socioeconomic status
Difficulty perceiving exacerbation severity of airway obstruction
The previous history of severe exacerbation led to ICU admission or intubation
Major psychiatric disorders
Refills of short-acting beta2 agonist two or more times per month
Three or more ED visits in the previous year

results are often normal as long as asthma is well controlled despite the key feature of the disease is variable in both symptoms and airflow limitation [10].

Asthmatic patients who initially present with more severe disease status may not show full reversibility in expiratory flow obstruction after inhaling the standard bronchodilator dose. The same can be noticed in chronically uncontrolled asthmatic patients because of airway remodeling [10].

The airflow limitation is simply described by a ratio of forced expiratory volume in one second (FEV_1) to forced vital capacity (FVC) less than 70% while positive bronchodilator responsiveness is indicated when the increase in FEV_1/FVC ratio is higher than 12% or 200 mL after administering bronchodilator. If the variability in airflow limitation isn't identified by reversibility testing with spirometry and asthma is still clinically suspected, in this case, the use of a peak flow meter may be recommended. The patient is asked to record peak expiratory flow twice daily for 2 weeks or more during the onset of respiratory symptoms. Variable airflow limitation can be also identified by excessive variable peak flows in the setting of normal spirometry which assures asthma diagnosis. The successful management of asthma depends on the continuous reassessment of the disease due to variability seen in symptoms and airflow limitation over time. This continual reassessment enables optimal control of the disease, treatment of underlying inflammation, and lowering the adverse effects from prescribed medication [10, 16]. Of note, lung functions are difficult to be assessed in preschoolers (age less than 6 years). Therefore, the diagnosis will be mainly dependent on the clinical history (involving the related risk factors for possible asthma development and the family history) in addition to physical examination. The purpose of that physical examination is to differentiate between asthma and other conditions with episodic respiratory symptoms [17]. As various preschool conditions exhibit an obstructive pattern presenting as asthma–like symptoms (e.g., cough, wheezing, and shortness of breath) which makes the diagnosis at such age represents a challenge [18, 19]. Therefore differential and correct diagnosis are essential to effectively manage and treat asthma and consequently the potential harm of misdiagnosis is lowered [19].

1.3.1.2 Asthma Phenotypes

Various disease phenotypes have been recognized. The most common examples are allergic asthma: this asthmatic phenotype often occurs among children. This phenotype is easily recognized. It is usually associated with family and/or past allergic history either allergic disease, e.g. allergic rhinitis, and eczema, or drug or food allergy [20]. Before treatment when the induced sputum is examined for these patients, it often shows eosinophilic airway inflammation. These patients show a better response to the inhaled corticosteroids (ICs) therapy [21].

Non-allergic asthma: this phenotype occurs among adults who exhibit asthma which is not accompanied by allergy. The inflammatory cells found in the patient sputum may be eosinophilic or neutrophilic in type or the sputum only contains a few cells. The response of patients with this phenotype to ICs therapy is less well [21].

Late-onset asthma: this phenotype is identified when some adults especially women complaining of asthma and it is the first time to have such symptoms in their lives. Also, this phenotype is non-allergic and patients may benefit from ICs in relatively higher doses or maybe somewhat refractory or insusceptible to ICs treatment [21].

Asthma with fixed airflow limitation: Persistent airway remodeling may be developed in patients suffering from long-standing asthma and consequently lead to fixed airflow limitation [21].

Asthma with obesity: this asthmatic phenotype is characterized by prominent respiratory symptoms in some obese patients and few eosinophilic inflammatory cells found in the sputum [21].

1.3.1.3 Asthma Management

Good symptom control, minimizing future exacerbation risk and fixed airflow limitations are the goals of asthma management in long term. The goals exhibited by the patient concerning their disease condition and its treatment is also needed to be identified [22].

Non-pharmacological Treatment

The cornerstone for asthma management is the avoidance of triggers. In patients with seasonal sensitivity or allergies to air pollutions, they should be advised to stay at home and close windows at times where the quality of outdoor air is poor or the air exhibit a high quantity of pollens [10, 11]. Smoking cessation and weight loss in obese patients are claimed to improve symptoms. Breathing exercise programs which are often delivered by a physiotherapist are encouraged as an adjunct to pharmacological treatment to decrease symptoms and improve life quality [23].

Pharmacological Treatment

For long term asthma treatment, the available pharmacological options are classified into three main groups:

- Controller medications: they are considered as regular maintenance treatment used to control symptoms, minimize airway inflammation and reduce the risk of both future exacerbations and the possible lung function decline. They mainly prevent the occurrence of persistent or irreversible airway remodeling [22]. For that, the controller medications are given to all patients with persistent asthma and even if mild disease status presents. Patients should know that they have a chronic disease and the absence of symptoms is due to the effective controller therapy. The wrong thought of '"no symptoms, no asthma" unfortunately leads to worse clinical outcomes [10, 24]. Inhaled corticosteroids (ICs) are the mainstay for controller therapy. They can result in common side effects as oral thrush and dysphonia. Oral thrush can be effectively lowered by the use of a spacer with pressurized metered-dose inhalers (pMDIs) and also by rinsing the mouth after receiving the dose. When to initiate ICs treatment is the key issue here. The early introduced ICs therapy has shown benefits in patients with very few symptoms or mild and intermittent asthma. The introduction of ICs therapy is recommended in patients who experience asthma symptoms more than two times in the last week (use albuterol inhaler more than two times per week for symptoms relief). Also, an exacerbation within the last year relieved by oral corticosteroid is often considered as a necessity for regular ICs therapy to decrease further exacerbation risk [25].

- Add-on therapies used for patients suffering from severe asthma. These medications can be prescribed for patients with persistent symptoms or having exacerbations despite optimized therapy with controller medications (ICs) [22]. Add-on therapies such as long-acting beta-agonists (LABA) or leukotriene modifiers can be given with concomitant ICs therapy if symptoms control is suboptimal where LABA is more effective than leukotriene modifiers [26, 27]. Long-acting muscarinic antagonists (LAMA) can also be used as an add-on therapy for asthma management showing the same effectiveness as LABA, and they are usually administered for patients with severe disease [27, 28]. Prescribing LABA only as monotherapy without concomitant ICs administration is contraindicated in asthmatic patients as they are associated with an increased risk of asthma-related deaths [10].
- Rescue or reliever medications: they are prescribed to all asthmatic patients to be administered as needed to relieve breakthrough symptoms. All patients who receive an initial diagnosis of asthma, usually prescribed short-acting bronchodilators to relieve asthma symptoms. Patients with intermittent asthma can be maintained only on short-acting bronchodilators. Also, these medications are recommended for prophylaxis from exercise-induced bronchoconstriction. A rescue inhaler containing albuterol is often offered to asthmatic patients where it can be used up to four times per day. Appropriately instructed adult patients can benefit from the drug delivered by pMDI with or without a spacer or by a nebulizer to the same extent but in practice, pMDI with a spacer and nebulizers deliver a more reliable drug dose. When the reliever treatment need is reduced or ideally eliminated is regarded as a success measure of asthma treatment and the main goal achieved in asthma management [22]. However, new 2019 GINA guidelines conclude that short-acting bronchodilators alone are no longer the preferred reliever agent and recommend the use of low dose ICs with Formoterol as a combination across all asthma severities to produce quick relieving of symptoms [29]. Treatment of asthma is performed in therapeutic steps with higher steps showing the excessive controller therapy (Fig. 1.1).

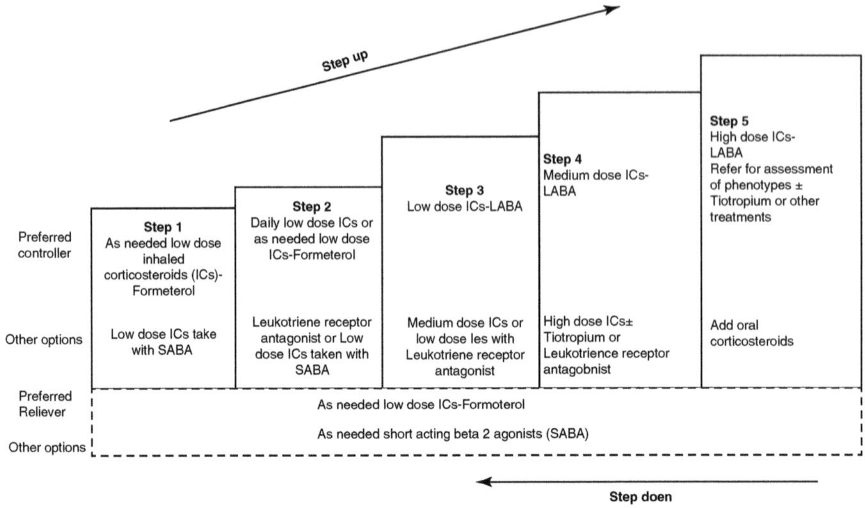

Fig. 1.1 Stepwise approach for asthma management

1.3.1.4 Asthma Exacerbations

Patients of all ages can experience signs and symptoms of respiratory distress causing them to enter the emergency department (ED). Initial assessment of those patients aims to determine respiratory distress severity and if an acute asthma exacerbation is a cause [30]. Unfortunately, severe asthma exacerbations can be fatal unless they are closely monitored for deterioration and promptly treated. Patient improvement can be assessed by serial pulmonary function measurement [31].

The National Asthma Education and Prevention Program (NAEPP) Expert Panel suggests that all clinicians dealing with asthmatic patients should be aware of the symptoms and signs of severe exacerbations, identifying risk factors associated with asthma-related mortality, and finally how to effectively treat an exacerbation [32]. Near-fatal asthma (NFA) risk factors are illustrated in Table 1.1. The increased use of B2-agonists administered either through pressurized metered-dose inhalers or nebulizers, oral corticosteroids, and theophylline and previous patient history of hospital stay or ICU admission due to asthma are strong predictors for NFA [33]. Patients experiencing an exacerbation should immediately be evaluated and started proper treatment based on the type of exacerbation: mild, moderate, severe, or life-threatening. Table 1.2 illustrates the difference in physical examination findings between various types of asthma exacerbations. The global ABC (airway, breathing, and circulation) concept must be maintained in severely symptomatic asthma patients while patients experiencing respiratory failure are in great need of ventilator support which requires detailed physical examination and history taking [30]. Clinicians should assess the pulmonary function of the patient unless he/she experiences a respiratory extremis and laboratory tests are performed as needed only [32].

Table 1.2 Physical examination findings based on the type of asthma exacerbation [8]

Classification	General examination	Respiratory examination	Vital signs
Mild	Complete sentences (+/−) Agitation	Moderate end-expiratory wheezing	Heart rate < 100 Elevated respiratory rate O_2 saturation > 95%
Moderate severe	Unable to speak in full sentences	(+/−) Use of accessory muscle Loud expiratory wheezing	Heart rate 100–120 Elevated respiratory rate O_2 saturation low 90 (+/−) paradoxical pulse
Severe	Unable to breathe at rest Unable to lie down agitated	Use of accessory muscle Loud biphasic wheezing	Heart rate > 120 Elevated respiratory rate O_2 saturation < 91% Paradoxical pulse
Imminent respiratory failure	Altered mental status Diaphoresis	Absent breath sounds Absent wheezing	Bradycardia Absent paradoxical pulse

The clinical patient presentation provides key information. For example, signs like high blood pressure, increased heart rate, and respiratory rate increase the likelihood for aggressive emergency treatment while signs of low blood pressure and heart rate indicating the decreased cardiac output are predictors for immediate resuscitative interventions and also increase the need for excluding the presence of other complications as pneumothorax and pneumomediastinum. Respiratory failure signs which necessitate the preparation for intubation include increased sweating, confusion or drowsiness, a silent chest, and paradoxical thoracoabdominal movement. The presence of severe exacerbations is assumed by the presence of speaking inability, taking tripod position and evidence of accessory muscles use. Additionally, pulse oximetry can be used as a guide for exacerbation severity. Oxygen saturation values lower than 90% on room air are an indication for severe exacerbation where supplemental oxygen is administered as urgent treatment and oxygen is regularly measured and followed in the emergency department. Measurement of arterial blood gases (ABG) is considered when a conflict presents between patient presentation and other clinical information. Also, ABG measurement is must be done to follow critically ill patients close to requiring respiratory support. The ABG measurement in case of mild and moderate exacerbations indicates the presence of respiratory alkalosis and has no role in guiding clinical care in such situations. Increased CO_2 serves as a sign for severe disease and possibly respiratory failure while metabolic acidosis is a strong predictor of very severe disease. More ever, chest auscultation can be used to evaluate the airway obstruction severity through listening for the quantity and quality of airflow and wheezing. Obstructions of the upper or large airway can be identified by monophasic wheezing or stridor heard over the central airways or generally over the neck. By using chest auscultation, one can determine the prolongation in the exhalation phase of the breathing cycle determining the severity of acute asthma. The inhalation to exhalation ratio is 1:1 in case of mild bronchospasm and 1:3 in case of severe obstruction while a silent chest is an indicator for very severe disease status and possibly respiratory failure. On the other hand, the accuracy of assessing the degree of bronchospasm in asthmatic patients based only on clinical examination is less reliable. So, the forced exhalation maneuver is usually used as a standard technique to achieve an accurate assessment of airflow limitation. The most common measurement device used for this reason is the peak expiratory flow meter while a spirometer is less commonly used. Peak expiratory flow meter measures peak expiratory flow rate (PEFR) while spirometer measures many pulmonary function parameters importantly forced expiratory volume in 1 s (FEV_1) here. These measurement devices have some advantages such as objectivity and having numerical value for the patient to follow him during therapy to evaluate the treatment course through comparing his current results with baseline or predicted values [30].

Manage a critically ill asthmatic patient is a challenge for the health care team as the patient exhibits many complications as hypoxemia, hypotension, dysthymia, pulmonary aspiration, pneumothorax, worsening bronchospasm, and dynamic hyperinflation. These devastating complications increase the need for mechanical ventilation but the reported outcomes are encouraging when compared with other diseases requiring respiratory support [34].

Prevention of Exacerbations

Asthma management has four essential components which include education of patients, symptoms and pulmonary function monitoring, control of risk factors and comorbidities, and monitoring of pharmacologic therapy. Patient education about asthma enables disease control and decreases the risk of future exacerbations. However, the severity of asthma varies among affected individuals, it is necessary to monitor the therapy effectiveness in controlling asthma to determine any required adjustments on treatment [35, 36].

Management of Asthma Exacerbations

Supplemental oxygen and inhaled short-acting bronchodilators should be administered to all patients who exhibited symptoms and signs of asthma exacerbation by emergency medical services providers. Patients can receive during transportation to the hospital up to three bronchodilator treatments within the first hour and after that one treatment per hour [35, 37]. However, mild asthma exacerbations are mostly treated at home and in some cases in the outpatient clinic by salbutamol delivered either by pMDI with a holding chamber or a nebulizer which is considered the first-line medication for management of a mild exacerbation [32]. It provides immediate symptomatic relief without affecting airway inflammation or exerting a sustained effect. Studies that investigated the delivery of salbutamol through either pMDI or nebulizer have shown the same effectiveness of both modalities to provide inhaled particles with the optimal diameter of 1–5 μm to the lower airways with no significant difference between them in hospital admission rate, hospital stay length, and

PEFR [38]. Preference of one modality over the other will be determined by patient factors as the respiratory distress degree which gives information on the ability of the patient to coordinate respiratory efforts with MDI use [38] Administering a short-acting B2-agonist (SABA) via a nebulizer is a good option for patients experiencing difficulties with pMDI use especially those with a more pronounced airflow limitation but data on whether continuous nebulization or intermittent nebulization being superior is so conflicted.

Generally, an exacerbation of mild severity is confirmed by the suitable and complete responsiveness to inhaled salbutamol or SABA with an improvement of existing symptoms like wheezing, dyspnea, and cough. These patients usually require no additional therapy and discharge from the hospital with a regular follow-up schedule [38]. They should be appropriately instructed on the proper use of inhaling devices and spacers. On the other hand, patients with a mild attack with improper and incomplete response to SABA or those with moderate exacerbation features should instantly administer supplemental oxygen, a SABA, and oral corticosteroids and during that initial and serial assessment of PEFR are carried out [30]. Systemic corticosteroids enhance the resolution of airflow limitation and decrease the post-ED relapse rate with their maximum benefit appeared when they administered as early as possible. They should be given to patients with moderate and severe exacerbations and those who do not initially respond to B2 agonists. Oral prednisone shows the same effectiveness as intravenous methylprednisolone. In mild exacerbations, systemic corticosteroids may be given as supplemental doses [39, 40]. The data is limited to support the use of inhaled corticosteroids as an alternative or adjunct to systemic corticosteroids when the patient is discharged from the emergency department. Inhaled corticosteroids in this context don't improve symptoms scores or quality of life and do not affect the recurrence of symptoms requiring hospital admission [15, 41]. Supplemental oxygen is usually administered through nasal prongs or even a mask to maintain oxygen saturation above 90 in all patients except for pregnant women or patients with cardiovascular comorbidities, the target oxygen saturation is greater than 95%. A mixture of oxygen and helium (heliox) has a lower density when compared with pure oxygen (100%) and also can flow easily through constricted patient airways and in turn improve clinical outcomes of exacerbated patients. However, insufficient data are available to support heliox-driven nebulization in the management of acute exacerbations [42]. Monitoring of oxygen saturation should be performed regularly until a clear response to therapy is reached. In ED, inhaled bronchodilators would reverse airflow limitation while three treatment doses are given each 20–30 min and then the frequency is adjusted based on the patient response. Most patients experiencing exacerbations significantly respond after the first dose and approximately 60–70% of patients fully respond to the three initial treatments [32, 43, 44]. Moreover, continuous administration of SABA is recommended over intermittent one in patients with severe exacerbations (FEV_1 or PEFR is less than 40% of predicted) as it is associated with better clinical outcomes as improved pulmonary function results and lower hospital admission rate with no obvious effect on the pulse, blood pressure or tremor [15]. The use of inhaled B2-agonists and muscarinic antagonists as combinations is compared with the use of B2-agonists alone in several studies performed on children (1–18 years) who exhibited mild, moderate, and severe exacerbations. The results showed that in children with severe exacerbations, the addition of several doses of inhaled muscarinic antagonists had improved lung function and lowered hospitalization. Adults with severe asthma exacerbations also can benefit from inhaled anticholinergics [45, 46]. Patients experiencing severe exacerbation can benefit from intravenous magnesium sulfate. Magnesium sulfate can be used in acute asthma inpatient cases that are refractory to bronchodilator and corticosteroid treatment and show suboptimal improvement or even clinical deterioration following therapy. Relaxation of bronchial smooth muscle is achieved by magnesium sulfate use by inhibiting the influx of calcium into smooth muscles and it is also thought to have anti-inflammatory effects. Parenteral magnesium sulfate is recommended over orally administered as it possesses higher bioavailability. Reduced hospital admissions and pulmonary function improvement were noticed with magnesium sulfate use in the emergency department. However, nebulized magnesium sulfate showed little effect on lung function and rate of hospital admissions in adults and approximately no impact on both outcomes in children [47].

Viral infections are the most common cause of asthma exacerbations so the use of antibiotics is not recommended in such situations [48]. So, antimicrobial treatment should be reserved for asthmatic patients with a clinical suspicion of bacterial infection causing the ongoing exacerbation [31]. Of note, severely exacerbated patients are in need to move to an area within the emergency department where respiratory failure and dynamic instability can be managed. Patient monitors are often used for continuous recording of pulse oximetry, blood pressure, and rhythm strip. The occurrence of respiratory failure can be predicted by using an end-tidal air stream CO_2 monitor. Tissue oxygenation is adequately maintained by supplemental oxygen delivery which also decreases the possibility of CO_2 narcosis in patients with significant hypoxemia. Two sites for intravenous excess are preferably established in those patients to administer intravenous fluids which are mostly needed for pediatrics and can be considered for adults [30, 49]. Unfortunately, the progression of respiratory failure occurs rapidly and its effects on the patient body are difficult to reverse so early recognition and suitable management are fundamental. Intubation is deemed necessary despite its possible complications when other treatments failed to control the patient's condition [32]. NAEPP sets the following recommendation regarding intubation [32, 50]:

- Patients with apnea or coma needed immediate intubation. Depressed mentality and the presence of increasing or sustained hypercapnia or exhaustion strongly advocate the need for respiratory support.
- Physicians should determine the urgent need of the patient for ventilation as it is very risky and complicated to ventilate patients with severe asthma. For that, intubation is performed in a semi-selective manner and before the occurrence of respiratory arrest. When intubation is the only available choice, it shouldn't be delayed and should be done in the emergency department with the possible transfer of the patient to an intensive care unit based on its age.

- At the time of intubation, hypotension may accompany the beginning of positive pressure ventilation hence intravascular volume should be preserved or replaced. Additionally, the use of high ventilator pressures should be avoided as they may subject the patient to barotrauma.
- The recommended ventilator approach to provide the required oxygen delivery with the lower air pressure used and barotrauma risk is called permissive hypercapnia or controlled hypoventilation.

Following discharge from the emergency department, patients go home with a systemic corticosteroid course consisting of 50–100 mg prednisone administered daily for 5–10 days which has proven efficacy in reducing the recurrence of asthma symptoms, future hospital admissions, and SABA use [51, 52]. In children with the age of 2–15 years, a 3 days course of corticosteroids with a prednisone dose of 1 mg/kg is sufficient for complete symptoms resolution within 1 week. On the other hand, data is insufficient to recommend the use of montelukast instead of oral corticosteroids or combining ICs with oral corticosteroids after patient discharge to prevent symptoms recurrence [15].

1.3.2 *Chronic Obstructive Pulmonary Disease*

Chronic obstructive pulmonary disease (COPD) is the third leading cause of mortality worldwide where it affects approximately 400 million individuals [53]. It is an inflammatory disorder that progressively affects the airways and the alveoli and is considered a preventable and treatable illness. The key characteristic of this disease is the irreversible and chronic nature of the existing airflow limitation. Two distinct processes are responsible for the occurrence of chronic inflammation: the first process is called small airway disease which involves obstructive bronchiolitis, narrowing or loss of peripheral airways and airway remodeling where the second process, emphysema, includes loss of alveoli formity due to parenchymal destruction, loss of elastic recoil, gas trapping and finally hyperinflation [54]. Figure 1.2 shows differences between healthy lung and obstructive one in COPD patients.

Pathological changes were seen in COPD result in a progressive decrease in FEV_1, incomplete lung emptying during expiration and consequently, dynamic and static hyperinflation may be developed [56, 57]. Exposure to inhaled causative agents for a long period with sufficient intensity is a key determinant for developing the disease so individuals below 40 years are rarely affected by such disease. About 80% of affected persons are former smokers while 15% of those persons are cited to have clinically significant disease. Other risk factors can account for developing the disease in nonsmokers as exposure to air pollution, biomass fuel, and secondhand smoke, occupational exposure to organic or inorganic fumes, vapors or dust, low birth weight, maternal smoking, asthma and reported respiratory infections in childhood Also, genetic causes as deficiency of alpha1 antitrypsin can account for disease development in some patients [53, 58, 59]. The clinical presentation of COPD

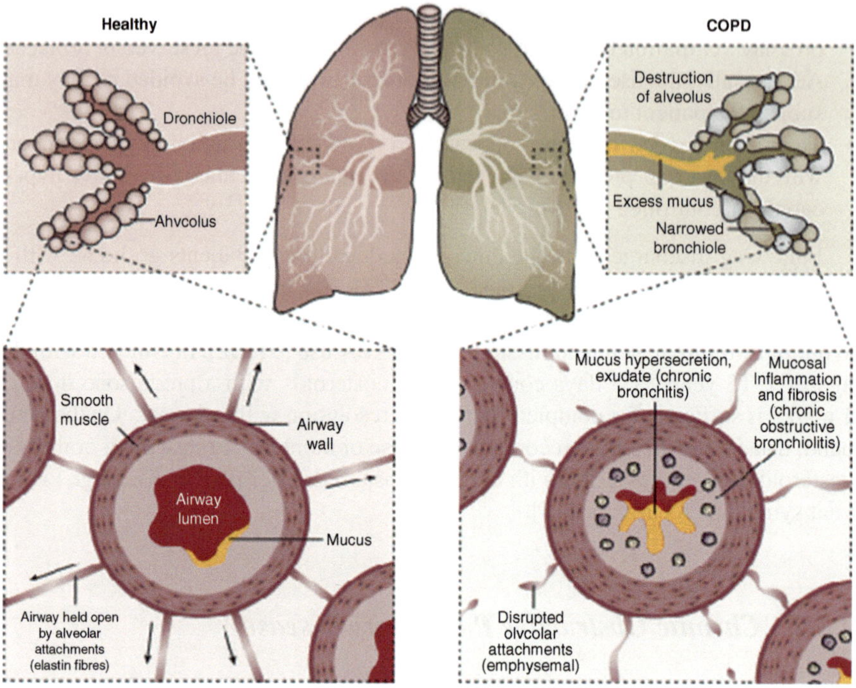

Fig. 1.2 Features of lungs in healthy individuals and COPD patients [55]

patients can greatly vary from one person to another but the commonly reported symptoms are Dyspnea or breathlessness which reported by greater than 70% of patients, and noticeably worse with physical activity; chronic cough which reported by 60% of patients and usually wrongly described by patients as “smoker’s cough”; mucus production or expectoration which reported by 63% of patients and may be an indicator of chronic bronchitis especially if lasts for longer than 3 months in two successive years. Chest tightness and Wheezing can also be reported by COPD patients. These symptoms are troublesome especially on awakening and are subject to variability from day-to-day. The diagnosis of mild or moderate COPD can’t be based on physical examination only where signs such as the use of accessory muscles, poor air movement, and muscle wasting are unclear till the patient reached an advanced disease stage [54, 60].

Other diseases that may affect COPD patients as muscle weakness, osteoporosis, cardiovascular diseases, lung cancer, and depression [61, 62]. The relation between COPD and lung cancer can be returned to DNA damage induced by the existing pulmonary inflammation and oxidative stress which lead to an imbalance between tissue repair and proliferation [63, 64]. Cardiovascular diseases and lung cancer are the predominant causes of death among COPD patients till the patients reached an advanced stage of the disease and in this case, respiratory causes may contribute to overall deaths [56, 62]. COPD mortality can be decreased if the patients with higher risks for lung cancer and cardiovascular diseases are early identified by diagnostic assessment. Additionally, phenotyping and grading severity of COPD patients are important predictors for the concomitant disease where patients with emphysematous phenotype are at a higher risk for lung cancer when compared with those with a predominant small airway disease phenotype [65, 66]. Risk for developing osteoporosis and loss of muscle mass is increased in patients with emphysema than those with a predominant airway phenotype. Also, cardiovascular risk is higher in patients with emphysema because of the increased stiffness of arteries. Generally, COPD patients with concomitant metabolic syndrome have a higher cardiovascular risk [67].

1.3.2.1 COPD Diagnosis

Clinical presentation of the patient and previous medical history has great importance in COPD diagnosis but spirometry is needed to confirm this finding. Spirometry is the best tool to identify airflow limitation in COPD patients where a post-bronchodilator FEV_1/FVC ratio below 0.7 identifies the presence of the disease. The severity of airflow limitation is used for COPD classification based on post-bronchodilator FEV_1: Grade I (mild; $FEV_1 \geq 80\%$ predicted), Grade II (moderate; $FEV_1 \geq 50\%$ and <80% predicted), Grade III (severe; FEV1 ≥ 30% and <50% predicted) and Grade IV (very severe; $FEV_1 < 30\%$ or <50% predicted) Recently, a classification based on the degree of airflow limitation, the severity of symptoms and history of exacerbation and/or hospitalization is recommended by GOLD guidelines as illustrated in Fig. 1.3 [68, 69].

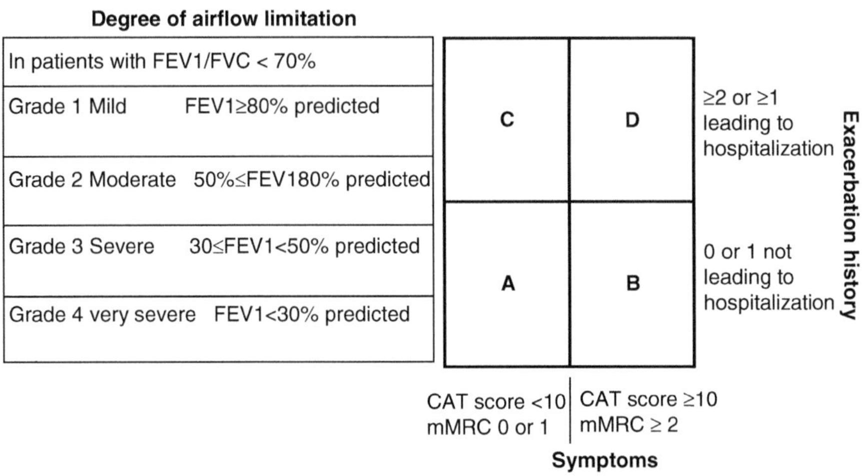

Fig. 1.3 Classification of COPD based on symptom severity, degree of airflow limitation, and exacerbation risk. *GOLD* Global Initiative for Chronic Obstructive Lung Disease, FEV_1 forced expiratory volume in 1 s, *FVC* forced vital capacity, *CAT* COPD Assessment Test, *mMRC* modified Medical Research Council score

1.3.2.2 Differences Between COPD and Asthma Diagnosis

Generally, Lung function is decreased in both diseases and the resistance of airways increases persistently in COPD while in asthma, the resistance increases only during an acute exacerbation. In asthmatic patients, inhaling B2-agonist can improve lung function and reduce airway resistance but such drug effect is limited in COPD patients [70]. Results of spirometry are usually normal in asthmatic patients during attack-free periods but such findings are rare in COPD patients who exhibit an FEV_1 lower than 70% of FVC at any time [71–73]. Peak flow measurement refers to measuring the exhaled air flow rate during forced exhalation maneuver by spirometry or peak flow meter and is highly dependent on airway resistance. The measurement of this parameter is beneficial in asthmatic patients than COPD patients [74, 75]. Asthma possesses no typical signs during the radiographic examination while in COPD, signs of emphysema are apparent. These radiological signs include extended intercostal spaces, flattened diaphragm, vascular paucity, rarefaction of pulmonary blood vessels and increased radiolucency of lungs [73] Signs of lung hyperinflation also occur in emphysema but one can't rely on them in the differential diagnosis as they can be found in asthma. In COPD, sputum produced by the patients contains eosinophils while in asthmatics, neutrophils are the predominant cells found [75, 76]. Also, asthmatics show a greater response to glucocorticoid therapy than COPD patients [77–79]. Tables 1.3 and 1.4 lists the differences between asthma and COPD in clinical presentation and diagnosis.

1.3.2.3 Management of Stable COPD

The goals for COPD treatment represent in relief of symptoms as decreased dyspnea, increased exercise tolerability, and improved quality of life besides preventing future risks of exacerbation, hospitalization, and premature death. The achievement

Table 1.3 Clinical differences between COPD and asthma [70]

	COPD	Asthma
Symptoms		
Dyspnea	First with exaggerated activity and later even at rest	During exacerbations
Cough	Productive cough especially in the morning	The dry cough usually at night
Mucus production	Clear, yellowish	Crystal clear, very tenacious
Age onset	Over 40 years	Very common during childhood and adulthood
Onset of disease	Slowly till reaching progressive chronic bronchitis	Often suddenly
Triggers or risk factors	Smoking, air pollution	Irritants as pollen, house dust mites, and animal hair, infection, cold, stress, exercise
Expectation of life	Significantly shortened	Life possible till reaching old age

Table 1.4 Differences between COPD and asthma in diagnosis and treatment [70]

	COPD	Asthma
Spirometry		
Pulmonary function	Decreased	Decreased
Airway resistance	Increased, hardly decreased by B2-agonists	Increased during exacerbations and improved by B2-agonists
Spirometry findings	The ratio of FEV_1/FVC is lower than the lower limit of normal	Often normal in attack-free periods
Peak flow rate	Exhibits very small fluctuations	Exhibits large fluctuations which decreased in the morning
Radiological examination	Signs of emphysema	No typical signs
Laboratory examination	Neutrophils	Immunoglobulin E, eosinophils
Sputum	Neutrophils	Eosinophils
Response to glucocorticoids	Little	Great

of such goals can provide some form of disease control [80, 81]. After setting the treatment goals, it is easy to identify the treatment strategies targeting certain mechanisms behind the impact of the disease. For example, bronchodilation is required to decrease the level of pulmonary hyperinflation and consequently relieve dyspnea which inturn fights muscle deconditioning. On the other hand, targeting inflammation and infection can result in reducing the exacerbation risk [82–84]. Nonpharmacological interventions as pulmonary rehabilitation can participate in disease management. Pulmonary rehabilitation refers to an individually designed and tailored care program directed to patients who suffered from chronic respiratory impairment aiming to enhance the social and physical ability of COPD patients. These programs provide individualized education and exercise programs that enable patients to have reduced dyspnea and improved health status, physical performance, exercise tolerance, and quality of life [55]. Therapeutic agents used to treat COPD are fallen into two main categories: inhaled bronchodilators and anti-inflammatory agents. Inhaled bronchodilators are either of short-acting or long-acting effect belonged to pharmacological classes of B2-agonists or antimuscarinic agents. Inhaled bronchodilators mainly manage symptoms and are given regularly to reduce or even prevent symptoms. Their mechanism of action depends on the alteration of airway smooth muscle tone and improving expiratory flow which indicates widening of the airways without affecting lung elastic recoil. They also reduce static and dynamic lung hyperinflation and improve exercise tolerance. B2- agonists produce airway muscle relaxation by stimulating B2-receptors which increase the level of Cyclic AMP and relieve the existing bronchoconstriction. Short-acting B2-agonists (SABAs) as albuterol, fenoterol, terbutaline act for approximately 4–6 h where long-acting B2-agonists(LABAs) as formoterol and salmeterol act up to 12 h. Antimuscarinic agents block the action of acetylcholine on M3-receptors which are abundantly found in airway smooth muscle preventing bronchoconstriction.

Short-acting muscarinic antagonists (SAMAs) as ipratropium and oxitropium can also block M2-receptors inhibiting the vagal induced bronchoconstriction. Long-acting muscarinic antagonists (LAMAs) such as tiotropium, aclidinium, umeclidinium, and glycopyrronium bromide have a prolonged bronchodilator action as they bind to M3-receptors for a relatively longer duration. Long-acting bronchodilators mainly exert their symptomatic action through their effect on lung volumes rather than reducing airflow obstruction. For that, the link between individual symptoms and the effect on FEV_1 is limited. Additionally, the positive response of an individual to a short-acting agent of a certain pharmacological class can't predict the same responsiveness to a long-acting agent of the same class [55]. Previous studies that compared the use of ipratropium alone or SABA alone or a combination of both agents in COPD patients demonstrated that a small benefit in lung function and oral steroids need was noticed with ipratropium over SABA. On the other hand, LAMAs are superior in reducing the exacerbations risk than LABA treatment [85]. Selecting the suitable drug for a patient will depend on several factors as patient preference, tolerability, drug availability, and cost. Antimuscurincs can cause dryness of the mouth (xerostomia) in COPD patients while the main side effects of B2- agonists are hypokalemia and tremor. The safety of long-acting bronchodilators in patients with cardiovascular comorbidities is still uncertain but recent studies indicated their safety as long as patients with stable disease status [86]. The use of LABA and LAMA as a combination demonstrates an additive or a synergistic effect on lung function [55]. Furthermore, the bronchodilation degree is increased when bronchodilators of different mechanisms and duration of action are combined over increasing the dose of one agent. Antiinflammatory agents include inhaled corticosteroids, phosphodiesterase-4 inhibitors, and macrolides. The responsiveness of COPD inflammation to ICs was found to be limited in in-vitro studies but the concomitant use of some drugs like B2-agonists can partially increase corticosteroid sensitivity in COPD patients. However, eosinophil count can predict the effectiveness of ICs therapy and in turn, can guide treatment decisions. Previous studies showed a reduction in exacerbation rate when a combination of ICs with LABA was used in patients with higher eosinophil count over the use of LABA alone or LAMA alone. GOLD guidelines indicated the relation between eosinophil count and the extent of ICs effect in COPD patients with the estimated benefit of adding this class of drugs to regular maintenance bronchodilator in preventing any future COPD exacerbation [69, 87]. Of note, this benefit is decreased or even disappeared in patients with lower eosinophil count [88]. When a LAMA is added to a combination of LABAs /ICs, one can predict improved pulmonary function especially in patients with a higher exacerbation risk. Generally, the administration of inhaled triple therapy which consists of LAMAs, LABAs, and ICs had proven better patient outcomes and improved lung function [85, 89, 90]. Theophylline belongs to methylxanthines and is also an example of PDE4 inhibitors with both modest bronchodilation and anti-inflammatory effects. It can be added to LABA to improve lung function but its use is limited because of its narrow therapeutic index and its various drug-drug and drug-food interactions which necessitate the close monitoring of the plasma level of the drug [81]. Roflumilast is also a second-generation PDE4 inhibitor that can be used only in GOLD group D patients with FEV_1 less than 50% predicted and chronic bronchitis (Fig. 1.4) [91, 92]. Macrolide antibiotics can play a role in reducing exacerbation risk in COPD patients with modest disease severity when administered continuously but the emerging bacterial resistance has the major concern with their use [93]. Also, mucolytic agents can decrease exacerbation rate and improve patient symptoms [94].

1.3.2.4 Management of COPD Exacerbations

A COPD exacerbation refers to an acute episode that is characterized by worsening of patients' symptoms beyond the normal day-to-day variations and requires a modification in regular patient therapy. Patients exhibit worsening breathlessness, increased sputum production or purulence, and cough but they can have other symptoms as cold symptoms and increased wheezing [95]. During a COPD exacerbation, patients have altered lung function but small variations in FEV_1 values are not beneficial in exacerbation prediction or even monitoring. The duration of an exacerbation can last for several days and almost 12 weeks are required for the patient to return to baseline status. Respiratory tract infections of viral or bacterial cause are mainly responsible for acute COPD exacerbation. So influenza and pneumococcal vaccinations are recommended to prevent exacerbations in COPD patients. Noninfectious causes as air pollution and patient comorbidities as heart failure and pulmonary embolism can participate to some extent in the occurrence of an exacerbation [96]. Unfortunately, 50% of COPD exacerbations defined by worsening of symptoms do not seek medical care and left untreated. Patients should be advised to

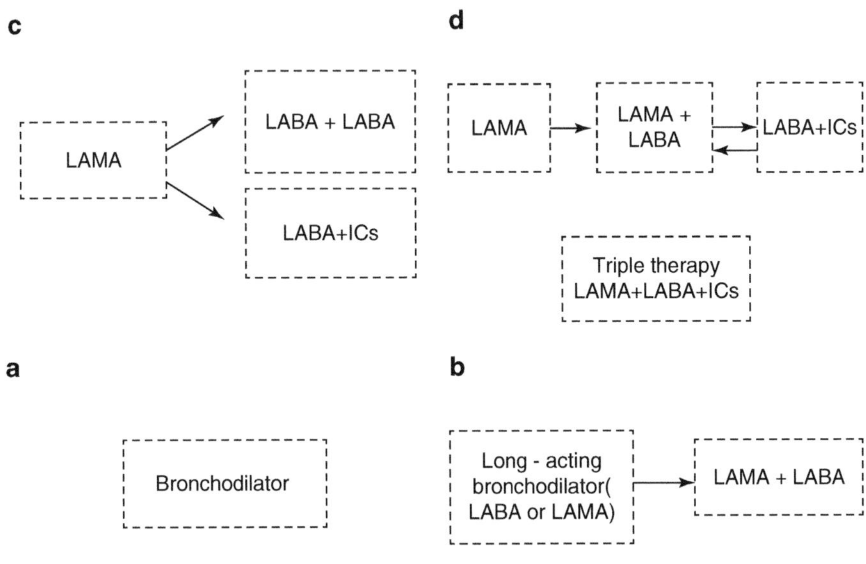

Fig. 1.4 Algorithm of COPD pharmacological treatment

consult their physicians if they have a worsened disease status despite treatment. Untreated COPD exacerbations are less severe than those seek medical care but they can eventually affect the health status of the patient [55, 97]. Exacerbations are the main cause for disease progression and hospital admissions besides they can independently predict death from COPD. Some trials returned the decrease in pulmonary function by 25% to the occurrence of an exacerbation [98, 99]. Any intervention which aims to reduce exacerbation risk, will positively affect health status. Also, patients with severe COPD exacerbations can be exposed to some cardiovascular events like myocardial infarction so they are in the need of hospital admissions [55, 100]. The initial management of a COPD exacerbation in the hospital includes an assessment of the severity of clinical signs and medical history, increasing the frequency and the dose of administered inhaled bronchodilator, administering supplemental oxygen therapy, adding a systemic corticosteroid (oral or intravenous) and finally administering oral or intravenous antibiotic if bacterial infection signs (increased sputum volume or purulence) are present [96]. Inhaled bronchodilators either SABA or SAMA are effective in managing an exacerbation where they can be administered in the acute setting by either a wet nebulizer or pMDI with a holding chamber. Both had proven equal efficiency in alleviating the acute airflow limitation and showed no difference in hospital stay length [101]. Systemic corticosteroids used during an exacerbation can suppress airway inflammation. Although a prolonged-high dose course of systemic corticosteroids can provide a better anti-inflammatory response, it is associated with many adverse effects returned to the cumulative dose especially with the relapsing nature of COPD exacerbation. A 5-day course of oral corticosteroids is similar to a conventional 14-day course in reducing the recurrence of exacerbations but with lower side effects [96, 102]. Moreover, broad-spectrum antibiotics such as amoxicillin alone or with clavulanic acid, tetracyclines, macrolides, and respiratory quinolones that cover the commonly known respiratory pathogens are recommended in the management of COPD exacerbations on either inpatient or outpatient basis. The use of these antibiotics depends on the presence of two or more signs of bacterial infection as increase sputum production or purulence and breathlessness [69]. In general, oral antibiotics are used for most patients while intravenous antibiotics are recommended if the patient experiences an impaired mental status, severe exacerbation, concomitant pneumonia, or swallowing difficulties. The optimal duration for antibiotic use is uncertain but antibiotics are often prescribed for 5 days [96]. Patients suffered from acute COPD exacerbations need oxygen therapy to maintain oxygen saturation between 88 and 92% and the oxygen, in this case, is needed to be titrated to avoid the occurrence of hypoxemia or hyperoxemia. Of note, Pulse oximetry should be routinely assessed in all clinical situations in which oxygen is administered. During oxygen therapy, air-driven nebulizers are frequently used to administer bronchodilators [103, 104]. Noninvasive ventilation (NIV) is recommended in acute respiratory acidosis (arterial pH $\leq$7.35 and/or partial arterial carbon dioxide concentration (PaCO) $\geq$45 mmHg or $\geq$6.0 kP), to improve dyspnea and reduce work of breathing, rate of respiration and hospital stay length. Also, NIV decreases intubation rate, complications as ventilator-associated pneumonia and mortality rate. The use of NIV with pharmacologically effective treatment will enable patients to rapidly recover and be weaned from NIV within a period of 2–10 days. The main adverse effects associated with NIV use are gastric distension, claustrophobia feeling especially with facemask interface, and risk of pneumonia. However, pneumonia risk is known to be lower with NIV than invasive ventilation [105, 106]. Invasive mechanical ventilation is recommended in case of NIV failure or patients cannot tolerate NIV. Generally, indications to start invasive ventilation are severe ventricular arrhythmia, cardiac or respiratory arrest, severe hemodynamic instability, loss of consciousness, massive aspiration, and inability to expel respiratory secretions [69]. During an exacerbation, nutrition, fluid balance, and heparin (subcutaneous or low molecular weight) should be monitored by health care providers. Also, patient comorbidities such as heart failure, arrhythmia must be monitored and treated [96, 107].

References

1. Ehrmann S, et al. Aerosol therapy in intensive and intermediate care units: prospective observation of 2808 critically ill patients. Intensive Care Med. 2016;42(2):192–201.
2. Laube BL, et al. What the pulmonary specialist should know about the new inhalation therapies. Eur Respir J. 2011;37(6):1308–31.
3. Dolovich MB, Dhand R. Aerosol drug delivery: developments in device design and clinical use. Lancet. 2011;377(9770):1032–45.
4. Hickey AJ, Mansour HM. Inhalation aerosols: physical and biological basis for therapy, vol. 1. Boca Raton: CRC Press; 2019.
5. Ari A. Aerosol therapy in pulmonary critical care. Respir Care. 2015;60(6):858–74; discussion 874–9.
6. Ari A, Fink JB. Guidelines for aerosol devices in infants, children and adults: which to choose, why and how to achieve effective aerosol therapy. Expert Rev Respir Med. 2011;5(4):561–72.
7. Loscalzo J. Harrison's pulmonary and critical care medicine. 2nd ed. New York: McGraw-Hill Education; 2013.
8. Patadia MO, Murrill LL, Corey J. Asthma: symptoms and presentation. Otolaryngol Clin North Am. 2014;47(1):23–32.
9. Rehman A, Amin F, Sadeeqa S. Prevalence of asthma and its management: a review. J Pak Med Assoc. 2018;68(12):1823–7.
10. Wu TD, Brigham EP, McCormack MC. Asthma in the primary care setting. Med Clin North Am. 2019;103(3):435–52.
11. Vernon MK, et al. What do we know about asthma triggers? A review of the literature. J Asthma. 2012;49(10):991–8.
12. Price D, et al. Asthma referrals: a key component of asthma management that needs to be addressed. J Asthma Allergy. 2017;10:209–23.
13. Boulet L-P, et al. The global initiative for asthma (GINA): 25 years later. Eur Respir J. 2019;54(2):1900598.
14. Cockcroft DW. Direct challenge tests: airway hyperresponsiveness in asthma: its measurement and clinical significance. Chest. 2010;138(2 Suppl):18S–24S.
15. Pollart SM, Compton RM, Elward KS. Management of acute asthma exacerbations. Am Fam Physician. 2011;84(1):40–7.
16. Pellegrino R, et al. Interpretative strategies for lung function tests. Eur Respir J. 2005;26(5):948–68.

17. Lougheed MD, et al. Canadian Thoracic Society 2012 guideline update: diagnosis and management of asthma in preschoolers, children and adults: executive summary. Can Respir J. 2012;19(6):e81–8.
18. Korang SK, et al. Non-invasive positive pressure ventilation for acute asthma in children. Cochrane Database Syst Rev. 2016;9:CD012067.
19. Cave AJ, Atkinson LL. Asthma in preschool children: a review of the diagnostic challenges. J Am Board Fam Med. 2014;27(4):538–48.
20. Papadopoulos NG, et al. International consensus on (ICON) pediatric asthma. Allergy. 2012;67(8):976–97.
21. FitzGerald M, et al. Global strategy for asthma management and prevention, Global Initiative for Asthma (GINA) [Internet]. 2015; 2016.
22. (GINA), G.I.f.A. Global strategy for asthma management and prevention; 2017. www.ginasthmas.org.
23. James DR, Lyttle MD. British guideline on the management of asthma: SIGN clinical guideline 141, 2014. Arch Dis Child Educ Pract Ed. 2016;101(6):319–22.
24. Winer RA, et al. Asthma incidence among children and adults: findings from the behavioral risk factor surveillance system asthma call-back survey—United States, 2006–2008. J Asthma. 2012;49(1):16–22.
25. Beasley R, et al. Asthma and Respiratory Foundation NZ adult asthma guidelines: a quick reference guide. NZ Med J. 2016;129:83–102.
26. Ducharme FM, Lasserson TJ, Cates CJ. Addition to inhaled corticosteroids of long-acting beta2-agonists versus anti-leukotrienes for chronic asthma. Cochrane Database Syst Rev. 2011;(5).
27. Chroinin MN, et al. Addition of long-acting beta2-agonists to inhaled steroids as first line therapy for persistent asthma in steroid-naive adults and children. Cochrane Database Syst Rev. 2009;(4).
28. Sobieraj DM, et al. Association of inhaled corticosteroids and long-acting muscarinic antagonists with asthma control in patients with uncontrolled, persistent asthma: a systematic review and meta-analysis. JAMA. 2018;319(14):1473–84.
29. GINA. Global strategy for asthma management and prevention; 2019. www.ginasthmas.org.
30. Adams JY, Sutter ME, Albertson TE. The patient with asthma in the emergency department. Clin Rev Allergy Immunol. 2012;43(1–2):14–29.
31. Rothe T, et al. Diagnosis and management of asthma—the Swiss guidelines. Respiration. 2018;95(5):364–80.
32. Camargo CA Jr, Rachelefsky G, Schatz M. Managing asthma exacerbations in the emergency department: summary of the National Asthma Education and Prevention Program Expert Panel Report 3 guidelines for the management of asthma exacerbations. Proc Am Thorac Soc. 2009;6(4):357–66.
33. Al-Dorzi HM, et al. Risk factors, management and outcomes of patients admitted with near fatal asthma to a tertiary care hospital in Riyadh. Ann Thorac Med. 2014;9(1):33–8.
34. Laher AE, Buchanan SK. Mechanically ventilating the severe asthmatic. J Intensive Care Med. 2018;33(9):491–501.
35. Castillo JR, Peters SP, Busse WW. Asthma exacerbations: pathogenesis, prevention, and treatment. J Allergy Clin Immunol Pract. 2017;5(4):918–27.
36. Janson SL, et al. Individualized asthma self-management improves medication adherence and markers of asthma control. J Allergy Clin Immunol. 2009;123(4):840–6.
37. Ortega HG, et al. Severe eosinophilic asthma treated with mepolizumab stratified by baseline eosinophil thresholds: a secondary analysis of the DREAM and MENSA studies. Lancet Respir Med. 2016;4(7):549–56.
38. Cates CJ, Welsh EJ, Rowe BH. Holding chambers (spacers) versus nebulisers for beta-agonist treatment of acute asthma. Cochrane Database Syst Rev. 2013;2013(9):CD000052.
39. Rowe B, et al. Corticosteroid therapy for acute asthma. Respir Med. 2004;98(4):275–84.

40. Edmonds ML, et al. Early use of inhaled corticosteroids in the emergency department treatment of acute asthma. Cochrane Database Syst Rev. 2012;(12).
41. Edmonds ML, et al. Inhaled steroids for acute asthma following emergency department discharge. Cochrane Database Syst Rev. 2012;(12).
42. Rodrigo GJ, et al. Heliox for non-intubated acute asthma patients. Cochrane Database Syst Rev. 2006;(4).
43. Camargo Jr C, Spooner C, Rowe B. Continuous versus intermittent b-agonists in the treatment of acute asthma (cochrane review). The Cochrane Library. 2003;(4).
44. National Asthma Education and Prevention Program. Expert Panel Report 3 (EPR-3): guidelines for the diagnosis and management of asthma-summary report 2007. J Allergy Clin Immunol. 2007;120(5 Suppl):S94.
45. Plotnick L, Ducharme F. Combined inhaled anticholinergics and beta2-agonists for initial treatment of acute asthma in children. Cochrane Database Syst Rev. 2000;(3).
46. Rodrigo GJ, Rodrigo C. First-line therapy for adult patients with acute asthma receiving a multiple-dose protocol of ipratropium bromide plus albuterol in the emergency department. Am J Respir Crit Care Med. 2000;161(6):1862–8.
47. Mohammed S, Goodacre S. Intravenous and nebulised magnesium sulphate for acute asthma: systematic review and meta-analysis. Emerg Med J. 2007;24(12):823–30.
48. Wark PA, et al. Viral and bacterial infection in acute asthma and chronic obstructive pulmonary disease increases the risk of readmission. Respirology. 2013;18(6):996–1002.
49. Ramsahai JM, Hansbro PM, Wark PAB. Mechanisms and management of asthma exacerbations. Am J Respir Crit Care Med. 2019;199(4):423–32.
50. Expert Panel Working Group of the National Heart, Lung, and Blood Institute (NHLBI) administered and coordinated National Asthma Education and Prevention Program Coordinating Committee (NAEPPCC), et al. 2020 focused updates to the asthma management guidelines: a report from the National Asthma Education and Prevention program coordinating committee expert panel working group. J Allergy Clin Immunol. 2020;146(6):1217–70.
51. Krishnan JA, et al. An umbrella review: corticosteroid therapy for adults with acute asthma. Am J Med. 2009;122(11):977–91.
52. Chang AB, et al. A 5-versus 3-day course of oral corticosteroids for children with asthma exacerbations who are not hospitalised: a randomised controlled trial. Med J Aust. 2008;189(6):306–10.
53. Labaki WW, Rosenberg SR. Chronic obstructive pulmonary disease. Ann Intern Med. 2020;173(3):ITC17–32.
54. Duffy SP, Criner GJ. Chronic obstructive pulmonary disease: evaluation and management. Med Clin North Am. 2019;103(3):453–61.
55. Barnes PJ, et al. Chronic obstructive pulmonary disease. Nat Rev Dis Primers. 2015;1:15076.
56. Rabe KF, Watz H. Chronic obstructive pulmonary disease. Lancet. 2017;389(10082):1931–40.
57. O'Donnell DE. Hyperinflation, dyspnea, and exercise intolerance in chronic obstructive pulmonary disease. Proc Am Thorac Soc. 2006;3(2):180–4.
58. Rennard SI, Vestbo J. COPD: the dangerous underestimate of 15%. Lancet. 2006;367(9518):1216–9.
59. Lamprecht B, et al. COPD in never smokers: results from the population-based burden of obstructive lung disease study. Chest. 2011;139(4):752–63.
60. Kessler R, et al. Symptom variability in patients with severe COPD: a pan-European cross-sectional study. Eur Respir J. 2011;37(2):264–72.
61. Nussbaumer-Ochsner Y, Rabe KF. Systemic manifestations of COPD. Chest. 2011;139(1):165–73.
62. Decramer M, Janssens W. Chronic obstructive pulmonary disease and comorbidities. Lancet Respir Med. 2013;1(1):73–83.
63. Houghton AM, Mouded M, Shapiro SD. Common origins of lung cancer and COPD. Nat Med. 2008;14(10):1023–4.

64. Houghton AM. Mechanistic links between COPD and lung cancer. Nat Rev Cancer. 2013;13(4):233–45.
65. de Torres JP, et al. Lung cancer in patients with chronic obstructive pulmonary disease. Development and validation of the COPD Lung Cancer Screening Score. Am J Respir Crit Care Med. 2015;191(3):285–91.
66. de Torres JP, et al. Lung cancer in patients with chronic obstructive pulmonary disease: incidence and predicting factors. Am J Respir Crit Care Med. 2011;184(8):913–9.
67. McAllister DA, et al. Arterial stiffness is independently associated with emphysema severity in patients with chronic obstructive pulmonary disease. Am J Respir Crit Care Med. 2007;176(12):1208–14.
68. Welte T, Vogelmeier C, Papi A. COPD: early diagnosis and treatment to slow disease progression. Int J Clin Pract. 2015;69(3):336–49.
69. GOLD. Pocket guide to COPD diagnosis,management and prevention. 2020 [cited 2020 1 April]. https://goldcopd.org/wp-content/uploads/2019/11/GOLD-2020-POCKET-GUIDE-FINAL-pgsized-wms.pdf.
70. Yayan J, Rasche K. Asthma and COPD: similarities and differences in the pathophysiology, diagnosis and therapy. In: Pokorski M, editor. Respiratory medicine and science. Cham: Springer International Publishing; 2016. p. 31–8.
71. Miravitlles M, et al. Difficulties in differential diagnosis of COPD and asthma in primary care. Br J Gen Pract. 2012;62(595):e68–75.
72. Oga T, et al. Multidimensional analyses of long-term clinical courses of asthma and chronic obstructive pulmonary disease. Allergol Int. 2010;59(3):257–65.
73. Chang J, Mosenifar Z. Differentiating COPD from asthma in clinical practice. J Intensive Care Med. 2007;22(5):300–9.
74. Mishima M. Physiological differences and similarities in asthma and COPD-based on respiratory function testing. Allergol Int. 2009;58(3):333–40.
75. Pauwels RA. Similarities and differences in asthma and chronic obstructive pulmonary disease exacerbations. Proc Am Thorac Soc. 2004;1(2):73–6.
76. Sutherland ER, Martin RJ. Airway inflammation in chronic obstructive pulmonary disease: comparisons with asthma. J Allergy Clin Immunol. 2003;112(5):819–27.
77. Bumbacea D, Bogdan MA. Update in pneumology–focus on asthma and COPD. Maedica. 2011;6(4):339.
78. Kaneko Y, et al. The search for common pathways underlying asthma and COPD. Int J Chron Obstruct Pulmon Dis. 2013;8:65.
79. Decramer M, Selroos O. Asthma and COPD: differences and similarities: with special reference to the usefulness of budesonide/formoterol in a single inhaler (Symbicort®) in both diseases. Int J Clin Pract. 2005;59(4):385–98.
80. Nibber A, et al. Validating the concept of COPD control: a real-world cohort study from the United Kingdom. COPD: J Chron Obstruct Pulmon Dis. 2017;14(5):504–12.
81. Roche N. Stable COPD treatment: where are we? COPD. 2018;15(2):123–9.
82. Aguilaniu B, Roche N. The difficulties of measuring and improving physical activity in COPD. npj Prim Care Respir Med. 2014;24(1):1–3.
83. Wedzicha JA, et al. Mechanisms and impact of the frequent exacerbator phenotype in chronic obstructive pulmonary disease. BMC Med. 2013;11(1):1–10.
84. Faner R, et al. The microbiome in respiratory medicine: current challenges and future perspectives. Eur Respir J. 2017;49(4):1602086.
85. O'Dell A, et al. CE: managing stable COPD: an evidence-based approach. Am J Nurs. 2018;118(9):36–47.
86. Calverley PM, et al. Cardiovascular events in patients with COPD: TORCH study results. Thorax. 2010;65(8):719–25.
87. GOLD. Pocket guide to COPD diagnosis,management and prevention. 2017 [cited 2017 12th December]. http://goldcopd.org/wp-content/uploads/2016/12/wms-GOLD-2017-Pocket-Guide-1.pdf.

88. Terry PD, Dhand R. Inhalation therapy for stable COPD: 20 years of GOLD reports. Adv Ther. 2020;37(5):1812–28.
89. Singh D, et al. Superiority of "triple" therapy with salmeterol/fluticasone propionate and tiotropium bromide versus individual components in moderate to severe COPD. Thorax. 2008;63(7):592–8.
90. Jung KS, et al. Comparison of tiotropium plus fluticasone propionate/salmeterol with tiotropium in COPD: a randomized controlled study. Respir Med. 2012;106(3):382–9.
91. Lipworth BJ. Phosphodiesterase-4 inhibitors for asthma and chronic obstructive pulmonary disease. Lancet. 2005;365(9454):167–75.
92. Vogelmeier CF, et al. Goals of COPD treatment: focus on symptoms and exacerbations. Respir Med. 2020;166:105938.
93. Herath SC, et al. Prophylactic antibiotic therapy for chronic obstructive pulmonary disease (COPD). Cochrane Database Syst Rev. 2018;(10).
94. Poole P, Chong J, Cates CJ. Mucolytic agents versus placebo for chronic bronchitis or chronic obstructive pulmonary disease. Cochrane Database Syst Rev. 2015;(7).
95. Seemungal T, et al. Detection of rhinovirus in induced sputum at exacerbation of chronic obstructive pulmonary disease. Eur Respir J. 2000;16(4):677–83.
96. Ko FW, et al. Acute exacerbation of COPD. Respirology. 2016;21(7):1152–65.
97. Wilkinson TM, et al. Early therapy improves outcomes of exacerbations of chronic obstructive pulmonary disease. Am J Respir Crit Care Med. 2004;169(12):1298–303.
98. Donaldson G, et al. Relationship between exacerbation frequency and lung function decline in chronic obstructive pulmonary disease. Thorax. 2002;57(10):847–52.
99. Kanner RE, Anthonisen NR, Connett JE. Lower respiratory illnesses promote FEV1 decline in current smokers but not ex-smokers with mild chronic obstructive pulmonary disease: results from the lung health study. Am J Respir Crit Care Med. 2001;164(3):358–64.
100. Zhou Y, et al. Lung function and incidence of chronic obstructive pulmonary disease after improved cooking fuels and kitchen ventilation: a 9-year prospective cohort study. PLoS Med. 2014;11(3):e1001621.
101. Dolovich MB, et al. Device selection and outcomes of aerosol therapy: evidence-based guidelines: American College of Chest Physicians/American College of Asthma, Allergy, and Immunology. Chest. 2005;127(1):335–71.
102. Leuppi JD, et al. Short-term vs conventional glucocorticoid therapy in acute exacerbations of chronic obstructive pulmonary disease: the REDUCE randomized clinical trial. JAMA. 2013;309(21):2223–31.
103. Beasley R, et al. Thoracic Society of Australia and New Zealand oxygen guidelines for acute oxygen use in adults: 'swimming between the flags'. Respirology. 2015;20(8):1182–91.
104. Edwards L, et al. Randomised controlled crossover trial of the effect on PtCO2 of oxygen-driven versus air-driven nebulisers in severe chronic obstructive pulmonary disease. Emerg Med J. 2012;29(11):894–8.
105. Verma AK, et al. Noninvasive mechanical ventilation: an 18-month experience of two tertiary care hospitals in North India. Lung India. 2013;30(4):307.
106. Lun CT, et al. A pilot randomized study comparing two methods of non-invasive ventilation withdrawal after acute respiratory failure in chronic obstructive pulmonary disease. Respirology. 2013;18(5):814–9.
107. Hillas G, Perlikos F, Tzanakis N. Acute exacerbation of COPD: is it the "stroke of the lungs"? Int J Chron Obstruct Pulmon Dis. 2016;11:1579.

Chapter 2
Types of Mechanical Ventilation

Contents

2.1 Mechanical Ventilation

Respiratory support is required for many patients suffering from obstructive lung diseases during acute exacerbations. As within this critical period, clinicians face major challenges as the presence of trapped air and dynamic overinflation [1]. Mechanical ventilation is external support for respiration to assist breathing in case of respiratory failure (either hypercapnic or hypoxemic). It aims at reducing the work of breathing by reducing the resistance of airways with a subsequent

M. E. A. Abdelrahim et al., *Essentials of Aerosol Therapy in Critically ill Patients*,
https://doi.org/10.1007/978-3-030-85026-5_2

improvement of oxygenation [2]. Mechanical ventilation need is considered a frequent reason for intensive care unit (ICU) admission. Invasive ventilation and non-invasive ventilation are the two main types of mechanical ventilation and the selection between them is based on patient severity and inclusion versus exclusion criteria [3, 4]. In invasive ventilation, the interface through which the air is given into the trachea is internal (e.g. intubation, tracheostomy).While non-invasive ventilation uses an interface that is external (e.g. facemask, nasal cannula, nasal mask) [5, 6].

2.2 Non-invasive Ventilation

Non-invasive ventilation (NIV) provides standard care to patients complaining of sleep apnoea, respiratory insufficiency, chronic obstructive pulmonary disease (COPD), and severely acute or chronic respiratory failure [7]. Over the past two decades, procedures for delivering NIV have gained enormous popularity over the invasive techniques as they offer the same physiologic usefulness, improving the gas exchange and reducing the work of breathing [8, 9]. In patients suffering from acute exacerbations of COPD, the successful use of NIV can eliminate the patient need for endotracheal intubation and do improve mortality [8, 9]. The well-known types of NIV differ mainly in the principle of work; negative-pressure and positive-pressure ventilation [7].

2.3 Non-invasive Negative Pressure Ventilation

Non-invasive negative pressure ventilation was the first mode of delivering NIV before positive pressure ventilation became the rule in the 1950s. The ventilation is achieved by reducing pressure surrounding the patient thorax to sub-atmospheric pressure so augmenting the work of respiratory muscles by facilitating chest expansion (lung inflation) followed by expiration [10]. Negative-pressure ventilators like an iron lung, portalung, pneumonia, and cuirass have the risk of upper airway obstruction, especially during sleep. Ventilator size varies from that could cover the whole patient body to that encases the thoracic case [11]. This, along with the practical considerations regarding their size complicating their use, they become virtually disused. Therefore, positive pressure ventilation replaced it and become the most commonly used NIV device [12].

2.4 Non-invasive Positive Pressure Ventilation

Non-invasive positive pressure ventilation (NIPPV) is the major ventilation technique used from the 1950s to the present. Positive ventilatory support delivers air to the patient's lung under the pressure produced from the ventilator either continuous or intermittent. This, in turn, decreases the breathing work of respiratory muscles, improves or even normalizes hypercapnia, and finally enhances better oxygenation. It is the most widespread ventilator due to its high efficiency and compliance [13]. They include simple non-invasive ventilators (like BiPAP and Auto-CPAP), advanced non-invasive ventilators (like Respironics Vision), home-care ventilators, and ICU ventilators. All are highly portable and efficient [14]. During NIV, gases could be delivered to patients by face mask, nasal mask, or nasal plugs, it was noted that in previous studies on COPD, a face mask made the higher physiologic improvement rate compared to nasal mask or plugs, but the nasal mask was the most tolerated by patients [15].

Facemask is recommended over nasal mask because of the possibility of gas leakage if the mouth is open during ventilation so that many patients are needed to be shifted to face mask from nasal mask [16, 17]. Another option is the use of a helmet interface which is more comfortable to patients than other interfaces, with low complication rates like irritation of eyes or necrosis of skin which can occur with both facemask and nasal mask. But also helmet interface has some disadvantages like hearing impairment caused by elevated levels of noise inside the helmet [18, 19].

Humidification of inspired air increased patient comfort during NIV, so humidifiers should be included during NIV [20]. Reduction of upper airway dryness is the main target of using heated humidification, which might reduce upper airway resistance and increase comfort, and might aid in the clearance of secretions [21].

Fortunately, NIV allows many of the complications associated with mechanical ventilation to be avoided, especially the occurrence of nosocomial infections (pneumonia and sinusitis), ventilator-associated lung injury, and barotrauma like pneumothorax [3]. Also, early use of NIV is associated with a marked reduction in the need for endotracheal intubation, a decrease in complication rate, a reduced duration of hospital stay, and a substantial reduction in-hospital mortality [22, 23]. On the other hand, NIV is involved in some milder complications (Table 2.1) [24].

Application of NIV is a safe and effective means of improving gas exchange in patients with many types of acute respiratory failure like; acute respiratory failure in immune-compromised patients, asphyxic forms of acute cardiogenic pulmonary

Table 2.1 Complications of NIV

Complication	Reason
Injury/ulceration of nose or above ears	Tight-fitting mask
Conjunctival irritation	Air leaks around the mask
Dry mucous membranes, nasal congestion, and thick secretions	A high flow of dry medical gas
Gastric distension	Insufflation of air at high flow
Claustrophobia	Tight-fitting mask with dyspnea
Aspiration pneumonia	Emesis with a decreased level of consciousness
Hemodynamic compromise and pneumothorax	Increased intra-thoracic pressure causing a decreased venous return

Table 2.2 Inclusion criteria for NIV

Inclusion criteria for NIV
• Moderate to severe dyspnea and tachypnea (≥25 breaths/min) with use of accessory muscles and paradoxical abdominal motion
• Moderate to severe acidosis (arterial pH (7.30–7.35) and hypercapnia ($PaCO_2$ (6.0–8.0 kPa, 45–60 mmHg))
• No excessive respiratory secretions
• Cooperative patient, not comatose or agitated and able to protect their airway

edema, and acute hypercapnic ventilatory failure. NIV is considered the first-line management of acute exacerbation of COPD [3]. Also, the addition of long-term NIV to standard treatment improves the survival of patients with hypercapnic stable COPD as NIV is targeted to reduce hypercapnia [13]. Also, it could act as an initial technique of ventilation or for weaning patients post-extubation [2]. Table 2.2 summarizes inclusion criteria for NIV [4, 25].

On the other hand, NIV is contraindicated in unconscious patients, in those with multiple organ failure or hemodynamic instability [2]. Moreover, it is contraindicated with impending cardiovascular collapse or respiratory arrest, high aspiration risk, viscous copious secretions, massive upper gastrointestinal bleeding, upper airway obstruction, head and neck tumors, recent facial or upper airway surgery, and with extreme obesity [4, 26].

2.5 Ventilation Modes

Generally, a breath is described as one cycle of positive flow (inhalation) and negative flow (exhalation). Ventilator mode is a pre-defined pattern of interaction between the patient and the ventilator that simply describes how the volume, pressure, and flow is controlled during a breath and how the breaths are sequenced (triggered "started" and cycled "stopped") [14]. A ventilatory mode possesses three essential components: breath sequence, ventilator breath control variable, and targeting scheme. Two types of breathing are available for ventilation; spontaneous breath, in which the inspiratory cycle is triggered and cycled by the patient, and mandatory breath, in which the inspiratory cycle is triggered and/or cycled by the ventilator. Therefore, there are only three possible breath sequences; continuous mandatory ventilation (CMV), intermittent mandatory ventilation (IMV), and continuous spontaneous ventilation (CSV) [14]. Mainly there are three ventilation modalities according to the control variable [27, 28]:

Volume-targeted ventilation (VTV), also named volume-controlled (VC), is the first ventilation modality in which the ventilator delivers a fixed volume in a given time regardless of the patient's contribution to ventilation. Therefore, airways pressure (Paw) is not constant. It has the advantage of the strict delivery of the present volume, in the absence of leaks but it does not account for patients' varying requirements, and if there is a leak, there will be no compensation leading to lower generated pressure and reduced delivered volume [27].

Pressure-targeted ventilation (PTV), also named pressure-controlled (PC), is the second ventilation modality in which the ventilator is set to deliver airflow by generating a pre-defined positive pressure for a given time while Paw is constant. Thus, for a given patient, the volume delivered is not fixed. It possesses the advantage of the ability to compensate for mild to moderate leaks [27].

Volume-targeted pressure ventilation, also named pressure-regulated volume control (PRVC), is the third ventilation modality which is a hybrid modality that combines features of VTV and PTV. The ventilator estimates the delivered tidal volume (TV) and adjusts its parameters to ensure a pre-determined target TV. Some ventilators adjust a target volume within each cycle but most of them progressively adjust the pressure level during several cycles to provide TV as close as possible to the target volume set by the clinician. However, some recent modes use a more physiological delivery of assistance following the spontaneous inspiratory signal coming from the patient (patient-triggered). Hence, they are supposed to improve patient-ventilator synchronism [27].

Finally, there are mainly five basic ventilatory patterns; volume-controlled continuous mandatory ventilation (VC-CMV), volume-controlled intermittent mandatory ventilation (VC-IMV), pressure-controlled continuous mandatory ventilation (PC-CMV), pressure-controlled intermittent mandatory ventilation (PC-IMV), pressure-controlled continuous spontaneous ventilation (PC-CSV) [14]. The most popular ventilator modes applied for NIV are summarized in Table 2.3 [27, 29, 30].

When NIV is initiated, the ventilator mode is determined based on a clinical evaluation of the patient besides diurnal blood gas variations [24]. Patients with acute respiratory failure due to acute COPD exacerbations require NIV. In those patients, AC mode achieves more reduction in work of breath than PSV but the latter is tolerable [31]. However, no difference was found between the two modes: CPAP and BiPAP in patients with cardiogenic pulmonary edema regarding mortality [32]. Also, PSV and proportional assist ventilation (PAV) were found to be similar regarding mortality and intubation rate [33].

2.6 Configuration of NIV Circuit

Mainly there are two main NIV circuit configurations; a single limb ventilation circuit and a dual limb ventilation circuit (Fig. 2.1). They extremely differ and would affect aerosol delivery. A dual limb ventilation circuit, consisting of inspiratory limb and expiratory limb, is pressure and volume controlled through a fixed valve at the expiration port that opens in response to patient expiration providing relatively high resistance to expiratory flow. On the other hand, a single limb ventilation circuit consists of only one limb supported with a small opened expiration port near the patient mask to prevent CO_2 rebreathing. It provides an advantage of

Table 2.3 Popular ventilation modes for NIV

Mode	Description
Pressure support ventilation (PSV)	• The patient triggers the ventilator assistance and the air is supplied from the ventilator in response to a certain predetermined pressure (PEEP) • The patient retains control of cycle length, depth, and flow profile
Continuous positive airway pressure (CPAP)	• All breaths are patient triggered and cycled • Constant mild positive pressure is continuously supplied throughout the respiratory cycle, not assist. • It could prevent obstructive sleep apnea
Proportional assist ventilation (PAV)	• It delivers patient-triggered and patient-cycled breaths, but it relies on the inspiratory flow of the patient's spontaneous breathing and adds fixed proportional assistance • It makes automatic synchrony between ventilator and patient • If the patient's flow increases, the assistance increases proportionally
Bi-level positive airway pressure (BiPAP)	• All breaths are patient-triggered • Ventilator supplies two different positive airway pressures; inspiratory and expiratory (IPAP and EPAP)
Assist mode	• The patient controls the onset of inspiration. However, the inspiratory length is regulated by the operator • The clinician must select a targeted volume or pressure and an inspiratory: Expiratory (I:E) ratio
Control mode "Timed mode"	• The entire work of breathing is performed by the ventilator • The clinician must select a targeted volume or pressure, a fixed respiratory rate (RR), and an I:E ratio
Assist control (AC)	• Similar to assist mode, patients initiate breathing not ventilator however, if the patient's spontaneous frequency is lower than a preset ventilator back-up RR, the system shifts to control mode in which the ventilator starts breathing
Synchronized intermittent mandatory ventilation (SIMV)	• Each inspiratory effort exceeding the threshold of trigger for a certain time leads to a mechanical breath • The limit for pressure, volume, and breathing rate is determined by the clinician

lower resistance to expiratory flow, so, reducing the expiratory effort by the patient. Also, the best place for the aerosol generator within the circuit is different; in the single limb ventilation circuit, it must be proximal to the patient. However, in the dual limb ventilation circuit, Jet nebulizers must be closer to the ventilator while pressurized metered-dose inhalers and vibrating and ultrasonic nebulizers must be located in the inspiratory limb 6 in from the Y adapter [27, 34, 35].

A dual limb ventilation circuit is typically used for invasive ventilation, for which an endotracheal tube, that limits aerosol leakage, is the patient interface. However, it is possible to use a dual limb system for NIV but with extreme disadvantages; it is not leaking tolerant as it cannot account for greater leaks from patient masks and would be bothersome to the patient due to high expiratory resistance [36].

Single limb ventilation is only available for NIV. It is referred to as "leak tolerant" systems because it accounts for the leak from the expiration port, as well as the

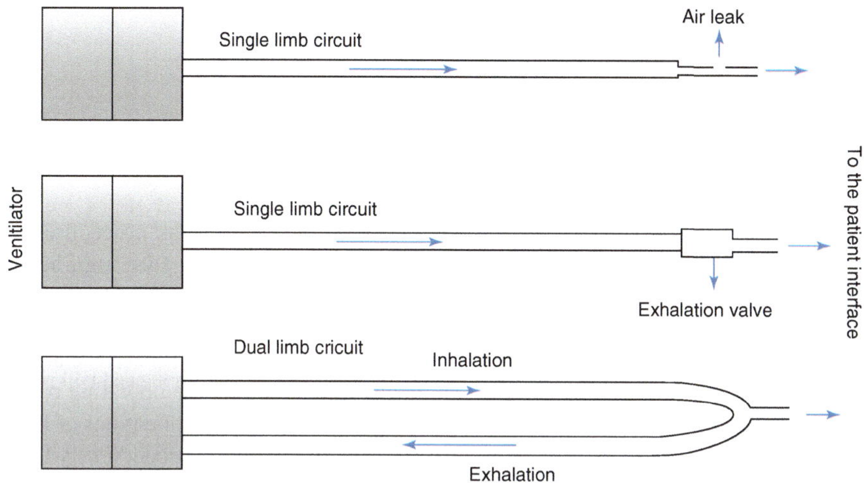

Fig. 2.1 NIV circuit configurations

unintentional leaks from the patient interface and finally the patient receives the desired pressure and/or flow. Also, they provide sufficient patient comfort due to low expiratory resistance. For this reason, dual limb ventilator systems are better suited for use in life support situations with invasive ventilation. Conversely, single limb ventilator systems are better suited with NIV [37]. Figure 2.1 shows the difference between single and dual limb configurations.

It is also known to provide NIV in a critical care ventilator by providing a single limb circuit having a proximal end coupled to the inspiratory limb portion of the ventilator and a distal end coupled to the patient interface with an actively controlled exhaust valve provided between breathing circuit and patient interface. Also, a hardwired connection must be provided between the ventilator and the actively controlled valve, so that the ventilator can control the operation of the valve. The valve is opened during an expiratory phase of a breathing cycle and closed during the inspiratory phase. This configuration is disadvantageous because it requires the relatively bulky and cumbersome actively controlled valve to be "hung" from the distal end of the single-limb circuit [36].

2.7 Invasive Ventilation

Invasive ventilation received either by endotracheal tube or tracheal cannula is considered an important therapy for patients suffered from acute respiratory insufficiency. These procedures enhance gas exchange in the lung during acute respiratory failure either of hypercapnic type with respiratory acidosis or hypoxemic type. Also, invasive ventilation is a beneficial therapy in the management of shocks that originate from any cause as it helps redistribution of blood flow to vital organs from working respiratory muscles.

2.8 Endotracheal Intubation

In the ICU, tracheal intubation is considered one of the highest-risk procedures to be performed. Approximately 40% of cases undergo intubation face significant complications because of the unstable respiratory and hemodynamic status of critically ill patients. These complications include severe hypoxemia which occurs in 25% of cases, severe hypotension occurring in 10–25% of cases, and cardiac arrest in 2% of patients [38, 39]. Intubation can be also carried out in the operating room (OR) but the risk of death or brain damage is higher following complications of ICU intubation [40]. ICU intubation and OR intubation are different procedures where OR intubation is performed in a suitable environment on a physiologically stable patient. On other hand, ICU intubation is performed in an environment that is often unsuitable for airway management on a hemodynamically unstable patient in a brief time to allow evaluation and planning [41]. The primary aim of OR intubation is to induce anesthesia where ICU intubation is considered a life-saving intervention with the main objective to sustain the airways in patients with respiratory failure. In anesthesia and pre-hospital practices, specific steps are included in intubation guidelines as pre-oxygenation, combined administration of a muscle-relaxing agent, and a sedative to obtain rapid sequence intubation and capnography to correctly check the tube placement where all of these steps are recommended to improve the safety of intubation [42]. Unfortunately, these standardized procedures are often unavailable in ICU practice [43]. The consideration of 'difficult airways' for all ICU intubations is the safest approach to use. Algorithms for difficult airways start with a 'forced to act' decision which includes an immediate best possible attempt for intubation or a decision of 'not forced to act' which mainly depends on an awake attempt. Although the awake attempt is considered the safest procedure for ICU intubation, the current clinical practice relies on deep sleep induction either with or without paralysis (apnea). During intubation, the induction of sedation and the neuromuscular blockade is thought to guarantee the success of first or second intubation attempts and lower the complications that occurred with several attempts [41]. However, the use of drug-induced apnea may be the reason for the failure of multiple intubation attempts because of the produced hypoxemia. Awake intubation is unsuitable for agitated patients [41]. When the trachea is successfully intubated and the endotracheal tube is properly placed by the healthcare giver then the settings of the ventilator (mode of ventilation) should be determined. Modes of ventilation are previously described where the most commonly used modes here are AC, PSV, and SIMV [44–46]. Intubation is indicated in an unconscious patient, those with initial clinical presentation very severe to conduct an NIV trial and patients with severe respiratory acidosis not improved by NIV therapy. The goals of mechanical ventilation in such cases can be divided into short-term and long-term goals. Short-term goals are represented in minimizing dynamic hyperinflation and obtaining acceptable values of the partial pressure of oxygen (PaO_2) and PH values but not normal partial pressure of CO_2 ($PaCO_2$). These goals can be achieved by using a controlled volume or pressure mode while minute ventilation is minimized and the inspiratory flow rate is increased to prolong the expiration period and enable the deflation of lung and the respiratory time is constant. A Long-term goal is set to allow the weaning of the patient from the ventilator while the work of breathing is decreased. During this period, spontaneous breathing efforts can be generated by the patient with the use of PSV while an external positive end-expiratory pressure (PEEP) only sufficient to counteract auto-PEEP may lower the added elastic load at the beginning of inhalation. Excessive levels of PSV are contraindicated as they can result in a prolonged time of inspiration and ineffective breathing efforts of the patient [47].

2.9 Tracheostomy

The use of a tracheostomy tube instead of a conventional endotracheal tube may result in improved patient safety and comfort. Table 2.4 illustrates the benefits of tracheostomy over endotracheal intubation. Generally, failure of manual ventilation and intubation attempts with gas exchange cessation recommend performing a tracheostomy. Tracheostomy is used for four main reasons: relieving obstruction of airways due to a foreign matter, infection, surgery, or tumor; providing a stable airway for patients needing prolonged respiratory support; preventing damage of larynges and upper airways because of prolonged intubation: facilitating removal of secretions from lower airways [48, 49].

Endotracheal intubation may affect many anatomical structures where it can cause edema or damage of vocal cords and laryngeal mucosa, stenosis and scarring of larynges, and recurrent damage of laryngeal nerve resulting in permanent disability. These injuries can't be recovered or surgically repaired with prolonged intubation. Removing the tube from the larynx and replacing it with a tracheostomy tube can cause a gradual improvement in the upper airways since these injuries are reversible [49]. Tracheostomy was recommended in older guidelines when

Table 2.4 Benefits of tracheostomy over endotracheal intubation

Benefits of tracheostomy
• Improving patient comfort
• Improved patient safety
• Lower sedation need
• Decreasing work of breathing
• Lower risk of ventilation association pneumonia
• Faster weaning of mechanical ventilation
• Shorter hospital stay length
• Earlier speaking ability
• Improved laryngeal function on long term

extubation wasn't expected after 21 days of intubation. Recently, a tracheostomy can be indicated within 2–10 days of intubation while a 14-day intubation need can be used as the procedure criterion. Tracheostomy in patients with head injury or trauma is beneficially recommended at an earlier time within only 3–4 days of intubation to avoid possible occurrence of laryngeal injury even with a short duration of intubation [49–51].

2.10 Complications of Mechanical Ventilation

Although Mechanical ventilation is a lifesaving technique, it can result in several ventilator-associated events (VAEs) caused by one of four conditions: acute respiratory syndrome (ARDS), ventilator-associated pneumonia (VAP), fluid overload, and atelectasis. Based on this classification, about 25–40% of VAEs are returned to pneumonia, 20–40% of VAEs caused by fluid overload (including pulmonary edema) while atelectasis represents 10–15% of VAEs and ARDS accounts for 10–20% of these events [52]. These complications can be returned to the type of patients using such procedure who are at a higher risk for lung or cardiac compromise, the direct effects of intrathoracic pressures created by the ventilator, and neural stimulation besides possible alveolar and systemic inflammation. However, these complications can be effectively minimized or even avoided which represents an important field for clinical studies [47, 53].

2.11 Acute Respiratory Distress Syndrome (ARDS)

Acute respiratory distress syndrome (ARDS) is defined as a new onset of respiratory symptoms or worsening of existing respiratory symptoms with opacities found bilaterally on chest x-rays and PaO_2/fraction of inspired oxygen (FiO_2) ratio equal to 300 mmHg or less while patients receive PEEP of 5 cm H_2O or higher [47]. In ARDs, impaired gas exchange is identified because of disruption of alveolar-capillary membrane and extensive pulmonary inflammation returned to diffuse lung injury. Also, the lungs are heavy, edematous, and exerting pressure to the dependent lung regions while normally aerated tissue is significantly decreased and in this case, the lung is described as 'baby lung' [47]. A lung-protective strategy of using lower than traditional TV of about 6 mL/kg and high PEEP guided by FiO_2 with limiting the plateau pressure lower than 30 cm H_2O was found to be beneficial in reducing mortality in patients with established ARDS [54]. Various studies showed the benefits of using low TV either with or without a certain degree of respiratory acidosis in limiting lung injury [55, 56]. Permissive hypoxemia also can be beneficial in ARDS patients and it refers to the concept of targeting lower than normal values of PaO_2 and oxygen saturation (SaO_2) to avoid the risks related to elevated FiO_2 [57]. While permissive hypercapnia and recruitment maneuvers together with supplying lower airway pressure were found to increase the mortality rate in ARDS patients [58]. Other adjunct interventions can be implemented in patients with moderately severe to severe ARDS (PaO_2/FiO_2 ratio below 150 mmHg) as early prone positioning and neuromuscular blockage in the first 48 h after severe ARDS onset [59]. Extracorporeal membrane oxygenation (ECMO) which involves direct oxygenation and removal of CO_2 from the blood is valuable in patients with the most severe ARDS in whom prone positioning is ineffective and still have refractory hypoxemia despite all efforts [60].

2.12 Ventilator-Associated Pneumonia (VAP)

Ventilator-associated pneumonia (VAP) can develop in ICU patients in whom mechanical ventilation has been implemented for at least 48 h. The higher risk of VAP in mechanically ventilated patients can be returned to the impaired host defense arising from lower cough efficiency and diminished mucociliary function besides microaspiration occurred from the oropharyngeal cavity [61]. VAP can be divided into two main classes: possible VAP can be identified in patients with a positive culture from the respiratory tract or those with quantitatively purulent respiratory secretions while probable VAP is characterized by both quantitatively purulent respiratory secretions and positive results from respiratory tract culture or pleural fluid culture or lung histopathology [62]. Also, VAP can occur within 4–5 days of intubation and in this case described as early-onset VAP which is mainly caused by bacteria having a favorable antibiotic sensitivity pattern as Streptococcus pneumoniae, H. influenza, and oral cavity anaerobes. While late-onset VAP is responsible for approximately two-thirds of cases and is caused by multidrug-resistant (MDR) bacteria like Pseudomonas aeruginosa, Staphylococcus aureus, Enterobacteriaceae, and Acinetobacter baumannii. This type of VAP is responsible for a longer duration of ventilation and ICU stay, higher mortality, and elevated therapy cost [63].

Generally, subglottic secretion suction results in lower VAP risk but it does not affect reducing the mechanical ventilation duration, the hospital stay length, other ventilator-associated events, antibiotic use, or mortality rate [64]. Oral care measures which include oral irrigation, tongue cleaning, and oropharyngeal suctioning can help the prevention of VAP. Additionally, the use of a silver-coated endotracheal tube is thought to decrease VAP risk but this measure is associated with limited clinical evidence. The selective decontamination of the digestive tract and oropharynx with topical non-absorbable antibiotics can participate in decreasing the occurrence of VAP but there is a great concern about the emerging bacterial resistance [62, 65]. Table 2.5 illustrates some measures that can be participated in the prevention of VAP in ventilated patients [62, 64, 66].

There are other strategies considered to be efficient to lower VAP risk and other VAEs like minimizing sedation (duration and depth), performing daily coordinated spontaneous awakening and breathing trials, initiating early exercise and mobility programs, the use of low tidal volume ventilation, and promoting conservative fluid management and conservative blood transfusion thresholds [52]. A sputum sample

Table 2.5 Preventive measures of VAP

Preventive measure	Reason
Spontaneous trials of awakening and breathing	To prepare patients for weaning and extubation and evaluate these trials before removal of mechanical ventilation
Head of the bed elevation by 30–45°	Prevention of aspiration from oropharyngeal cavity or stomach
Subglottic secretion suction and tube cuff pressure above 20 cm H_2O	To prevent aspiration over the endotracheal tube
The change of ventilator and suction tubes is limited unless there is a certain clinical indication	To prevent the introduction of new pathogens from the surrounding environment to the patient

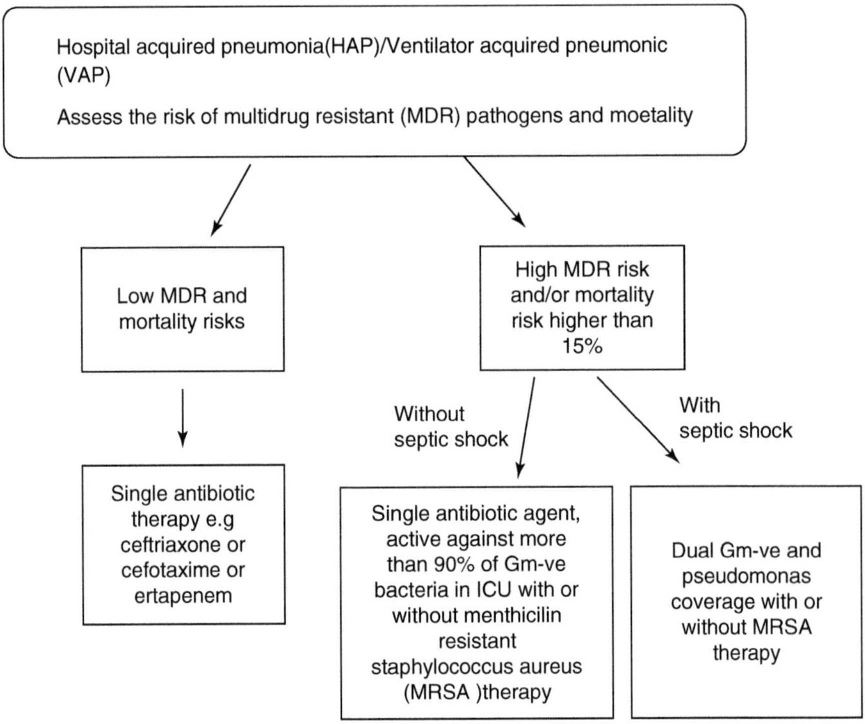

Fig. 2.2 Empiric antimicrobial therapy algorithm for Hospital-acquired pneumonia (HAP) and Ventilator acquired pneumonia (VAP)

should be taken from the patient and sent for laboratory investigation if VAP is clinically suspected. The initial selection of antibiotics should be appropriate and adequate and for that, some criteria should be considered as episode timing, most likely causative bacteria, existing co-morbidities, previous antibiotic history, and category of patients developing VAP. The empirical antibiotic therapy is recommended to be initiated as soon as possible while awaiting the laboratory findings [67, 68] (Fig. 2.2).

Patients suffered from VAP require close monitoring to identify any sign of sepsis while sepsis signs according to the Quick Sequential Organ Failure Assessment tool include altered mental status, hypotension, and tachypnea. Patients are thought to have a septic episode if they experience at least two of these mentioned signs. This screening tool is inappropriate in sedated patients on a mandatory ventilation mode and in this case, the change in baseline of two or more signs can guide the accurate sepsis screening [62].

2.13 Pneumothorax

Pneumothorax can be defined as the presence of air in the pleural cavity because of weak tissues or lung injury that occurred and associated with higher morbidity and mortality [69]. Pneumothorax can be classified into primary, secondary, traumatic, or iatrogenic based on the cause. The most common cause for iatrogenic pneumothorax is mechanical ventilation. This serious complication is noticed when high PEEP values are used during mechanical ventilation. Underlying respiratory illness as ARDS, COPD, asthma, or pneumonia is identified in most ICU patients who develop pneumothorax while intubated patients with normal lungs are rarely exhibited such disease [70]. Chest tube thoracostomy is the recommended treatment for pneumothorax where an image-guided small catheter is used with a size of 7–10 Fr to enable the air trapped in the pleural cavity to leave to avoid the progression to a tension pneumothorax. A previous study used small-bore chest tube drainage in 62 ventilated patients with pneumothorax, demonstrated that no residual air was found in the next chest radiograph in about 68.6% of cases with no major complications. Thoracic surgical consultation is often required in patients experiencing therapy failure or persistent air leakage within 3–5 days as surgical intervention is very safe and effective but it lacks evidence in critically ill patients. Also, the occurrence of pneumothorax can be minimized in ARDS patients by administering muscle relaxants [70].

2.14 Atelectasis

This term is used to describe collapsed and non-aerated regions of the lung parenchyma which could affect alveoli, a small part of the lower lungs, a full lobe, or the whole lung causing loss of lung volume [71]. The development of atelectasis can be returned to the use of high oxygen concentration as a few minutes of oxygen (100%) can produce absorption atelectasis [72]. Also, the use of lower TV during mechanical ventilation in the absence of ARDS or lung injury can result in atelectasis. Generally, the risk of alveolar collapse and in turn atelectasis is increased in postoperative patients as they spent a prolonged time in the supine position [73]. High PEEP can prevent and alleviate atelectasis besides decreasing the risk of lung injury and ARDS development. Also, the use of sufficient tidal volumes and lower FiO_2 during mechanical ventilation can resolve atelectasis by encouraging patient mobilization.

2.15 Pulmonary Edema

Mechanical ventilation is thought to be indirectly related to the accumulation of excess fluids in the lungs. The fluid status of ventilated patients must be frequently monitored as this status can participate in the development of various VAEs as VAP and ARDS. Therefore, conservative fluid management decreases such events and successfully improves weaning. Diuretic therapy with or without renal replacement therapy can be beneficial in the management of pulmonary edema to drain excess fluids [52, 74, 75].

2.16 Pleural Effusion

Pleural effusion occurs in about 62% of ICU patients who have underlying conditions as fluid overload, pneumonia, atelectasis, malignancies, or postoperative complications, and in this case, mechanical ventilation is an indirect cause of such effusion. However, the use of PEEP during mechanical ventilation improves oxygenation and lowers work of breathing which is affected greatly by the presence of large or bilateral effusions. Small pleural effusions need only monitoring while diuretic therapy may be used for the treatment of significant effusions [62, 76].

References

1. Caramez MP, et al. Paradoxical responses to positive end-expiratory pressure in patients with airway obstruction during controlled ventilation. Crit Care Med. 2005;33(7):1519.
2. Brochard L. Mechanical ventilation: invasive versus noninvasive. Eur Respir J. 2003;22(47 suppl):31s–7s.
3. Antonelli M, et al. A comparison of noninvasive positive-pressure ventilation and conventional mechanical ventilation in patients with acute respiratory failure. N Engl J Med. 1998;339(7):429–35.
4. Pauwels RA, et al. Global strategy for the diagnosis, management, and prevention of chronic obstructive pulmonary disease: NHLBI/WHO global initiative for chronic obstructive lung disease (GOLD) workshop summary. Am J Respir Crit Care Med. 2001;163(5):1256–76.
5. Korang SK, et al. Non-invasive positive pressure ventilation for acute asthma in children. Cochrane Database Syst Rev. 2016;9:CD012067.
6. Pavone M, et al. Non-invasive positive pressure ventilation in children. Early Hum Dev. 2013;89(Suppl 3):S25–31.

7. Longest PW, Tian G, Hindle M. Improving the lung delivery of nasally administered aerosols during noninvasive ventilation-an application of enhanced condensational growth (ECG). J Aerosol Med Pulm Drug Deliv. 2011;24(2):103–18.
8. Dhand R. Aerosol therapy in patients receiving noninvasive positive pressure ventilation. J Aerosol Med Pulm Drug Deliv. 2012;25(2):63–78.
9. Brochard L, et al. Noninvasive ventilation for acute exacerbations of chronic obstructive pulmonary disease. N Engl J Med. 1995;333(13):817–22.
10. Slutsky AS. History of mechanical ventilation. From vesalius to ventilator-induced lung injury. Am J Respir Crit Care Med. 2015;191(10):1106–15.
11. Hoo G, Byrd Jr R. Noninvasive ventilation. Methods of delivery medscape. [Updated 2014 April, 4].
12. Hess DR. Noninvasive ventilation in neuromuscular disease: equipment and application. Respir Care. 2006;51(8):896–912.
13. Köhnlein T, et al. Non-invasive positive pressure ventilation for the treatment of severe stable chronic obstructive pulmonary disease: a prospective, multicentre, randomised, controlled clinical trial. Lancet Respir Med. 2014;2(9):698–705.
14. Chatburn RL. Which ventilators and modes can be used to deliver noninvasive ventilation? Respir Care. 2009;54(1):85–101.
15. Navalesi P, et al. Physiologic evaluation of noninvasive mechanical ventilation delivered with three types of masks in patients with chronic hypercapnic respiratory failure. Crit Care Med. 2000;28(6):1785–90.
16. Erickson SE, et al. Racial and ethnic disparities in mortality from acute lung injury. Crit Care Med. 2009;37(1):1.
17. Liesching T, Kwok H, Hill NS. Acute applications of noninvasive positive pressure ventilation. Chest J. 2003;124(2):699–713.
18. Navalesi P, et al. Non-invasive ventilation in chronic obstructive pulmonary disease patients: helmet versus facial mask. Intensive Care Med. 2007;33(1):74–81.
19. Racca F, et al. Helmet ventilation and carbon dioxide rebreathing: effects of adding a leak at the helmet ports. Intensive Care Med. 2008;34(8):1461–8.
20. Holland AE, et al. Efficacy of a heated passover humidifier during noninvasive ventilation: a bench study. Respir Care. 2007;52(1):38–44.
21. Tuggey JM, Delmastro M, Elliott MW. The effect of mouth leak and humidification during nasal non-invasive ventilation. Respir Med. 2007;101(9):1874–9.
22. Plant PK, Owen JL, Elliott MW. Early use of non-invasive ventilation for acute exacerbations of chronic obstructive pulmonary disease on general respiratory wards: a multicentre randomised controlled trial. Lancet. 2000;355(9219):1931–5.
23. Brochard L, et al. Reversal of acute exacerbations of chronic obstructive lung disease by inspiratory assistance with a face mask. N Engl J Med. 1990;323(22):1523–30.
24. Rose L. Management of critically ill patients receiving noninvasive and invasive mechanical ventilation in the emergency department. Open Access Emerg Med. 2012;4:5.
25. Vestbo J, et al. Global strategy for the diagnosis, management, and prevention of chronic obstructive pulmonary disease: GOLD executive summary. Am J Respir Crit Care Med. 2013;187(4):347–65.
26. Calfee CS, Matthay MA. Recent advances in mechanical ventilation. Am J Med. 2005;118(6):584–91.
27. Rabec C, et al. Ventilator modes and settings during non-invasive ventilation: effects on respiratory events and implications for their identification. Thorax. 2011;66(2): 170–8.
28. Fichtner F, et al. Clinical guideline for treating acute respiratory insufficiency with invasive ventilation and extracorporeal membrane oxygenation: evidence-based recommendations for choosing modes and setting parameters of mechanical ventilation. Respiration. 2019;98(4):357–72.

29. Pennock BE, et al. Pressure support ventilation with a simplified ventilatory support system administered with a nasal mask in patients with respiratory failure. Chest. 1991;100(5):v1371–6.
30. Ramanathan R. Synchronized intermittent mandatory ventilation and pressure support: to sync or not to sync? Pressure support or no pressure support? J Perinatol. 2005;25(Suppl 2):S23–5; discussion S26–7.
31. Girault C, et al. Comparative physiologic effects of noninvasive assist-control and pressure support ventilation in acute hypercapnic respiratory failure. Chest. 1997;111(6):1639–48.
32. Peter JV, et al. Effect of non-invasive positive pressure ventilation (NIPPV) on mortality in patients with acute cardiogenic pulmonary oedema: a meta-analysis. Lancet. 2006;367(9517):1155–63.
33. Fernández-Vivas M, et al. Noninvasive pressure support versus proportional assist ventilation in acute respiratory failure. Intensive Care Med. 2003;29(7):1126–33.
34. Dhand R. Inhalation therapy in invasive and noninvasive mechanical ventilation. Curr Opin Crit Care. 2007;13(1):27–38.
35. Ari A, Fink JB. Factors affecting bronchodilator delivery in mechanically ventilated adults. Nurs Crit Care. 2010;15(4):192–203.
36. Doyle PR. Ventilator adaptable for use with either a dual-limb circuit or a single-limb circuit; 2009. Google Patents.
37. Hess DR. Noninvasive ventilation for acute respiratory failure. Respir Care. 2013;58(6):950–72.
38. Chatburn RL, Mireles-Cabodevila E, Tobin MJ Basic principles of ventilator design. Principles and practice of mechanical ventilation; 2013.
39. Jaber S, et al. An intervention to decrease complications related to endotracheal intubation in the intensive care unit: a prospective, multiple-center study. Intensive Care Med. 2010;36(2):248–55.
40. Cook TM, et al. Major complications of airway management in the UK: results of the Fourth National Audit Project of the Royal College of Anaesthetists and the Difficult Airway Society. Part 1: anaesthesia. Br J Anaesth. 2011;106(5):617–31.
41. Lapinsky SE. Endotracheal intubation in the ICU. Crit Care. 2015;19:258.
42. Smith DC, et al. A trial of etomidate for rapid sequence intubation in the emergency department. J Emerg Med. 2000;18(1):13–6.
43. Leibowitz AB. Tracheal intubation in the intensive care unit: extremely hazardous even in the best of hands. Crit Care Med. 2006;34(9):2497–8.
44. Gali B, Goyal DG. Positive pressure mechanical ventilation. Emerg Med Clin. 2003;21(2):453–73.
45. Chiumello D, et al. Different modes of assisted ventilation in patients with acute respiratory failure. Eur Respir J. 2002;20(4):925–33.
46. Singer BD, Corbridge TC. Basic invasive mechanical ventilation. South Med J. 2009;102(12):1238–45.
47. Pham T, Brochard LJ, Slutsky AS. Mechanical ventilation: state of the art. Mayo Clin Proc. 2017;92(9):1382–400.
48. Caplan R et al. American Society of Anesthesiologists Task Force on Management of the Difficult Airway. Practice guidelines for management of the difficult airway. An updated report by the American Society of Anesthesiologists Task Force on Management of the Difficult Airway. Anesthesiology. 2003;98(5):1269–77.
49. Durbin CG. Tracheostomy: why, when, and how? Respir Care. 2010;55(8):1056–68.
50. Mitchell RB, et al. Clinical consensus statement: tracheostomy care. Otolaryngol Head Neck Surg. 2013;148(1):6–20.
51. McWhorter AJ. Tracheotomy: timing and techniques. Curr Opin Otolaryngol Head Neck Surg. 2003;11(6):473–9.
52. Klompas M. Potential strategies to prevent ventilator-associated events. Am J Respir Crit Care Med. 2015;192(12):1420–30.
53. Klompas M. Ventilator-associated events: what they are and what they are not. Respir Care. 2019;64(8):953–61.

54. Meade MO, et al. Ventilation strategy using low tidal volumes, recruitment maneuvers, and high positive end-expiratory pressure for acute lung injury and acute respiratory distress syndrome: a randomized controlled trial. JAMA. 2008;299(6):637–45.
55. Needham DM, et al. Timing of low tidal volume ventilation and intensive care unit mortality in acute respiratory distress syndrome. A prospective cohort study. Am J Respir Crit Care Med. 2015;191(2):177–85.
56. Jardin F. Tidal volume reduction in patients with acute lung injury when plateau pressures are not high. Am J Respir Crit Care Med. 2006;173(6):685–6.
57. Gonzalez S. Permissive hypoxemia versus normoxemia for critically ill patients receiving mechanical ventilation. Crit Care Nurse. 2015;35(2):80–1.
58. Wang C, et al. Lung ventilation strategies for acute respiratory distress syndrome: a systematic review and network meta-analysis. Sci Rep. 2016;6:22855.
59. Papazian L, et al. Neuromuscular blockers in early acute respiratory distress syndrome. N Engl J Med. 2010;363(12):1107–16.
60. Brodie D, Bacchetta M. Extracorporeal membrane oxygenation for ARDS in adults. N Engl J Med. 2011;365(20):1905–14.
61. Kalil AC, et al. Management of adults with hospital-acquired and ventilator-associated pneumonia: 2016 clinical practice guidelines by the Infectious Diseases Society of America and the American Thoracic Society. Clin Infect Dis. 2016;63(5):e61–e111.
62. Baid H. Patient safety: identifying and managing complications of mechanical ventilation. Crit Care Nurs Clin North Am. 2016;28(4):451–62.
63. Bassetti M, et al. Management of ventilator-associated pneumonia: epidemiology, diagnosis and antimicrobial therapy. Expert Rev Anti Infect Ther. 2012;10(5):585–96.
64. Caroff DA, et al. Subglottic secretion drainage and objective outcomes: a systematic review and meta-analysis. Crit Care Med. 2016;44(4):830–40.
65. Torres A, et al. International ERS/ESICM/ESCMID/ALAT guidelines for the management of hospital-acquired pneumonia and ventilator-associated pneumonia: guidelines for the management of hospital-acquired pneumonia (HAP)/ventilator-associated pneumonia (VAP) of the European Respiratory Society (ERS), European Society of Intensive Care Medicine (ESICM), European Society of Clinical Microbiology and Infectious Diseases (ESCMID) and Asociacion Latinoamericana del Torax (ALAT). Eur Respir J. 2017;50(3): 1700582.
66. Klompas M, et al. The preventability of ventilator-associated events. The CDC prevention epicenters wake up and breathe collaborative. Am J Respir Crit Care Med. 2015;191(3): 292–301.
67. Vandana Kalwaje E, Rello J. Management of ventilator-associated pneumonia: need for a personalized approach. Expert Rev Anti Infect Ther. 2018;16(8):641–53.
68. Metersky ML, Kalil AC. Management of ventilator-associated pneumonia: guidelines. Clin Chest Med. 2018;39(4):797–808.
69. Noppen M, De Keukeleire T. Pneumothorax. Respiration. 2008;76(2):121–7.
70. Hsu CW, Sun SF. Iatrogenic pneumothorax related to mechanical ventilation. World J Crit Care Med. 2014;3(1):8–14.
71. Ray K, Bodenham A, Paramasivam E. Pulmonary atelectasis in anaesthesia and critical care. Contin Educ Anaesth Crit Care Pain. 2014;14(5):236–45.
72. Suzuki S, et al. Atelectasis and mechanical ventilation mode during conservative oxygen therapy: a before-and-after study. J Crit Care. 2015;30(6):1232–7.
73. Duggan M, Kavanagh BP, Warltier DC. Pulmonary atelectasis: a pathogenic perioperative entity. J Am Soc Anesthesiol. 2005;102(4):838–54.
74. Lewis SC, et al. Risk factors for ventilator-associated events: a case-control multivariable analysis. Crit Care Med. 2014;42(8):1839.
75. Dessap AM, et al. Ventilator-associated pneumonia during weaning from mechanical ventilation: role of fluid management. Chest. 2014;146(1):58–65.
76. Mekontso Dessap A, et al. Ventilator-associated pneumonia during weaning from mechanical ventilation: role of fluid management. Chest. 2014;146(1):58–65.

Chapter 3
Oxygen Delivery Systems and Nasally Ventilated Patients

Contents

3.1 Introduction

In clinical settings, oxygen is the most common drug to be used which remarkably saves patient lives. However, its inappropriate use can expose the patients to great harm. The misconception that "oxygen couldn't hurt" had led to the delivery of high

M. E. A. Abdelrahim et al., *Essentials of Aerosol Therapy in Critically ill Patients*,
https://doi.org/10.1007/978-3-030-85026-5_3

oxygen levels to critically unwell patients or those who even complain of dyspnea which causes a noticeable increase in the duration of hospitalization, the probability of high dependency unit admission, and mortality rate [1, 2]. In acute exacerbations of chronic obstructive pulmonary disease (COPD), supplemental oxygen therapy is widely given to patients while uncontrolled delivery especially that with high oxygen concentrations can lead to a worsened hypercapnia [3, 4]. Where high oxygen concentrations could inhibit pulmonary vasoconstriction which results in a worsening mismatch of ventilation/perfusion and an increased partial pressure of CO_2 due to the right-hand shift of the dissociation curve of CO_2. Also, the high density of oxygen can increase work of breathing and the existing absorption atelectasis can add a further increase in ventilation/perfusion mismatch [4–6].

3.2 Oxygen Device

Low flow oxygen delivery devices as a nasal cannula, bag valve masks, and non-rebreathing masks can deliver a medical gas up to 15 L/min where the fraction of inspired oxygen (FiO_2) can vary with the delivered gas flow, peak inspiratory flow of the patient and characteristics of the delivery system and device used [7]. These devices provide 100% oxygen concentration at a maximum flow of 15 L/min while the inspiratory flow of the patient even at quiet breathing is approximately 30 L/min exceeding that maximum flow of supplemental oxygen. Thus, the room air which contains 21% oxygen is entrained to match the patient's inspiratory demand resulting in a diluted total FiO_2. Similarly, during respiratory distress, more entrainment of large volumes of air is observed resulting in a much lower FiO_2. One of the major benefits of low flow devices is their use for providing oxygen at home (home oxygen therapy) which will be discussed in detail later in this chapter. Air entrainment mask or venturi mask is an example of intermediate oxygen flow systems where its principle depends on pumping pressurized oxygen at a constant flow through a small orifice and at an adjusted air/oxygen ratio; room air enters through entrainment ports. Venturi masks are considered to supply a predictable FiO_2 by adjusting the ratio of oxygen to room air [8]. When the requirements for FiO_2 are low, these masks supply higher gas flow rates because of the more entrained air through large ports e.g. a total flow of 44 L/min approximately provides 28% FiO_2. To achieve a higher FiO_2, the ratio of supplemental oxygen to room air is proposed to be increased so less air is entrained and the total flow is decreased e.g. a total flow of 24 L/min provides 60% FiO_2. On the other hand, if the patient exhibits a high inspiratory flow rate, additional air is expected to be entrained around the mask which dilutes the oxygen and decreases the delivered FiO_2 [8, 9].

Several limitations can be identified with the use of conventional oxygen systems. These devices provide insufficient heated and humidified medical gas resulting in poor tolerance and patient discomfort. Also, the FiO_2 provided by these systems is not constant and in most cases is unknown as the maximum oxygen flow supplied is no more than 15 L/min where the patient's inspiratory flow during respiratory failure can vary between 30 and 120 L/min. This difference between the delivered flow and the inspiratory flow of the patient leads to oxygen dilution with room air and lower oxygen concentration to reach the patient (below 10%) [9, 10].

By contrast, high flow nasal cannula (HFNC) oxygen therapy can allow the delivery of FiO2 in a range of 21–100% and generates gas flows up to 60 L/min [11]. The gas is heated and humidified when passes over an active heated humidifier (Fig. 3.1). Then, this heated and humidified gas is delivered through a single limb heated circuit to keep the moisture and the heat of the delivered gas until reaching the patient through a large diameter nasal cannula [12].

Typically, a high-flow system consists of a flow generator, a heated humidifier, a heated circuit, and a nasal interface. Flow generators are of three popular types: air-oxygen blenders, entrainment flow systems, and built-in flow generators. For that, HFNC systems can be classified into three clinically available types: the air-oxygen blender (HFNC/blender), the Venturi (HFNC/Venturi), and the turbine (HFNC/turbine) [13]. Air-oxygen blender is the common type used where the wall supply is responsible for providing both air and oxygen passing through a flow meter which ensures the stable delivery of gas flow and FiO_2. Built-in flow generators are usually precise and incorporated into devices manufactured by Vapotherm and Fisher & Paykel Healthcare companies. Their principle depends on using turbines to entrain room air to deliver high flow and oxygen can be provided only through low-pressure systems so the delivery of high oxygen concentration can't be established by these generators. Oxygen concentration is monitored by the device. However, the air-entrainment system (Max–Venturi) can provide a high gas flow rate with a higher oxygen concentration by using a flow meter to titrate oxygen concentration. An Air-entrainment system is usually used when the outlet for the medical gas is unavailable as in patients receiving physical therapy or transfer and those recovered

Fig. 3.1 High flow oxygen system

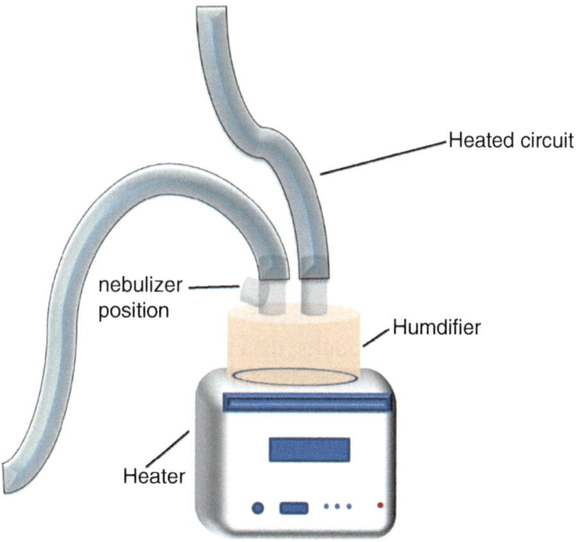

after minimally invasive surgeries. Noise is the common problem noticed while the use of various types of flow generators greatly increases with increasing the gas flow or FiO_2. Patients feel uncomfortable during HFNC due to the noise generated [13, 14]. The noise levels of HFNC/venturi are higher than that created by either the HFNC/blender or the HFNC/turbine. A previous study comparing three HFNC types had found that the noise level of the Venturi type might be reduced by adding a filter to the air intake side of the device [13].

Heated humidifiers incorporated into the HFNC delivery system are of two types: active (pass-over) humidifiers and passive (filter-type) humidifiers. Inactive humidifiers, medical gas is directly passed overheated water from which it acquires its heat and becomes saturated with water vapor. In filter-type humidifiers as those found in Vapotherm, the blended gas acquires its humidification by passing through a bundle of narrow tubes with a pore size of 0.005 μm. For that, passive humidifiers require a large evaporative surface if compared with active humidifiers. Two cartridge sizes are supplied by Vapotherm: one for low flows (1–8 L/min) and the other for high flows (5–40 L/min). The performance of active and passive humidifiers is considered satisfactory until the gas flow exceeds 60 L/min. Also, the performance of humidification depends on patient characteristics as tidal volume and inspiratory flow [14–16]. The third component of the high flow system is the heated wire circuit which has a main role to avoid vapor loss and ensuring the delivery of adequately heated and humidified gas [17]. Vapotherm doesn't use a heated wire circuit but the warm water passes between the inner and outer lumens of tubes through which the gas is supplied. Generally, by the use of this system, cooling by room air and condensation in the inspiratory limb is minimized.it resembles systems used for blood and infusion fluids warming [14, 18]. Condensation can also occur in the nasal prongs beyond the circuit which leads to the accumulation of water droplets in the nose and it can be increased by decreasing the ambient temperature. This water condensate affects the patients in different ways through disturbing sleep, causing discomfort, and inducing cough, aspiration, and desaturation. The final component of the HFNC system is the patient interface. The nasal cannula is the most tolerated interface and is considered the great advantage offered by this system over non-invasive ventilation (NIV).In the high-velocity nasal insufflation Vapotherm system (Hi-VNI), the nasal cannula used resembles that of regular or standard nasal prongs which have a narrow internal diameter and nasal bores and can deliver high flows [19]. Meanwhile, the Optiflow cannula supplied by Fisher & Paykel has both wide-bore nasal prongs and tubing while the gas flow is delivered only from one side, unlike standard nasal prongs.

The use of HFNC has been well studied in various conditions affecting neonates and pediatrics but in adults, data are still limited [20]. Of note, HFNC can provide a constant FiO_2 and lowers the dilution of oxygen. Also, it offers several advantages regarding oxygenation and ventilation over conventional oxygen devices as flushing out of CO_2 from anatomical dead space, providing a lower level of positive end-expiratory pressure (PEEP) and it facilitates secretions mobility and clearance, relieves bronchospasm, and maintains the integrity of mucosa by the supplied heated and humidified gas [21, 22].

3.3 Clinical Benefits Offered by HFNC

3.3.1 Improvement of Mucociliary Clearance

The respiratory epithelium is covered by a thin layer of liquid consisting of two films which are SOL (aqueous) and Gel (mucus). Globet cells are responsible for the production of the gel layer in which the cilia are located. The correct movement of cilia to remove the mucus depends on this existing layer. The epithelial cells have to perform their normal function to absorb sodium and eliminate chlorine since secretions contain an adequate amount of water and need mobilization. Since mucus viscosity is dependent on its water content which plays the main role in secretion transport. Increased airway secretions are predominately seen in patients who experience respiratory distress which requires a great effort from the patients to expel them. This can lead to fatigue of respiratory muscles and the development of respiratory failure, especially with thick and immobilized secretions [23]. Conditions required for maintaining the normal function of epithelial cells are indicated by providing air in the main bronchi which are completely saturated with water vapor (100%) and have a temperature of 37 °C. HFNC can effectively provide these optimal conditions [24]. On the other hand, dry gas breathing can desiccate and damage epithelial cells by altering mucus characteristics. Therefore, humidification of inspired gases is beneficial to maintain and optimize the functions of epithelial cells through improving gas exchange, maintaining host defense, and limiting the metabolic cost of respiration [25]. In patients with bronchiectasis, HFNC was used to facilitate the removal of secretions because of its ability to hydrate airways. Similarly, conditions like COPD, cystic fibrosis, pneumonia, and acute and chronic bronchitis can benefit from the use of HFNC as one of the main goals for treating such diseases is the adequate removal of secretions [23].

3.3.2 Anatomical Dead Space Washout

When gas is supplied at high flow, it causes the washout of CO_2 eliminating the dead space attributed to this flushed-out volume which in turn allows a higher minute ventilation fraction to take part in gas exchange. However, HFNC doesn't cause any active improvement in tidal volume as it is an open system [26]. The precise mechanism for dead space washout can't be determined because of the inability to measure in-vivo gas flow and the complexity of the pharyngeal airway. Higher flows were found to decrease the dead space but the relationship is not determined yet. A previous study compared the effects of high flow systems with that of conventional low flow devices in COPD patients had demonstrated that patients using HFNC tolerated exercising for a longer duration than those using conventional oxygen devices [27, 28]. Also, patients who used HFNC had experienced less dyspnea, improved pulmonary function, and decreased arterial tension through enhancing oxygenation [27, 28]. Generally, exercise intolerance in COPD patients is returned to the high dead space volume of the upper airways which results in a compensatory increase in minute ventilation. HFNC participates in improving the exercise performance in those patients by washing out the residual gas and in turn, reduces the increase in ineffective ventilation [29, 30]. Additionally, in a previous study performed on animals, partial pressure of CO_2 ($PaCO_2$) was found to decrease with increasing gas flow which greatly suggested the effective washout of CO_2 by using HFNC. When FiO_2 was compared in volunteers breathing with open and closed mouth, the higher FiO_2 was noticed with mouth-open breathing. This may be returned to the reservoir function of the oral cavity, the nose, and the pharynx. During exhalation, oxygen is allowed to completely suffuse the nasal cavity with mouth-open breathing which effectively washes out CO_2. With inhalation, oxygen is entrained within the nose and results in higher FIO_2 [31, 32].

Furthermore, the nasal cannula is considered the only interface which does not affect increasing the dead space as it possesses the lowest instrumental death space while oxygen mask can lead to rebreathing of carbon dioxide especially at low flow. Also, non-invasive ventilation (NIV) interfaces increase dead space [24].

3.3.3 Positive End-Expiratory Pressure (PEEP) Effect

A mild distending pressure can be provided by HFNC. HFNC is known as an open system but high gas flow rates can oppose to some extent the resistance of expiratory flow and also increase airway pressure by about 3 cm H_2O based on the gas flow rate and the size of nasal prongs in proportion to the nostrils [33]. In a previous study, the pharyngeal pressure was measured while delivering oxygen inflow rates range from 0 to 60 L/min, the expiratory pressure was found to be significantly higher with closed mouth breathing than with open mouth. As HFNC therapy produces a certain degree of continuous positive airway pressure (CPAP) which is dependent on both gas flow rate and open or closed-mouth breathing [27, 34]. When the mouth is closed during breathing, high flows can perform resistance to exhalation. Parke et al. conducted a study in post-cardiac surgery patients to measure the nasopharyngeal pressure where both HFNC and facemask were compared at a flow rate of 35 L/min. HFNC was found to increase nasopharyngeal pressure by 2.7 ± 1.04 cmH_2O with closed mouth breathing and by 1.2 ± 0.76 cmH_2O with open mouth while zero increase in nasopharyngeal pressure was noticed with facemask [33]. Generally, Each increase in gas flow rate by 10 L/min may result in an increase in mean airway pressure by 0.69 cmH_2O with closed-mouth breathing and by 0.35 cmH_2O with open-mouth breathing [33]. This created pressure counterbalance auto-PEEP and inspiratory pressure which contributes to the reduction of work of breathing and effort of respiratory muscles seen with HFNC therapy [35].

3.3.4 Provision of the Stable Fraction of Inspired Oxygen

As known, conventional low oxygen devices provide unstable FiO_2 which is much lower than the values predicted by the equipment algorithm [36]. The patient-breathing pattern generally determines the FiO_2 value. FiO_2 is in a range of 0.26–0.54 with quiet breathing at a gas flow of 1–6 L/min while with rapid breathing, FiO2 ranges from 0.24 to 0.45 [32]. At a flow of 6–15 L/min, FiO_2 increases to reach 0.54–0.75 with quiet breathing and 0.49–0.72 with rapid breathing. Also, FiO_2 increases with open-mouth breathing than with closed mouth. On the other hand, HFNC systems can deliver actual FiO_2 close to predicted or calculated FiO_2. A previous study conducted by Ritchie et al. had demonstrated that when the flow rate of delivered gas exceeded the peak inspiratory flow rate (PIFR) of the patient, the measured FiO_2 was approximately equal to the delivered FiO_2, and also the increase in PIFR during exercise resulted in lower FiO_2 than that measured during rest. Open mouth breathing decreases delivered FiO_2 than closed-mouth due to mixing of the high oxygen flow with room air which inhaled through the mouth. Additionally, PIFR can reach 90 L/min or more during exercise which exceeds the flow capacity of HFNC but under these circumstances, HFNC can perform better than traditional oxygen devices [23]. Finally, it can be concluded that high gas flow rates together with closed mouth breathing produce an actual FiO_2 close to the predicted or calculated FiO_2 where the delivered gas is much higher than the inspiratory flow of the patient [24, 31, 37].

3.4 Attenuation of Inspiratory Resistance (Work of Breathing)

The inspiratory resistance is attenuated through two essential mechanisms:

3.4.1 By Providing Adequate Flow

No active inspiratory support is provided by HFNC in contrast to NIV devices which can deliver inspiratory pressure support. However, HFNC can increase tidal volume (TV), decrease both breathing rate and minute ventilation when compared with spontaneous breathing [38]. These changes in breathing pattern and lung volumes may help in patients with pulmonary edema where flooded alveoli can be opened with enhanced oxygenation, improved pulmonary compliance, and reduced left ventricular afterload which mimics the same effects produced by CPAP [23]. Also, Chatila et al. demonstrated that COPD patients who received HFNC tolerated exercising for a longer duration with improved oxygenation, better breathing pattern, less breathlessness, and lower arterial pressure than those who received their oxygen therapy by conventional low flow devices. So, HFNC is considered an acceptable choice for COPD patients who experience exercise intolerance by using conventional ways [28, 30]. Of note, the nasopharynx has distinct expandability that creates an alterable resistance. One of the main effects of HFNC is to reduce the nasopharyngeal airflow resistance by providing higher inspiratory flows than other means of respiratory support [27].

3.4.2 *By Supplying Adequately Heated and Humidified Gas*

In the nasal mucosa, the inhaled air is normally conditioned where it is heated and humidified due to its highly vascular sinusoid tissue. Humidification of oxygen at flow rates greater than 4 L/min is required since the normal conditioning function of the nasal mucosa may be insufficient in this case. Poor patient tolerance to oxygen therapy is identified if the delivered gas is dry and unwarmed. So, one can notice the lower adherence to long-term oxygen therapy (LTOT) despite its improved patient outcomes. Under-humidification results in dryness of nasal mucosa, throat, and mouth, frequent nasal bleeding, eye irritation, and high cost of oxygen therapy. Also, breathing cold air by healthy individuals can activate osmoreceptors that present in the nasal mucosa resulting in bronchoconstriction. The same is noticed in COPD patients when inhaling dry and cold air but through the activation of muscarinic receptors which induces bronchospasm. For conventional low flow oxygen devices, bubble humidifiers are used to humidify oxygen but they produce a low absolute humidity. However, an active humidification system is used within the HFNC system to warm the medical gas at 37 °C with an absolute humidity close to the recommended values while the presence of a heated wire circuit connected to this humidification system prevents the loss of water vapor by condensation [17]. The metabolic cost for warming and heating the inhaled gas is not negligible especially in patients with acute respiratory failure who experience tachypnea. For example, if the inspired air is at room temperature (21 °C) and with 50% relative humidity containing 9 mg of water per liter. Then, each liter of air requires 107.5 J (26 Calories) to raise its temperature by 21 °C and vaporize 35 mg of water into it. This means 156 calories/min is required for gas conditioning in an adult with a typical tidal volume of 500 mL and a breathing rate of 12 breaths/min in addition to the metabolic cost of mucus formation and moving the water. So, patients can benefit from the energy-saving effects of HFNC therapy [23, 39]. These benefits are proven by clinical studies in infants who showed more weight gain on using the Vapotherm device when compared with those who used conventional CPAP [24, 39, 40].

3.4.2.1 Potential Clinical HFNC Applications

As HFNC can improve many clinical and physiological parameters which are previously mentioned, this encourages the researchers to assess this therapy in many situations facing them in the clinical settings [10].

3.5 Obstructive Airways Diseases

Frequent exacerbation and decline in pulmonary function can occur in patients with obstructive airway disease as COPD because of the persistent inflammation of airways and mucus retention. Various studies illustrated the relation between airway surface dehydration and pulmonary damage seen in chronic obstructive airway diseases. HFNC therapy was found to improve lung function and quality of life of COPD patients if compared with more traditional techniques of respiratory support [41]. Also, a disease like obstructive sleep apnea (OSA) can benefit from HFNC therapy. This disease is caused as a result of upper airway destruction occurred due to discontinuous hypoxemia, neurocognitive dysfunction, and a cardiovascular problem. CPAP is considered the standard and highly effective therapy of OSA but suboptimal adherence is the major limitation of its use [42]. the higher tolerability of HFNC therapy with its ability to deliver heated, humidified and pressurized oxygen at a high flow can help the management of OSA [43]. A study conducted by Hawkins et al. on ten OSA patients with an age range of 1–18 years. Authors found that HFNC therapy resulted in decreased respiratory events and heart rate and improved oxygenation. So, HFNC might be beneficial with children who couldn't tolerate CPAP therapy and had moderate to severe OSA [44]. Also, McGinley et al. had proven the efficacy of HFNC therapy in relieving the obstruction of airways in both children and adults where it reduced apnea-hypopnea index (AHI) [45, 46].

3.6 Hypoxemic Respiratory Failure

Acute hypoxemic respiratory failure is considered a primary reason for initiating HFNC therapy but the evidence of its effects on intubation and mortality rates is still unclear. Several trials of HFNC were identified in patients experiencing different hypoxemic respiratory failure types. Some studies focused on the oxygenation and comfort effects of HFNC in respiratory failure. Roca et al. compared oxygen therapy via HFNC and a traditional face mask in 20 patients with acute respiratory failure to demonstrate which is more comfortable. Facemask was connected to nasal cannula where the sum of gas flow was 20 L/min and is considered a high flow facemask. Results came to encourage the use of HFNC in those patients as it was associated with less dryness of mouth, reduced dyspnea and respiratory rate, and a higher PaO_2 [47]. Another prospective observational study conducted by Sztrymf et al. showed the same beneficial effects of HFNC in lowering the respiratory rate and increasing oxygen saturation and PaO_2 when compared with traditional oxygen therapy [48].

Patients with hypoxemic respiratory failure mostly received HFNC therapy in high dependency units or emergency departments (ED). Several clinical parameters were measured during HFNC therapy in a retrospective study carried on 75 patients with acute respiratory failure to assess the success of therapy. The baseline characteristics of patients before receiving the therapy and respiratory parameters at 1 and 24 h after receiving HFNC were measured. Authors found that about 63% of included patients avoided intubation and HFNC therapy significantly improved respiratory parameters like PaO_2, oxygen saturation (SaO_2), heart rate, and respiration rate during the first 24 h of receiving the therapy [49]. Also, Lenglet et al. evaluated the use of HFNC in ED where they found oxygenation, respiratory rate, and dyspnea score were improved after 15 min of receiving the therapy. HFNC was found to be the preferred oxygenation method over conventional methods by 75% of ED patients [50]. However, the positive effects of HFNC especially over non-invasive ventilation are still debated. During invasive procedures as bronchoscopy, hypoxemia is a common complication so that supplemental oxygen is needed. Lucangelo et al. had compared two oxygen delivery systems which were air-entrainment masks at a flow rate of 40 L/min and HFNC at two different flows: 40 and 60 L/min. They demonstrated that HFNC at 60 L/min caused better oxygenation than both HFNC at 40 L/min and air entrainment mask at 40 L/min [51]. A study was performed to compare the effects of HFNC via NIV in hypoxemic patients who were subjected to flexible bronchoscopy. Authors randomly placed the patients in one of two groups: the first group received HFNC and the other received NIV. NIV group was found to have a higher oxygen level when compared with the HFNC group. Also, NIV had resulted in improved oxygenation outcomes before, during, and after the bronchoscopic procedure [52]. Also, Kang et al. reported the failure of HFNC therapy in improving the symptoms of patients with respiratory failure which led to delayed intubations and worsened patient outcomes [53]. For that, HFNC therapy can be used to safely manage the patient with hypoxemic respiratory failure at the early disease stages while its extended use before intubation can significantly harm the patients [47, 53]. Generally, HFNC is an effective means for respiratory support in hypoxemic patients with mild to moderate disease status [31].

Clinicians should be aware of the selection criteria as respiratory rate, SaO_2, and PaO_2/FiO_2. After recognizing the signs of HFNC failure, clinicians should have access to established protocols to determine the patient's need for initiating NIV or invasive ventilation (intubation) [27]. Distressed thoracoabdominal asynchrony, the use of accessory respiratory muscles, and persistence of higher respiration rates are predictors for an inadequate response for HFNC therapy and the need to consider intubation [9]. Also, patients experiencing other organ failures like hemodynamic instability besides the worsened respiratory disease can highly be subjected to HFNC failure [9].

Additionally, large multi-center randomized trials are needed to assess the oxygenation capability of HFNC compared with conventional oxygen therapy, NIV since all available data were only reported from small-scale studies. These large-scale trials can determine which type and severity level of acute hypoxemic respiratory failure may benefit from HFNC therapy [23].

3.7 Hypercapnic Respiratory Failure

Management of patients with hypercapnic respiratory failure represents a challenge for health care providers as mechanical ventilation is unsuitable for many of them who may exhibit multiple comorbidities. So, NIV has been known as the standard respiratory support technique in hypercapnic patients [31]. The use of NIV is troublesome in certain patients due to the poor tolerability of traditional facemasks. Thus, HFNC can be beneficial in those patients who are unable to withstand NIV [54]. A previous study was conducted on COPD patients who had chronic hypercapnic respiratory failure to demonstrate the effects of using HFNC. Authors found that the response of patients to HFNC was varied after receiving of 22 L/min air/oxygen mixture (sum of 20 L/min air and 2 L/min oxygen) for 45 min given through nasal cannula while some patients experienced decreased respiratory rate and some had a reduced PaO_2 [55]. Rittayamai et al. demonstrated that the implementation of HFNC therapy for a short duration at a gas flow rate of 30 L/min had reduced the inspiratory effort in hypercapnic COPD patients experiencing mild to moderate exacerbations similar to the effect of NIV given at modest pressure levels. Also, high flow rates had reduced inspiration rate and improved oxygenation but had no significant effect on $PaCO_2$ [56]. So, in the management of certain types of hypercapnic respiratory failure, HFNC is considered a highly promising therapy [31].

3.8 Acute Cardiogenic Pulmonary Edema (ACPE)

High flow therapy is applied for the treatment of acute cardiogenic pulmonary edema (ACPE) because of its ability to provide low levels of PEEP and improve oxygenation. It can also open flooded alveoli and enhance pulmonary compliance similar to CPAP. The cardiac function of ACPE patients can be improved by using HFNC through reducing cardiac afterload by the produced PEEP effect. Perales et al. used HFNC therapy in ACPE patients who had dyspnea and hypoxemia refractory to conventional oxygen therapy after NIV treatment and observed that clinical and gasometric parameters as dyspnea grade, PaO_2, and PH were significantly improved after 24 h of HFNC therapy [57]. Also, Moriyama et al. found that HFNC therapy was able to maintain oxygenation in patients complaining of life-threatening pulmonary edema [58].

3.9 Respiratory Infection

In acute respiratory infections, HFNC can be used to provide respiratory support to manage ongoing hypoxemic respiratory failure as its extensive use has recently been seen in severe cases of COVID-19 patients who develop acute hypoxemic failure secondary to existing acute respiratory distress syndrome. In these cases, the use of HFNC aims to avoid the development of severe respiratory failure and to reduce the need for invasive techniques (endotracheal intubation). Additionally, HFNC and NIV can be used in patients exhibiting a mild respiratory failure which defined by the ratio of PaO_2/FiO_2 being equal to 200–300 and also in those with moderate respiratory failure with PaO_2/FiO_2 ratio equal to 150–200 and the work of breathing is low. Close monitoring of COVID-19 patients on HFNC for 1–2 h is needed to early identify the failure of therapy and consider invasive ventilation [59].

3.10 Post-extubation

After prolonged mechanical ventilation or surgical procedures, respiratory failure can occur following extubation and often require re-intubation [60]. The risk of mortality and the length of hospital stay are thought to be increased with re-intubation which can be decreased with the use of HFNC. A previous work comparing the effects of HFNC and Venturi mask on post-intubated patients regarding oxygenation and other clinical outcomes demonstrating that HFNC increased PaO_2/FIO_2 ratio than Venturi mask. Also, only fewer patients receiving HFNC are not improved and required NIV or re-intubation [61, 62].

3.11 Do-Not-Intubate Patients and Palliative Care

In do-not-intubate patients, HFNC therapy can serve as palliative therapy for respiratory distress or hypoxemia. The use of NIV in those patients can cause discomfort and interference with normal activities as eating and speaking so that HFNC is considered a suitable option [54]. Epstein et al. performed a retrospective study on "do-not-intubate" cancer patients who exhibited respiratory distress. Authors demonstrated that the majority of included patients treated with HFNC were improved or even remained stable [63, 64].

3.12 Home Oxygen Therapy or Long Term Oxygen Therapy (LTOT)

In COPD patients and those with complicated hypoxemia, the use of oxygen has been expanded from inpatient to outpatient settings. They should have access to home oxygen devices with high clinical effectiveness to meet their needs outside the hospital [65]. In COPD patients, pulmonary rehabilitation with LTOT enables the patient to perform physical activities with the existing chronic lung disease besides providing proper patient education and counseling can reduce the disease complications and improve the patient's quality of life [66]. Of note, oxygen is a drug that needs a prescription, therapeutic dosing, effective delivery system, and continuous monitoring for efficacy. The domiciliary use of oxygen is mainly recommended by a study performed by the British Medical Research Council and the Nocturnal Oxygen Trial [67, 68]. Females highly use Long term oxygen therapy (LTOT) with a possible increase in the future because of the extensive spread of smoking within middle-aged females [69]. LTOT is required for certain patients: patients with PaO_2 less than or equal 55 mmHg in non-recumbent position at rest despite the use of optimal therapy, patients with the observed decline of PaO_2 lower than 55 mmHg with desaturation occurred during sleeping and/ or exercise, and those with PaO_2 higher than 55 mmHg with central nervous system dysfunction, secondary pulmonary hypertension, cor pulmonale, or polycythemia [70, 71]. Oxygen-conserving devices available for LTOT are variable while the optimal selection and prescribing of the device, its cost, and impact on the patient's quality of life are issues needed to be considered [70]. Three classes of LTOT oxygen delivery devices are well known: oxygen concentrators, gaseous oxygen systems, and liquid oxygen systems.

3.13 Oxygen Concentrators

An oxygen concentrator or provider represents a safe device for providing oxygen-enriched air. Its principle depends on passing the room air through filters to remove any bacteria or dust or particulate matter from the entrained air. Also, oxygen concentrators remove nitrogen from the entrained air to deliver gas with oxygen concentration equal to or exceeds 90% [72]. Generally, in clinical practice, oxygen concentrations of 85% or higher can be considered equivalent to 100% oxygen. A typical oxygen concentrator can provide oxygen flows range from 0.5 to 5 L/min which is known as a low flow oxygen concentrator while some devices (high flow oxygen concentrators) can deliver oxygen flow up to 10–15 L/min [72]. Two types of oxygen concentrators are available: portable oxygen concentrators and stationary oxygen concentrators.

Stationary or home oxygen concentrators uninterruptedly deliver oxygen while the gas flow is in a range of 0.5 to 10–15 L/min. Most devices now have the capability for monitoring oxygen concentration where the device is provided with alarm signals to notify the user when the delivery is inadequate. These devices are electrically powered with a backup compressed cylinder to be used in case of power failure. They are considered safe and with lower cost when compared with compressed gas cylinders. Solar energy may be used to concentrate oxygen from room air in clinical settings [72]. Noise and vibrations produced while the device is operating are the main problems reported by users but recent models have reduced such problems [73]. Recently, portable oxygen concentrators are developed for LTOT users while they are small in size with a portable oxygen solution placed in a compact and mobile unit. Different types of portable concentrators vary in weight, battery life, oxygen flow settings, and the range of flow that can be provided. Intermittent and continuous oxygen flow can be delivered by portable concentrators while devices with the smallest size are with limited oxygen production capability and are designed only to supply oxygen in an intermittent flow [65]. Oxygen output, size, power option, and cost are the main differences between stationary and portable devices. Stationary oxygen concentrators are of lower price and higher oxygen output while portable devices offer smaller sizes with greater flexibility for power sources. Patients with active lives can benefit more from portable oxygen concentrators where the wall socket for power supply is unavailable [74]. Lithium-ion batteries are used within portable oxygen concentrators where they degrade over time with approximately 300 times use before a significant degradation occurs. Two types of oxygen delivery are identified with the use of oxygen concentrators: pulse mode delivery and continuous flow delivery. The continuous flow dose delivery provides a steady and reliable flow of oxygen based on the oxygen setting of the devices so it is associated with gas wastage as inspiration constitutes only a part of the respiration cycle.

A consistent saving of oxygen is achieved by only providing the gas during early inhalation where the inhaled gas is mostly utilized for alveolar ventilation. So, Pulse mode delivery provides a bolus of oxygen gas when the subject starts inhalation [70]. Newer devices have been developed to only provide oxygen during inhalation and they are mainly classified into active and passive intermittent flow devices. Active devices are activated by the negative pressure of inhalation (trigger) and automatically cycle after delivering a set volume of oxygen. On the other hand, intermittent flow devices of passive-type can store oxygen during expiration into a reservoir while it will be released during the subsequent inhalation as a pulse [72].

In most cases, portable concentrators with the pulsed or intermittent flow have proven efficacy as other oxygen delivery devices and have shown certain oxygen delivery efficiency in COPD patients at rest with eliminating the waste of oxygen during exhalation. However, during sleeping, they may have a limited efficiency when the patient breathing is little. Also, they may exhibit insufficient oxygen release in patients with higher respiration rates as during exercise [72]. A randomized study was performed on 13 COPD patients to compare the efficacy of the continuous delivery device and four intermittent flow delivery devices where they found that all intermittent flow devices adequately performed at rest but not with physical activity [72]. Some models of portable devices have a mode option that enables the device to automatically turn to continuous mode during sleep when no breathing is detected and others can be used with the ventilator equipment [75]. The use of oxygen concentrators is recommended in the patient requiring oxygen more than 1.4 h/day [74]. No guideline recommends the choice of certain oxygen delivery devices but the use of portable devices may be suggested in LTOT patients who regularly go outside. Also, portable oxygen concentrators can be used for ambulatory oxygen delivery in subjects who are already on LTOT and want to use oxygen outside as it can improve breathlessness and exercise tolerability. Several studies suggest that the appropriate use of oxygen concentrators is associated with a higher survival rate of respiratory diseases, increased tolerance, improved mental attentiveness, and improved mood [70, 72].

3.14 Compressed Gas Cylinders

Oxygen in a gaseous form is stored in cylinders which are usually made of steel but recently aluminum cylinders with carbon fibers and are used for oxygen storage which leads to a significant decrease in the system weight by about 50%. For a long time, oxygen cylinders were the main source of oxygen in hospitals until the piped oxygen system was developed which is capable of supplying large gas volumes from the bulk that is stored in cryogenic dewars. For patient transport within the hospital, oxygen cylinders are mainly used for this purpose. Patients need cylinders with lightweight in the home which operates for a longer time to facilitate the daily activity of the patient [65]. Also, the use of gaseous oxygen is considered the first choice for delivering occasional oxygen therapy. The safe adjustment of oxygen flow is guaranteed by a regulator which is placed on the top of the cylinder and works as a tap. Oxygen will move toward an oxygen delivery device as a nasal cannula or a mask to the patient when the tape is opened. Cylinders are of variable sizes where the cylinder size and fill pressure determine how much the content of oxygen gas in the cylinder. Trans-filling of small cylinders can be done through the use of large cylinders by specific delivery devices to reduce the cost of using newer equipment. Also, home cylinders may be refilled via an oxygen concentrator. The amount of oxygen in the cylinder available for supply is estimated by a pressure reading [76]. An oxygen conserving device can be used instead of a gas regulator attached to the cylinder to supply pulsed oxygen rather than continuous oxygen flow while mainly released during only the inhalation phase of the patient respiratory cycle. The use of such a device will reduce gas wastage during exhalation which causes the cylinder to last for a longer time and reduce the overall cost of therapy [76]. Compressed gas cylinders are used for patients who need supplemental oxygen therapy at home and are usually combined with oxygen concentrators. The users of compressed gas cylinders are commonly less mobile as they spent most of their lives within the home without the need for mobile oxygen and in this case oxygen cylinder represents a backup strategy when there is a power cut or failure of the stationary oxygen concentrator. Their use in the hospital is limited to patient transport as when invasively ventilated patients need to leave ICU to perform diagnostic procedures or others [77].

3.15 Liquid Oxygen Systems

Liquid oxygen refers to the conversion of oxygen gas to a liquid state at of temperature equal to or below −240 °C. Liquid oxygen has the advantage of storing large quantities of gaseous oxygen at a given volume since 1 L of liquid oxygen can produce about 860 L of oxygen gas. A reservoir of liquid oxygen that contains 30–40 L can provide a gas flow of 2 L/min for 8–10 days [72]. Before the patient receives oxygen through the nasal cannula, the liquid oxygen must be converted back to compressed gas through evaporation and warmed to the room temperature inside the device. Also, liquid oxygen systems are classified into portable and stationary systems. High-flow liquid oxygen systems can provide oxygen flow up to 15 L/min at a purity of 99% consequently they are suitable for patients requiring ambulatory high flow oxygen. So, liquid oxygen may be indicated for patients who have chronic respiratory disabilities who require gas flow above 5 L/min to go work and carry out normal daily activities [75].

However, high flow liquid systems have a major problem as there is a possibility of ice formation on the portable device because of freezing of ambient humidity at the heat exchange coils. Such limitation can be minimized by using 2 high-flow liquid oxygen systems where there is an opportunity for one unit to de-ice while the patient uses the other.

The interface used commonly with the previously mentioned LTOT oxygen delivery devices is nasal cannula as it is easy to use, of low cost, doesn't interfere with eating or speaking, and has lower rebreathing risk. The nasal cannula is connected to the oxygen delivery system through the tubing of 2–2.5 m long. Longer extensions up to 30 m may be needed to improve the mobility of the device except for portable concentrators with intermittent flow delivery which has a manufacture's recommendation of not using tubes longer than 7 m with them [78, 79]. Standard nasal prongs connected to any of the home oxygen systems have the same limitations of low flow devices discussed earlier in this chapter.

Most patients receiving LTOT are on gas flow rates of 2–4 L/min without any need for external humidification but in real life, humidifiers may be independently used irrespective of the driven flow rate. However, portable devices don't need humidifiers [72, 78].

References

1. Kane B, Decalmer S, O'Driscoll BR. Emergency oxygen therapy: from guideline to implementation. Breathe. 2013;9(4):246–53.
2. Joosten SA, et al. The effects of oxygen therapy in patients presenting to an emergency department with exacerbation of chronic obstructive pulmonary disease. Med J Aust. 2007;186(5):235–8.
3. Brill SE, Wedzicha JA. Oxygen therapy in acute exacerbations of chronic obstructive pulmonary disease. Int J Chron Obstruct Pulmon Dis. 2014;9:1241.
4. Cousins JL, Wark PA, McDonald VM. Acute oxygen therapy: a review of prescribing and delivery practices. Int J Chron Obstruct Pulmon Dis. 2016;11:1067–75.
5. Littleton SW. Hypercapnia from hyperoxia in COPD: another piece of the puzzle or another puzzle entirely? Respir Care. 2015;60(3):473–5.
6. Abdo WF, Heunks LM. Oxygen-induced hypercapnia in COPD: myths and facts. Crit Care. 2012;16(5):1–4.
7. Bazuaye E, et al. Variability of inspired oxygen concentration with nasal cannulas. Thorax. 1992;47(8):609–11.
8. Drake MG. High-flow nasal cannula oxygen in adults: an evidence-based assessment. Ann Am Thorac Soc. 2018;15(2):145–55.

9. Papazian L, et al. Use of high-flow nasal cannula oxygenation in ICU adults: a narrative review. Intensive Care Med. 2016;42(9):1336–49.
10. Gotera C, et al. Clinical evidence on high flow oxygen therapy and active humidification in adults. Rev Port Pneumol. 2013;19(5):217–27.
11. Dugernier J, et al. Nasal high-flow nebulization for lung drug delivery: theoretical, experimental, and clinical application. J Aerosol Med Pulm Drug Deliv. 2019;32(6):341–51.
12. Ricard J. High flow nasal oxygen in acute respiratory failure. Minerva Anestesiol. 2012;78(7):836–41.
13. Kubo T, et al. Noise exposure from high-flow nasal cannula oxygen therapy: a bench study on noise reduction. Respir Care. 2018;63(3):267–73.
14. Nishimura M. High-flow nasal cannula oxygen therapy devices. Respir Care. 2019;64(6):735–42.
15. Calvano TP, et al. Use of a high-flow oxygen delivery system in a critically ill patient with dementia. Respir Care. 2008;53(12):1739–43.
16. McQueen M, et al. Safety and long term outcomes with high flow nasal cannula therapy in neonatology: a large retrospective cohort study. J Pulm Respir Med. 2014;4(6):216.
17. Chikata Y, et al. Inspiratory tube condensation during high-flow nasal cannula therapy: a bench study. Respir Care. 2016;61(3):300–5.
18. Tero R, et al. Risks associated with conventional humidifiers adapted for high-flow nasal cannula therapy in human infants: results of a time and motion study. Int J Clin Pediatr. 2015;3(4):99–104.
19. Miller T, Saberi B, Saberi S. Computational fluid dynamics modeling of extrathoracic airway flush: evaluation of high flow nasal cannula design elements. J Pulm Respir Med. 2016;6(5):376.
20. Wilkinson D, et al. High flow nasal cannula for respiratory support in preterm infants. Cochrane Database Syst Rev. 2016;(2).
21. Parke R, et al. Open-label, phase II study of routine high-flow nasal oxygen therapy in cardiac surgical patients. Br J Anaesth. 2013;111(6):925–31.
22. Lee CC, et al. High flow nasal cannula versus conventional oxygen therapy and non-invasive ventilation in adults with acute hypoxemic respiratory failure: a systematic review. Respir Med. 2016;121:100–8.
23. Spoletini G, et al. Heated humidified high-flow nasal oxygen in adults: mechanisms of action and clinical implications. Chest. 2015;148(1):253–61.
24. Pisani L, Vega ML. Use of nasal high flow in stable COPD: rationale and physiology. J Chron Obstruct Pulm Dis. 2017;14(3):346–50.
25. Rodriguez AME, et al. Clinical review: humidifiers during non-invasive ventilation-key topics and practical implications. Crit Care. 2012;16(1):1–7.
26. Möller W, et al. Nasal high flow reduces dead space. J Appl Physiol. 2017;122(1):191–7.
27. Zhang J, et al. High-flow nasal cannula therapy for adult patients. J Int Med Res. 2016;44(6):1200–11.
28. Chatila W, et al. The effects of high-flow vs low-flow oxygen on exercise in advanced obstructive airways disease. Chest. 2004;126(4):1108–15.
29. Elbehairy AF, et al. Pulmonary gas exchange abnormalities in mild chronic obstructive pulmonary disease. Implications for dyspnea and exercise intolerance. Am J Respir Crit Care Med. 2015;191(12):1384–94.
30. Cirio S, et al. Effects of heated and humidified high flow gases during high-intensity constant-load exercise on severe COPD patients with ventilatory limitation. Respir Med. 2016;118:128–32.
31. Nishimura M. High-flow nasal cannula oxygen therapy in adults. J Intensive Care. 2015;3(1):15.
32. Wettstein RB, Shelledy DC, Peters JI. Delivered oxygen concentrations using low-flow and high-flow nasal cannulas. Respir Care. 2005;50(5):604–9.
33. Parke R, McGuinness S, Eccleston M. Nasal high-flow therapy delivers low level positive airway pressure. Br J Anaesth. 2009;103(6):886–90.

34. Groves N, Tobin A. High flow nasal oxygen generates positive airway pressure in adult volunteers. Aust Crit Care. 2007;20(4):126–31.
35. Pisani L, Vega ML. Use of nasal high flow in stable COPD: rationale and physiology. COPD: J Chron Obstruct Pulmon Dis. 2017;14(3):346–50.
36. Markovitz GH, et al. Effective inspired oxygen concentration measured via transtracheal and oral gas analysis. Respir Care. 2010;55(4):453–9.
37. Ritchie J, et al. Evaluation of a humidified nasal high-flow oxygen system, using oxygraphy, capnography and measurement of upper airway pressures. Anaesth Intensive Care. 2011;39(6):1103–10.
38. Fraser JF, et al. Nasal high flow oxygen therapy in patients with COPD reduces respiratory rate and tissue carbon dioxide while increasing tidal and end-expiratory lung volumes: a randomised crossover trial. Thorax. 2016;71(8):759–61.
39. Dysart K, et al. Research in high flow therapy: mechanisms of action. Respir Med. 2009;103(10):1400–5.
40. Holleman-Duray D, Kaupie D, Weiss M. Heated humidified high-flow nasal cannula: use and a neonatal early extubation protocol. J Perinatol. 2007;27(12):776–81.
41. Rea H, et al. The clinical utility of long-term humidification therapy in chronic airway disease. Respir Med. 2010;104(4):525–33.
42. Marcus CL, et al. Adherence to and effectiveness of positive airway pressure therapy in children with obstructive sleep apnea. Pediatrics. 2006;117(3):e442–51.
43. Perlstrom J, Macmillan NJ, Miller TL. Heated humidified high flow nasal cannula (HFNC) in the treatment of obstructive sleep apnea (OSA), in D29. Treatment of sleep disordered breathing. American Thoracic Society; 2010. p. A5572.
44. Hawkins S, et al. High-flow, heated, humidified air via nasal cannula treats CPAP-intolerant children with obstructive sleep apnea. J Clin Sleep Med. 2017;13(8):981–9.
45. McGinley BM, et al. A nasal cannula can be used to treat obstructive sleep apnea. Am J Respir Crit Care Med. 2007;176(2):194–200.
46. Nishimura M. High-flow nasal cannula oxygen therapy in adults: physiological benefits, indication, clinical benefits, and adverse effects. Respir Care. 2016;61(4):529–41.
47. Roca O, et al. High-flow oxygen therapy in acute respiratory failure. Respir Care. 2010;55(4):408–13.
48. Sztrymf B, et al. Impact of high-flow nasal cannula oxygen therapy on intensive care unit patients with acute respiratory failure: a prospective observational study. J Crit Care. 2012;27(3):324.e9–324.e13.
49. Cho WH, et al. High-flow nasal cannula therapy for acute hypoxemic respiratory failure in adults: a retrospective analysis. Intern Med. 2015;54(18):2307–13.
50. Lenglet H, et al. Humidified high flow nasal oxygen during respiratory failure in the emergency department: feasibility and efficacy. Respir Care. 2012;57(11):1873–8.
51. Lucangelo U, et al. High-flow nasal interface improves oxygenation in patients undergoing bronchoscopy. Crit Care Res Prac. 2012;2012:506382.
52. Simon M, et al. High-flow nasal cannula oxygen versus non-invasive ventilation in patients with acute hypoxaemic respiratory failure undergoing flexible bronchoscopy-a prospective randomised trial. Crit Care. 2014;18(6):1–9.
53. Kang BJ, et al. Failure of high-flow nasal cannula therapy may delay intubation and increase mortality. Intensive Care Med. 2015;41(4):623–32.
54. Millar J, Lutton S, O'Connor P. The use of high-flow nasal oxygen therapy in the management of hypercarbic respiratory failure. Ther Adv Respir Dis. 2014;8(2):63–4.
55. Nilius G, et al. Effects of nasal insufflation on arterial gas exchange and breathing pattern in patients with chronic obstructive pulmonary disease and hypercapnic respiratory failure. In: Respiratory regulation-clinical advances. Springer; 2013. p. 27–34.
56. Rittayamai N, et al. Effects of high-flow nasal cannula and non-invasive ventilation on inspiratory effort in hypercapnic patients with chronic obstructive pulmonary disease: a preliminary study. Ann Intensive Care. 2019;9(1):122.

57. Perales JMC, et al. High-flow therapy via nasal cannula in acute heart failure. Rev Esp Cardiol. 2011;64(8):723–5.
58. Moriyama K, et al. High-flow nasal cannula therapy in a patient with reperfusion pulmonary edema following percutaneous transluminal pulmonary angioplasty. Case Rep Pulmonol. 2014;2014:837612.
59. Harb HS, et al. The role of non-invasive ventilation. In: Covid-19 airway management and ventilation strategy for critically ill older patients. Cham: Springer; 2020. p. 141–3.
60. Dries DJ. High-flow nasal cannula: where does it fit? Respir Care. 2018;63(3):367–70.
61. Maggiore SM, et al. Nasal high-flow versus Venturi mask oxygen therapy after extubation. Effects on oxygenation, comfort, and clinical outcome. Am J Respir Crit Care Med. 2014;190(3):282–8.
62. Esteban A, et al. Characteristics and outcomes in adult patients receiving mechanical ventilation: a 28-day international study. JAMA. 2002;287(3):345–55.
63. Spoletini G, et al. Heated humidified high-flow nasal oxygen in adults. Chest. 2015;148(1):253–61.
64. Epstein AS, et al. Humidified high-flow nasal oxygen utilization in patients with cancer at Memorial Sloan-Kettering Cancer Center. J Palliat Med. 2011;14(7):835–9.
65. McCoy RW. Options for home oxygen therapy equipment: storage and metering of oxygen in the home. Respir Care. 2013;58(1):65–85.
66. Ries AL, et al. Pulmonary rehabilitation: joint ACCP/AACVPR evidence-based clinical practice guidelines. Chest. 2007;131(5):4S–42S.
67. Continuous or nocturnal oxygen therapy in hypoxemic chronic obstructive lung disease: a clinical trial. Nocturnal Oxygen Therapy Trial Group. Ann Intern Med. 1980;93(3):391–8.
68. Stuart H, et al. Long term domiciliary oxygen therapy in chronic hypoxic cor pulmonale complicating chronic bronchitis and emphysema: report of the Medical Research Council Working Party; 1981.
69. Franklin KA, et al. Survival and future need of long-term oxygen therapy for chronic obstructive pulmonary disease—gender differences. Respir Med. 2007;101(7):1506–11.
70. Hardavella G, et al. Oxygen devices and delivery systems. Breathe (Sheff). 2019;15(3):e108–16.
71. O'Driscoll B, et al. BTS guideline for oxygen use in adults in healthcare and emergency settings. Thorax. 2017;72(Suppl 1):ii1–ii90.
72. Melani AS, Sestini P, Rottoli P. Home oxygen therapy: re-thinking the role of devices. Expert Rev Clin Pharmacol. 2018;11(3):279–89.
73. Diego González EG, Méndez Lanza A, Mosquera Pestaña JA. Noise and machine failures: determining factors in the acceptance and behavior of O2 concentrator. The Asturias project. An Med Interna. 1996;13(9):430–3.
74. Jackson M, Shneerson J. An evaluation of the use of concentrators for domiciliary oxygen supply for less than 8 h day−1. Respir Med. 1998;92(2):250–5.
75. Lobato SD, González JLG, Alises SM. The debate on continuous home oxygen therapy. Arch Bronconeumol. 2015;51(1):31–7.
76. Hardinge M, et al. British Thoracic Society guidelines for home oxygen use in adults: accredited by NICE. Thorax. 2015;70(Suppl 1):i1–i43.
77. Magnussen H, et al. Guidelines for long-term oxygen therapy. German Society for Pneumology and Respiratory Medicine. Pneumologie. 2008;62(12):748–56.
78. Godoy I, et al. The importance of knowing the home conditions of patients receiving long-term oxygen therapy. Int J Chron Obstruct Pulmon Dis. 2012;7:421.
79. Aguiar C, et al. Tubing length for long-term oxygen therapy. Respir Care. 2015;60(2):179–82.

Chapter 4
Special Needs for Neonates, Infants, and Toddler

Contents

4.1 Introduction

Inhaled medications are used with young patients who suffer from respiratory disorders such as asthma. Besides the management of respiratory disorders, aerosol therapy is used for the management of cardiovascular and infective diseases. Bronchodilators, corticosteroids, mucolytics, and antibiotics are among the most commonly used inhaled medications.

The main advantage of aerosol therapy compared with systemic drug delivery is the high safety margin of the therapy due to local drug delivery. Inhaled medications

M. E. A. Abdelrahim et al., *Essentials of Aerosol Therapy in Critically ill Patients*,
https://doi.org/10.1007/978-3-030-85026-5_4

are delivered and deposited in the lung to exert their role either as an anti-inflammatory, bronchodilator, or antibacterial action. Besides the safety, rapid onset of action is another advantage for aerosol therapy compared with systemic drug delivery. Local drug deposition (lung) reduces the systemic absorption and the probability of developing adverse effects. On the other hand, aerosol therapy efficacy could be influenced by several factors that could be related to the aerosol-generating devices, drug formulations, and patient. The main drawback related to aerosol efficacy is the low amount of inhaled medication that reach and deposit in the lung, especially peripheral airways. Clinical studies showed that the actual amount of inhaled medication that reached the infant lung after the end of drug nebulization is less than 3% of the total amount, this percentage increased to be 4% and more than 10% for young children and adults, respectively [1–3]. The reported percentages during these studies are related to the traditional jet nebulizers. There are more efficient nebulizers that could deliver higher amounts of aerosol such as ultrasonic and vibrating mesh nebulizers, as there is no sufficient in-vivo data available regarding the pediatric patients.

There are several common problems and nuanced concerns related to aerosol distribution and deposition in children that are not present in adults. These issues raise from the physiological, anatomical, and mental differences between children and adults [4].

In the scope of treatment for critically ill children, it is not rare for a patient to receive several inhaled medications with many different delivery options during a hospitalization time. These choices include the use of aerosol masks or mouthpieces, a heated high-flow nasal cannula (HFNC), non-invasive ventilation (NIV), or mechanical ventilation. Different aerosol-generating devices are connected to mechanical ventilation circuits of critically ill children through specific connections, some of these connections could combine more than one device.

4.2 Differences Between Pediatric and Adult Patients in the Delivery of Inhaled Medications

The main difference between pediatric and adult patients is the low amount of aerosol that reaches pediatric lung with significantly low peripheral deposition. The younger the patient the lower the peripheral aerosol deposition hence lower aerosol delivery and efficacy. For a pediatric patient with an age less than 1.5 years the major portion of the emitted aerosol would be deposited in the upper airway. Also, this problem could be significant for pediatric patients at an age of fewer than 4 years [4].

Medication deposition and accumulation in peripheral airways and alveoli is decreased in infants and young children, possibly due to narrowed airways, lower tidal volumes, and faster respiratory rates which combine to minimize the residence time of small aerosol particles in airways. In addition to the strong resistance due to the airways' limited cross-sectional diameter. High resistance and short inspiratory time of pediatric patient which shorten the time for an aerosol to deposit in the airways. A large portion of nebulized medication to pediatric patients is lost with the exhaled gases as a result of short inspiratory to expiratory time. This significantly occurs with the continuous nebulization of inhaled medications. Another critical factor related to young patients is the behavioral aspect. They cannot use aerosol-generating devices that require coordination and which depend mainly on patient intervention. Also, infants and toddlers did not accept some devices or tools that require fit mouth closure (mouthpiece) or that make them not comfortable (tight mask).

The oral cavity of the infant is relatively less suitable for aerosol passage compared with adults. The reason behind that is the proximity of epiglottis and larynx to the tongue base, also the large tongue size of infants compared with the oral cavity hence, the infants are breathing obligatory from the nose. Besides, there are smaller nostrils, a shorter turbinate area, a narrower nasopharynx, a narrower pharynx-larynx, and a comparatively larger anatomical dead space for younger patients than adults, making delivery of drugs a challenge [5]. Nasal airway resistance is a common cause of healthy infant respiratory resistance, amounts of the drug that deposit inside the nose during nasal aerosol delivery for young children is mainly due to the turbulent flow of air at this region that led to aerosol particles impaction. The efficacy of nasal aerosol delivery for infants and toddlers is similar to that of mouth aerosol delivery, but it is not the same for older children and adult patients, who have more well-developed nasal turbinate and less complex airway structures [6]. The nasal drug delivery to an infant is lower than that of the mouth in case of nasal obstruction as a result of inflammation or secretions.

4.3 Age Is a Factor for Choosing the Best Aerosol-Generating Device

Selecting the appropriate aerosol-generating devices for pediatric patients should meet certain criteria that ensure the safety and efficacy of aerosol therapy. These criteria involve the suitability of the device using a technique with the patient's age and mentality. Also, other factors related to the cost, availability, and compatibility with the ventilation type such as spontaneous breathing, NIV, and mechanical ventilation.

For nebulizers, children aged less than 4 years could use a small volume nebulizer, however, the type of connection that is connected to the nebulizer differ according to the age, for infants, a small mask or hood could be used, in general for children less than or equal to 3 years facial mask is suitable for aerosol delivery. For pediatric patients aged less than 4 years, the pressurized metered-dose inhaler (pMDI) could be used with a spacer or valved holding chamber connected to a facial mask, and it could be used without a mask for patient equal to or more than 4 years.

Also, at age of 4 years or more, the pediatric patient would be able to use dry powder inhalers (DPIs). pMDI alone without other connections, breath-actuated pMDI, breath-actuated nebulizers could be used with older children aged 5 years or more because they can follow the specific instruction of the device usage technique [7].

4.4 Patient-Related Factors

Selecting a suitable device for a certain age is not the only step to ensure effective aerosol delivery to pediatric patients, but also patient education by health care professionals is a significant and critical step for optimizing aerosol therapy for the pediatric patient. Education and demonstration for the aerosol-generating device technique are important to enhance the ability of the child or the family to correctly used the device. There are many ways for patient counseling, some of these techniques could be suitable for a specific age. Examples of counseling methods are verbal counseling, physical demonstration, using a training device, using written and visual brochures, and mobile applications [8, 9].

Not only patient education but also some interventions that induce strong cough for a pediatric patient that has secretions of his lung, sitting patients upright during aerosol delivery, and training the patient on deep breathing.

Follow-up for pediatric patients who receive aerosol therapy is very important to assess the suitability of the selected device with the patient through asking the family about the adherence to the therapy by this device. Also, the efficacy and safety of the therapy should be monitored after initiation of the therapy to determine whether the selected device will be replaced, or the dose of the drug will be changed. For older patients, aerosol therapy monitoring using spirometry could provide good guidance on the aerosol therapy efficacy.

The respiratory support type for pediatric patients could also influence the device selection and the type of connections that sometimes will be attached to more than one aerosol-generating device such as a MinimHal that combines both nebulizer and pMDI.

4.5 Selection of Aerosol-Generating Devices

Aerosol generating devices produce particles of different sizes, the inhalable range of the produced aerosol is between 1 and 5 μm of the mass median aerodynamic diameter (MMAD) [10]. Aerosol particles less than 1 μm would be exhaled out of the lung without deposition, while particles with a diameter larger than 5 μm would be deposited on the upper respiratory airways (oropharynx). Large aerosol particles that deposit in the upper airways are absorbed systemically and may lead to more adverse effects.

The most commonly used devices to deliver aerosol in pediatric subjects are pMDI plus spacer or valved holding chamber (VHC), jet nebulizers, breath-actuated nebulizer, vibrating mesh nebulizer, dry powder inhaler. pMDI and nebulizers are suitable to be used during mechanical ventilation.

Using jet nebulizers and pMDIs for bronchodilators delivery in pediatric patients suffering from bronchiolitis was not effective in delivering sufficient amounts of the inhaled medications which resulted in poor management of viral bronchiolitis. Hence, the use of vibrating mesh nebulizers or pMDI/spacer could be more effective for aerosol delivery in pediatric patients. These devices are commonly used in pediatric subjects to deliver most inhalable medications. Small-volume nebulizers are the most commonly used type (jet or vibrating mesh). Nebulizers could deliver different types of medications while pMDI is used for limited medications. Using nebulizers is easier than pMDI and does not require coordination during aerosol emissions. Breath actuated nebulizers and dry powder inhalers require the application of strong inhalation by the pediatric subjects during the process of aerosol emission.

4.6 Aerosol Generating Devices

Several aerosol-generating devices could be used with pediatric patients such as nebulizers, pMDIs, and DPIs, which are different in operating mechanisms and hence the efficacy of aerosol delivery. Besides, several factors influence the selection of the appropriate device for aerosol delivery to pediatrics (Fig. 4.1). Also, there are other factors related to the ventilator circuit that could influence the aerosol therapy (Table 4.1).

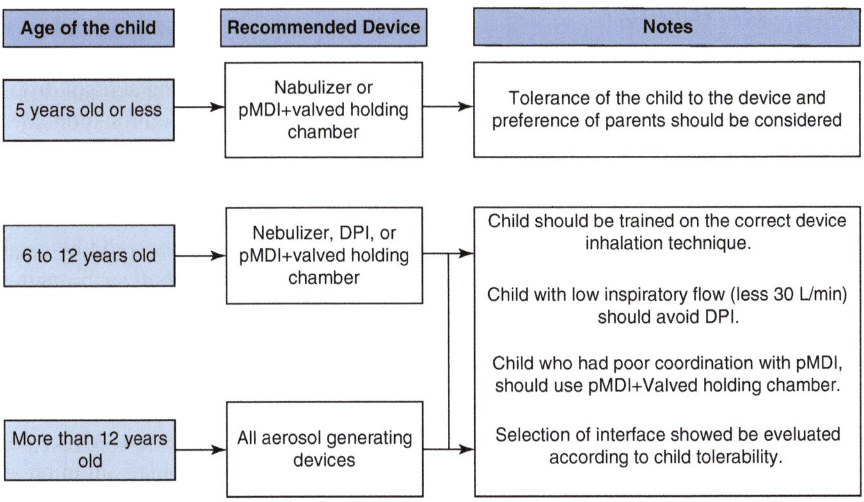

Fig. 4.1 Criteria for selection of an aerosol-generating device for pediatric patients

Table 4.1 Ventilator circuit factors affecting aerosol delivery during mechanical ventilation and recommendations for improving aerosol delivery for mechanically ventilated patients [11, 12]

Factor	Effects	Recommendations
Heat and humidity	The heat and moisture exchange (HME) filter decrease drug delivery as it acts as a barrier to inhaled drugs Humidification prevents mucosal dryness but also reduces nebulized drug deposition by increasing particle size	Previously it was recommended HME should be removed during the nebulization process and back again after finishing However, it was found recently that removing a humidifier is not necessary not recommended during nebulization [13, 14]
The density of inhaled gas	Using gases with low density as an operator of JN decreases aerosol output for mechanically ventilated patients But using heliox to deliver aerosol generated from nebulizer head increases lung deposition of inhaled drugs	Operating JN using oxygen rather than heliox is recommended Using heliox as inspired gas to carry aerosol is recommended

4.7 Nebulizers

Nebulization is a process through which liquid drugs are converted to droplets by using certain devices [15]. Devices of nebulization were classified into three main types JN, VMN, and ultrasonic nebulizers, they differ in the mechanism by which drug converts to fine droplets, and also the efficacy of drug delivery differ from one type to another, this efficacy is influenced by different factors (Table 4.2).

4.7.1 *Jet Nebulizer*

The jet nebulizer is the most commonly used nebulizer for producing aerosol droplets used for the treatment of pediatric patients [16]. JN could be used for spontaneous breathing child or who is mechanically ventilated.

In general, during mechanical ventilation, nebulizers are connected to the ventilator inspiratory limb. JN can be operated continuously or intermittently. Continuous operation by using a separated air compressor or from gas cylinders could be used with all pediatric subjects. While the intermittent operation of nebulizer by using gas produced from a ventilator machine. In general, JN is the least expensive compared to ultrasonic and VMN, but also it had the least efficacy [11, 16, 17]. Intermittent nebulization delivers a high drug amount to the patient compared with continuous nebulization, as the amount of the drug lost during exhalation was limited, while in continuous operation great amount of drugs would be lost. Also, synchronization of nebulizer operation with mechanical ventilator would result in great drug delivery [18, 19].

Table 4.2 Nebulizers factors affecting aerosol delivery during mechanical ventilation and recommendation for improving aerosol delivery [11]

Factor	Effects	Recommendations
Position of the nebulizer in circuit	Different positions of nebulizers in ventilator circuits result in different aerosol lung deposition	Ultrasonic and VMN should be placed 15 cm away from the Y adapter JN should be placed close to the ventilator
Nebulizer type	JN is less effective than ultrasonic and VMNs	If available use VMN for aerosol delivery during mechanical ventilation
Intermittent and continuous nebulization	Intermittent operation of nebulizer and to be synchronized with patient inspiration result in higher lung deposition of aerosol than is a continuous operation	Intermittent operation of jet nebulizer is recommended If this option not available on the ventilator, use gas flow 6–8 L/min or as recommended by the nebulizer manufacturer
Residual dead volume	The dead volume that remains in the nebulizer chamber influences amounts of aerosol that could be delivered to the patient	VMN is recommended if available
Gas flow	Effect of gas flow only on JNs because ultrasonic and VMNs are electrically operated The lower the gas flow of JN the higher the particle size and lower lung deposition	VMN or ultrasonic nebulizers are recommended if available For JN use a high flow rate of 6–8 L/min or as recommended by the nebulizer manufacturer

Many brands of JNs are available, but all of them had different aerosol production rates from each other's [20–22]. Not only rate of aerosol production differed among different brands, but also particle size of produced aerosol could be different. Hence, resulted in different lung deposition [22, 23].

Factors like gas flow rate and ventilator setting affecting the efficacy of nebulizers [24]. Also, the distance between the endotracheal tube and nebulizer could affect the efficacy of the nebulizer, placing the nebulizer head at distance from the tube was better than placing it between the endotracheal tube and Y tube of the patient [25].

In a previous study demonstrating the effect of nebulizer position and type of operation on the delivered amount of the drug by nebulizer [19], it was noted that position of nebulizer had a great effect on delivered drug amount than nebulization mode. It was demonstrated that placing a nebulizer near the ventilator 90 cm from the Y adapter resulted in higher drug delivery than placing a nebulizer at the Y adapter.

Disposable JN is easy to use and relatively inexpensive compared with other types of nebulizers, but aerosol delivery is extremely inefficient and variable due to the highly variable particle size of the emitted aerosol and large dead volume of the drug remain inside the nebulizer chamber at the end of the nebulization. In some cases, the dead volume can account for about 75% of the inhalable medication placed in the nebulizer chamber [26]. Integrating jet nebulizers into a ventilator circuit or respiratory support devices may accidentally increase pressure and volume and affect triggering due to the additional flow.

4.7.2 *Ultrasonic Nebulizers*

The main disadvantage of this type of nebulizer was the increasing temperature of the nebulized solution about 10 °C above the normal temperature of liquid drugs at the start of nebulization. Temperature rising of respirable solution occurred after 5–10 min from the start of nebulization, [27, 28] for this reason ultrasonic nebulizer was not recommended to be used with heat-sensitive drugs. Also, it is not effective in the delivery of viscous material, so it was not recommended for the delivery of proteins and suspension [29–32].

Comparing ultrasonic to JN regarding the time of nebulization, ultrasonic nebulizers had a higher nebulization rate at a shorter time than JNs, the shorter the time of nebulization the more suitable the nebulizer for pediatric subjects [18]. The particle size of produced aerosol was larger than that of JN. Position of nebulizers in ventilation circuit did not affect the delivered dose of drugs, placing ultrasonic nebulizer proximal to Y adapter did not change the efficacy of nebulizer drug deliver compared to distal position [25, 33]. Also, it was indicated that placing nebulizer away from Y adapter (50 cm) or at Y adapter had no difference on the efficacy of nebulizer [33].

Ultrasonic nebulizers and small-particle aerosol generators are typically approved to deliver specialty inhalable medications and are generally bulky, so they are not used frequently in the clinical setting that requires aerosol delivery to pediatric patients.

4.7.3 *Vibrating Mesh Nebulizers*

There are two main types of VMN, first is passive VMN in which electric energy converts to vibration by piezoelectric crystals then vibration transfers to transducer horn, which in contact with the liquid drug in nebulizer reservoir, so wave travel through liquid drug placed in nebulizer reservoir toward a plate with aperture, leading to the production of aerosol droplets coming out from plate aperture [34, 35]. An example of passive VMN is the Omron MicroAir nebulizer.

The second type is active VMN, in which the perforated mesh or plate vibrate after the electric supply producing aerosol droplets coming out from the aperture with a small diameter of about 4 microns [36, 37].

Nebulized liquid temperature elevation was less than that of ultrasonic nebulizer, about 3 °C in 5-min nebulization [27]. Characteristics of drug formulation are the main factor controlling the efficacy of VMNs, it was indicated that increasing viscosity of nebulized drug would decrease nebulizer output, so it was not recommended for drugs with a viscosity of more than 2 cP [38, 39]. Also, viscosity affects the aerodynamic diameter of produced aerosol droplets, increased viscosity resulted in decreased aerodynamic diameter and decreased output rate of drugs, but increasing electrolyte concentration would result in increasing total output, and also decreasing the aerodynamic diameter of produced drugs [40, 41]. The efficacy of VMNs in delivering drugs with low viscosity was higher than that of JN [17, 42–44]. Regarding delivery of protein solution, passive VMNs were superior to JN [45, 46].

The VMN is unique in that it does not need a gas source, making it extremely effective and safe during NIV or invasive mechanical ventilation. The high efficiency of VMN is based on a very low residual drug volume (about 0.1 mL) remaining in the nebulizer chamber after the end of nebulization.

Specifically signed for premature infants, an investigational next-generation VMN (eFlow, PARI Medical, Starnberg, Germany) demonstrated approximately 20-time greater aerosol delivery to a neonatal model in comparison with JNs and pMDIs/VHCs [47]. This could have important clinical consequences for patients receiving aerosolized artificial surfactant or not responding to bronchodilators (i.e., bronchiolitis). While these results are fascinating from a study point of view, suggesting VMN or ultrasonic nebulizers over JN for routine delivery of drugs is irrational from a cost standpoint.

The dead volume also called residual volume is the remaining amount of drug after the nebulization process, this amount differs from one nebulizer to another and it ranges from 0.1 to 2.4 mL. The greater the dead volume of nebulizers the less the amount of drug delivered to the patient's lung, dead volume was higher in JN, but also variable so small fill volume for jet nebulizers resulted in a low delivered amount of drug to the patient [11, 48]. So, increasing fill volume may result in a higher output of liquid drugs, but no accurate volume is determined to be used, also the effect of fill volume on VMN is not demonstrated.

4.8 Pressurized Metered-Dose Inhalers

Pressurized metered-dose inhalers (pMDIs) (Fig. 4.2) are the most commonly used aerosol-generating devices that have a high degree of suitability for many patients due to their portability and multi-dosing system [49]. pMDIs could be used in combination with an extension (spacers) that would add additional space and time for drug inhalation by younger children because they can not use the pMDIs correctly [47].

The inhaled drug is present in a canister in the form of solution or suspension with other ingredients like a lubricant, surfactant, and propellant at a pressure. The canister contains a metering valve and lodged downside in the actuator. The aerosol pre-metered dose would be released from the pMDI after pressing the bottom of the

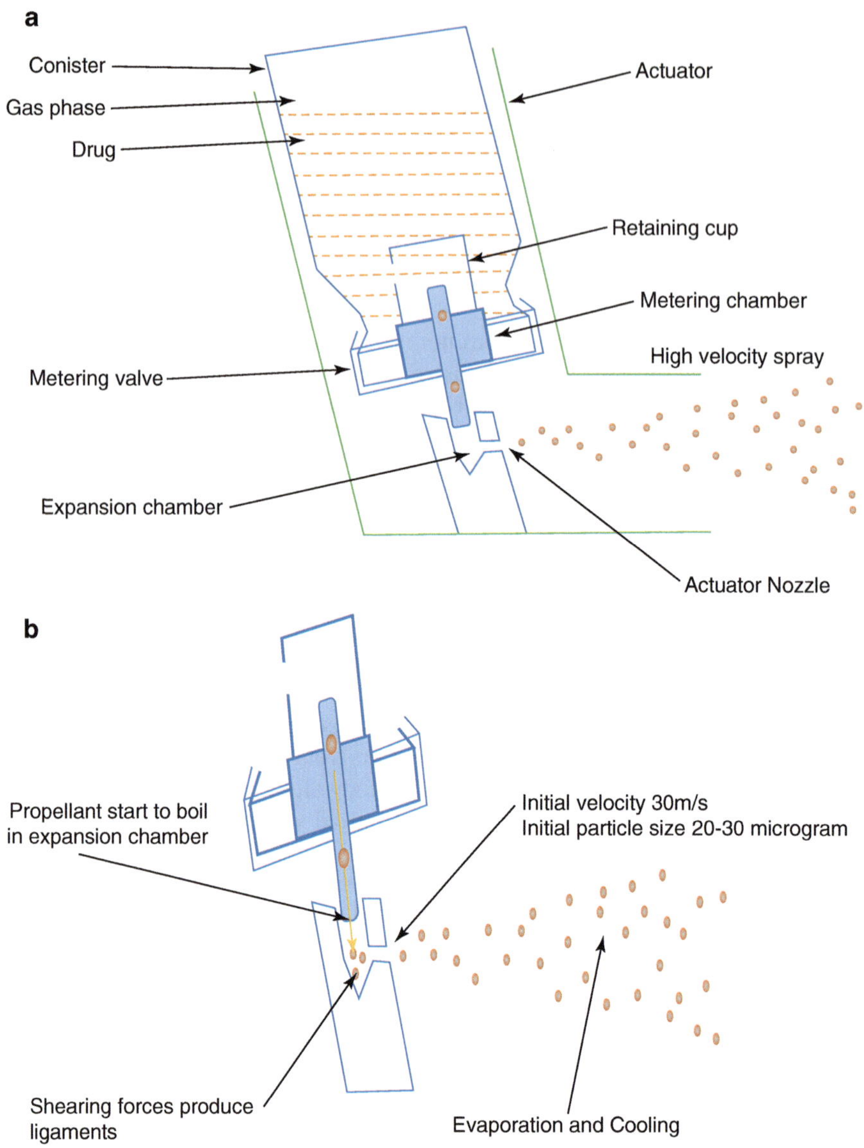

Fig. 4.2 Schematic design of pressurized metered-dose inhaler (**a**) and its nozzle (**b**)

canister. The propellant carrying the inhaled drug will pass through the actuator nozzle under the gas pressure resulting in the formation of fine droplets cloud. Released aerosol from the pMDI contains particles of different sizes, large particles will deposit in the oropharynx as shown by previous studies [50, 51]. From a buff containing 100 μg of the inhaled drug such as salbutamol sulfate in the Ventolin, approximately 10% of the drug remains in the pMDI actuator and the mouthpiece,

75–80% is deposited in the upper part of the respiratory system and about 10–15% reaches the deep part of the patients' respiratory system [50, 51].

The aerosol particle size produced from the pMDI is influenced by many factors, including; the properties of the propellant including the physical and chemical characteristics, the pressure produced by the gas inside the pMDI canister, the design of the valve and the outlet nozzle, the drug formulation and the mouthpiece attached to the pMDI [52, 53]. Two main factors could affect the aerosol particle size, the first is the time of propellant evaporation, the second is the distance that the aerosol will travel after the release from the pMDI [54].

Chlorofluorocarbons (CFCs) were the predominant propellants that had been used in the pMDIs. CFCs were reported in 1974 to be increasingly added to the environment and cause damage to the ozone layer [55]. The use of CFCs was prevented in all forms including the pMDI in 1987 by the Montreal Protocol to protect the ozone layer from being damaged. In the pharmaceutical industry, the hydrofluorocarbons (HFCs) were used instead of CFCs propellants due to the safety of HFAs on the ozone layer [56].

The major drawback to pMDI-delivered therapy is the sub-optimal inhalation technique resulting from a lack of coordination between the patient inhaling and the aerosol discharge from the device as shown in Table 4.3 [57]. Effective patient education about correct pMDI inhalation technique is an urgent requirement because less than 10% of patients use their pMDI correctly [58–60]. Traditionally, verbal training includes 11 steps to ensure the correct use of the pMDI [59, 60] most of which, in theory at least, are easily executed by the patient and easily checked by the trainer. These include shaking the device, exhaling before inhalation of the aerosol, and positioning the pMDI in the patient's mouth [59]. Unfortunately, teaching the correct pMDI technique via verbal instruction at chest clinics and to elderly patients is not adequate for correcting coordination errors [61, 62].

Inhaling the emitted aerosol slowly and deeply for at least 5 s is a critical step in pMDI use because fast inhalation results in reduced lung deposition and increased oropharyngeal deposition of the drug [63]. Hence, fast inhalation reduces the

Table 4.3 Main drawbacks related to the use of pressurized metered-dose inhalers

Item	Drawbacks
Device	pMDI canister that contains the drug is not shaken well before the aerosol delivery The cap of the device mouthpiece is not removed before inhalation
Patient	The patient inhales the air before or after aerosol delivery or breaths through the nose The patient exhales out during the aerosol delivery or before completing the inhalation The patient presses the canister multiple times and that leads to the release of more than one dose during the same breath Aerosol delivery from the device and inhalation from the patient are not simultaneous and there is no coordination. The lack of coordination is a major issue, especially in young children Too fast inhalation flow by the patient Interruption of the patient inhalation as a result of 'Freon effect' (early breath cut-off due to a cold sensation caused by the propellant in the upper airways (the mouth and the pharynx))

efficacy of the pMDI and results in poor disease control [64–66]. Optimal lung deposition of the emitted drug is achieved at an inspiratory flow rate (IFR), through the pMDI, of 30–60 L/min; unfortunately, basic verbal counseling cannot ensure that the patient IFR is within this range [58, 59].

Counseling conducted regularly has been shown to enhance therapy outcomes and improve the control of obstructive lung diseases [67, 68]. Monitoring the effect of counseling on asthma control could be done by measuring lung function and with asthma control tests [59, 69, 70]. Recently, training devices have been introduced to aid the counseling process by addressing the most important drawback of the inhalation technique, the IFR. These training devices can be considered an add-on device to traditional pMDI verbal counseling; they guide the patient because they produce an audible sound when the IFR is in the required range. Duration of inhalation is also important to ensure the delivery of a high portion of the emitted dose to the lungs. A newly available smartphone application could solve this by determining the duration of correct inhalation flow.

4.9 Dry Powder Inhalers

DPI is an efficient aerosol delivery method for obstructive lung disease patients (Fig. 4.3). However, the DPI overcomes the pMDI coordination drawback also requires the subject to be able to inhale the aerosol released from the device as fast and as deep as possible [71]. Different types of DPIs are available with different degrees of resistance [72]. Each DPI has a special technique to load the dose and needed critical inhalation flow to deliver the aerosolized dose [73–75]. They also have different patient preferences and several handling errors. The easier the DPI to be handled the more preferred it is by asthma and COPD patients, also the health care profession [76].

DPIs have a critical step in dose delivery which is to inhale the released dose as fast and as deep as possible [73–75]. Some chronic obstructive lung disease (COPD) patients cannot reach an inhalation flow of 30 L/min or inhalation volume of 2 L which hinders them from receiving the needed dose from the DPI by inhaling as fast as deep as possible [66, 77]. Also, the patient might inhale double the needed dose if he loaded the DPI twice [78]. This could put the patients at risk of unneeded side effects.

Ellipta® is a new multi-dose DPI with a medium resistance that was shown to be very efficient for pulmonary drug delivery [79–82]. It consists of two rolled-up blister strips in which the drug is formulated in 30 individual doses of inhaled medications ready for administration once the dose is prepared [83]. The design of the Ellipta® decreases the possibility of drug interactions since the blisters containing the medication are separated and open only when the dose is to be inhaled [83].

There were some, previously found, handling errors of the DPI that could result in inconsistency of delivered dose or possibly double dosing e.g. failure to hold device in the right position [79] turning the inhaler upside down after loading a dose

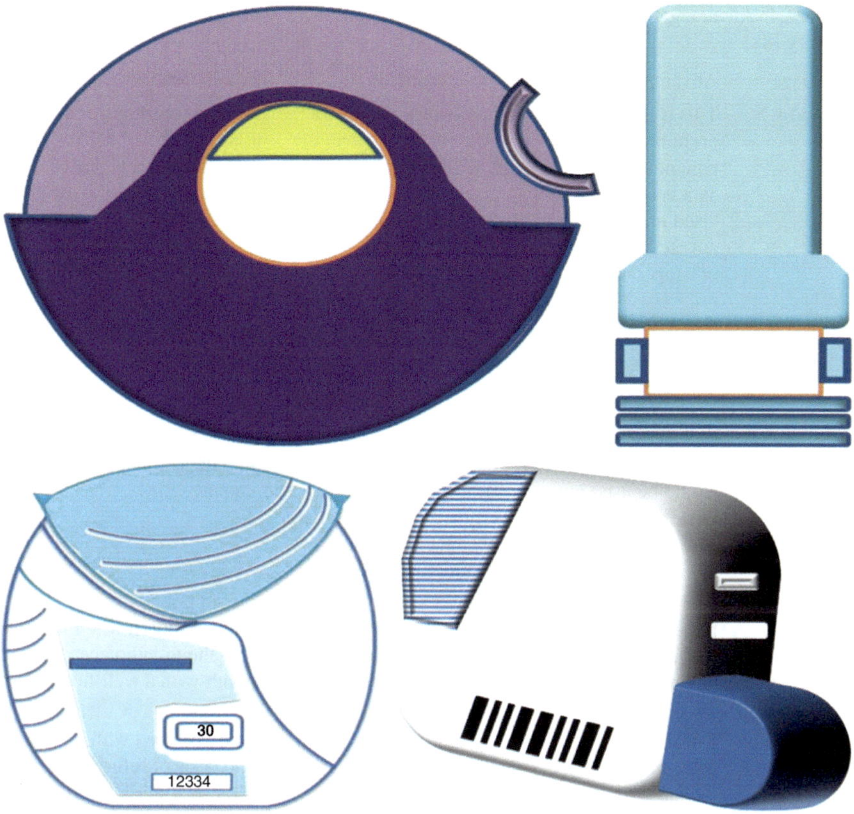

Fig. 4.3 Different dry powder inhalers

[82] or even playing with the cover. Those DPIs handling errors cannot be considered as device errors but they could be considered as human or patient errors. These human errors could result in the patient having the medication in his hand but cannot properly receive his therapy [84]. These human errors are a very hard obstacle in inpatient counseling of inhaled medication e.g. inhaling slowly when using pMDI and inhaling fast when using DPI [85–87].

4.10 Selection of Aerosol Therapy Interface

There are several types of interfaces or accessory devices that could be used for aerosol delivery and they are different in their characteristics (Table 4.4 and Fig. 4.4).

The mouthpiece is the most effective connection that has been used with aerosol therapy in older spontaneously breathing pediatric patients [47]. A mouthpiece could provide high amounts of inhaled medications that could be two folds that

Table 4.4 Advantage and disadvantage of different interfaces that could be used for aerosol delivery [88]

Interface	Advantages	Disadvantages	Recommendations
Blow-by	This technique is preferred by the patient and his parents as it is comfortable Used in case of an agitated, crying, or uncooperative child	Its efficacy in aerosol delivery is less than the traditional mask by about 50–80% It cannot be used with a certain aerosol-generating device such as a breath-actuated nebulizer, pMDI, and VMN	It is not recommended to be used for aerosol delivery in pediatric patients due to lack of efficacy
Facemask	Effective interface for aerosol delivery compared with the mouthpiece Could be used with a wide range of aerosol-generating devices	Its efficacy of aerosol delivery could be affected by a lack of well-fit contact with the skin without leakage Cause skin irritation and enhance children's agitation and crying	The selected mask should be with small dead space and has a good seal with the face to provide a sufficient inhaled amount
Mouthpiece	More effective in aerosol delivery than the traditional facemask by 2 folds	Requires well fit closure of the mouth around it. Hence, could not be used with young children less than 3 years	Should not be used with young children who unable to keep the mouthpiece in the mouth with a well-fit closure
Pacifier mask	Enhance the compliance of pediatric patients though keeping the child calm during aerosol delivery		Could be used with an infant who cries or refuses the traditional mask
Nasal mask	Its tolerability is better than the traditional face mask. Besides, being easier to be used with a child	Its efficacy for aerosol delivery is lower than that of the traditional face mask	
Hood	It is more tolerated by pediatric patients because it does not stimulate crying compared with a face mask Could be used with an infant who cannot use the mouthpiece correctly	Its setup is not easier than other interfaces and requires specific training to provide a proper efficacy of delivering aerosol	Should be used for pediatric patients if they can not use the mouthpiece or the facial mask The infant should be placed in a face-side position to avoid an ocular aerosol deposition

(continued)

Table 4.4 (continued)

Interface	Advantages	Disadvantages	Recommendations
Valved holding chamber	Enhance aerosol deposition through reduction of drug amount that deposits in upper airways Does not require coordination between the patient and pMDI	The aerosol delivery from VHC is largely affected by electrostatic charges and the size of the chamber	It is preferred to use the non-electrostatic VHCs which are coated with an antistatic coat In case of non-availability of the antistatic VHC, wash the VHC with a soapy solution and let it dry in the air to mask the static charges Another option to decrease the effect of the static charges is by releasing two buffs of the inhaled drug before initiation of the therapy
High flow nasal cannula	HFNC has good tolerability for neonates and infants compared with a nasal or facial mask	Cannot be used with pMDI devices The deposition of large amounts of aerosol inside the tube could have a negative impact that requires more investigations	VMN, when used with HFNC, should be placed before the humidifier for effective aerosol delivery

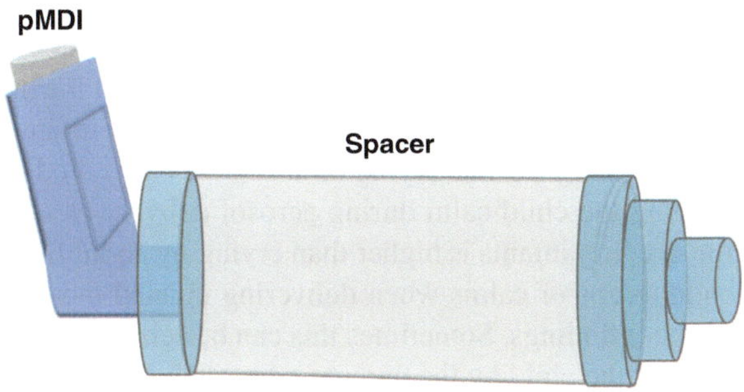

Fig. 4.4 Criteria for selection of interface for aerosol delivery for pediatric patients

could be delivered using a facial mask [16]. A slow deep inhalation accompanied by a breath-holding for a few seconds could also help boost the delivery of inhaled medication to the lungs. Most children are not able to open and close their mouth to achieve a suitable seal around the mouthpiece, nor are they capable of breathing deeply and keeping their breath in command. Hence, for uncooperative young patients, toddlers, and infants who are unable to use a mouthpiece, a well-fitted mask could be used instead. The facial mask should be properly fitted with the child's face to prevent the emission of fugitive aerosol to the surrounding area, also to prevent eye irritation as a result of aerosolized drug deposition. For different types of nebulizers used with small children, the design of the mask is an essential element that controls the aerosol delivery [89]. It is preferably to be made of flexible and soft material. The facial masks are available in different sizes that are suitable for patients of different ages. The smaller the patient receiving aerosol therapy, the smaller the mask that should be used. Small masks have a small dead space which allows delivery of high aerosol fraction to the lung [90, 91]. This is particularly true in the case of the use of pMDIs/VHCs or other devices that insert gas into the system such as VMN. While, in the case of jet nebulizers, the design of the mask is especially necessary since gas flows of 6–10 L/min result in high flux velocities, particulate inertia, and deposition in the mask. Regarding the mask design, it was proved through several studies that the front-loaded masks deliver high portions of inhaled medications compared with masks that are bottom-loaded. This difference in efficacy could be explained by the effect of mask design, as the bottom-loaded one deliver aerosol particles to the wall of the mask which lead to the deposition of a large portion of aerosol particles, while the front-loaded mask delivers the aerosol directly to the patient nose which facilitates the drug inhalation and deposition. Nasal masks could be used with pediatric subjects especially with jet nebulizers, [92] while for VMN, this type of mask would deliver a low amount of inhaled medication due to the absence of a gas source that aids in delivering aerosol particles [4]. For young children who do not tolerate face or nasal masks, the hood attached to the nebulizer could be the preferred option. Hoods result in less agitation by the infant compared with the facial mask which stimulates crying and discomfort. Regarding the efficacy of aerosol delivery, both mask and hood have a comparable efficacy while the selection point between them is the tolerability and the low nebulization time that would be in favor of hoods [93–95]. Infant crying during aerosol therapy is a common aspect especially related to using the facial mask attached to nebulizers, the effect of crying on aerosol delivery efficacy is controversial. It was thought that crying would increase the inhaled amount of the inhaled medication while clinical studies showed the opposite results, calm infants inhaled aerosol medication four folds higher than crying infants [96]. Other studies indicated the importance of keeping the child calm during aerosol delivery as it reported that aerosol delivery for sleeping infants is higher than crying by about five folds [97]. It is better when a child sleeps or calms when delivering inhaled medication using a nebulizer based on these findings. Sometimes this can be achieved by hanging the child down, or by holding the child by the parent and providing care to alleviate the patient.

Blow-by is a technique that is used with a JN placed within a distance from the child's face and directs emitted aerosol plume towards the subject's face. This technique was introduced to solve the problem of aerosol delivery to agitated children and crying infants, caused by placing the nebulizer away from the skin, the child will be less stimulated and become calm during aerosol delivery. Also, this technique is highly suitable and preferred by parents to avoid children agitation.

But this strategy has a variety of drawbacks. One of these drawbacks is the inability to be used with devices that require the application of inhalation force to open a valve that allows the release of aerosol particles. Hence blow-by cannot be used with pMDI/VHD or breath-actuated nebulizer [7]. Consequently, using blow-by techniques for aerosol therapy in young children is not recommended.

Problems associated with blow-by highlight not only the importance of interface selection in inhalation therapy but also finding a better alternative for delivering aerosolized medications to neonates and pediatrics. Mouthpiece, facemask, nasal mask, pacifier mask, hood, high flow nasal cannula, and VHCs may be viable choices of the interface in children and the following sections will describe each interface more in detail. Facemask is a suitable interface for young children who are unable to use the mouthpiece for inhaling emitted aerosol during treatment. The selected mask should be compatible with the patient regarding the size of the mask, young children require small-size masks with small dead volumes with fit contact with the skin to provide a high portion of aerosol to the child's lung. This is specifically true when the aerosol-generating device is VMN or pMDI that do not involve gas production during the aerosol generation when used for the treatment of neonates [88].

The pacifier mask was developed to achieve higher aerosol deposition that led to therapeutic lung deposition in children as a modern and revolutionary advancement of the children-oriented drug delivery interface by removing their irritation, anxiety, and crying caused by using the traditional facemask and keeping them relaxed through a pacifier.

This requires the infant's pacifier to be connected to the mask's anterior wall. By sucking the pacifier by the young child during treatment while nasally inhaling the generated aerosolized medications produced by pMDIs/VHCs or nebulizers during aerosol therapy, the infant holds the Soother mask sealed to his face [98]. In 12 infants less than 1 year of age, Amirav et al. [99] compared Soother's mask with a traditional bottom-loaded face mask for bronchodilator delivery through imaging technique (scintigraphy imaging). The finding indicated that both masks have comparable efficacy for delivering bronchodilators, but the tolerability for the pacifier mask was higher among the recruited infants [99].

A high flow nasal cannula (HFNC) is a heated and humidified system that allows the delivery of different fractions of inspired oxygen levels at very high flow rates [100, 101]. A high flow of gas is considered when the flow is more than 2 liters per minute, in the case of children high gas flows were used ranging from 6 to 30 liters per minute [102, 103]. The need for high flow is not only to deliver higher portions of the inspired oxygen but also, to provide respiratory support through the continuous positive pressure [101, 104]. For a critically ill child, there are several options for the administration of aerosolized medications such as using traditional interfaces (masks) with nebulizers or spacers with pMDI. Another option is to deliver aerosol without removing HFNC and using it as the interface that delivers inhaled medication nasally [105].

Delivery of aerosol through HFNC has become popular in the field of aerosol therapy related to pulmonary diseases of pediatric patients based on the reported efficacy of several studies which indicated the effectiveness of this interface to deliver higher aerosol amount compared with oral delivery [6, 106]. The type of gas and more specifically its density is an important factor that controls the delivery of the aerosol. It was reported that heliox was able of delivering higher amounts of aerosol compared with oxygen only through HFNC used for the treatment of pediatric patients [107].

According to a previous study, the amount of aerosol deposition found with different cannula sizes of flows used with HFNC was lower than the amount needed for optimum clinical response [105]. Besides, the inhaled medication accumulates inside the cannula and could be a potential issue with HFNC.

4.11 Valved Holding Chamber and Spacers

The accessory device (VHC or spacer) is a type of add-on device that is attached to pMDIs to provide additional space for aerosol particles to travel in as shown in Fig. 4.5. It is a tube connected from one end to the pMDI and the other end provides the aerosol particles to the patient. The spacer end that provides aerosol to the patient could be attached to a face mask or mouthpiece. The aim of using accessory devices is to solve the breath actuation problem in which the patient cannot inhale the aerosol released from the pMDI correctly [108, 109].

Accessory devices affect factors that enhance aerosol delivery; first is the velocity of the aerosol which will be reduced and the second is the particle size of aerosol droplets which will be reduced. It is difficult to teach patients to use pMDI in an emergency where they need drugs to be administered very rapidly. Teaching children and elderly patients is similarly challenging [59, 60]. In these cases, placing accessory devices (reservoir) between the pMDI and the patient allows more time for drug inhalation (Fig. 4.5) [110, 111]. Accessory devices enhance aerosol delivery to the patient because large particles emitted by the pMDI settle inside the accessory device rather than being deposited in the mouth and throat. This increases the dose of fine particles [111, 112].

The construction of the accessory device can affect the emitted dose of inhaled medications and also influences its cost, which is important when considering the

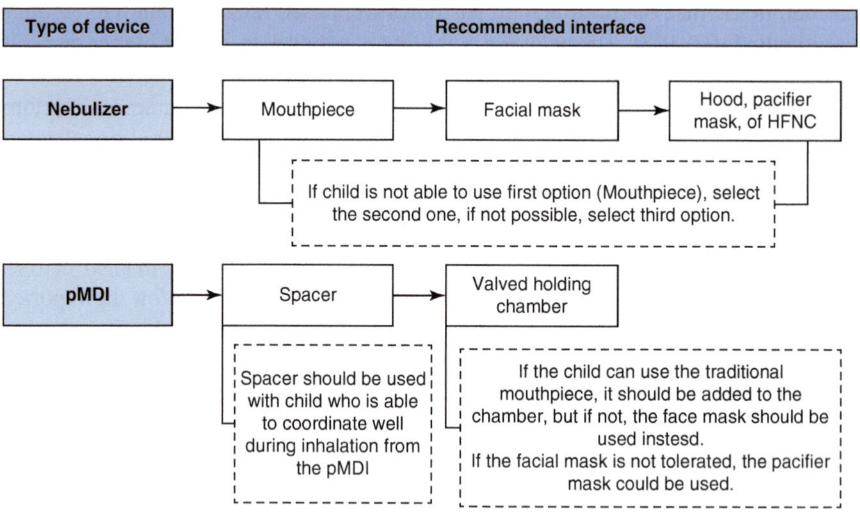

Fig. 4.5 Valved holding chamber attached to pressurized metered-dose inhale

pharmacoeconomic aspects of accessory devices. The material from which the accessory devices are made is an important factor affecting aerosol delivery [113]. Most traditional accessory devices on the market are made from lightweight plastic for greater durability and enhanced spacer portability [114, 115]. Polypropylene and polycarbonate are the most commonly used materials for making a plastic accessory device; however, their non-conducting nature leads to the accumulation of electrostatic charges on the wall of the accessory device [116–118]. As drugs released from pMDIs also are electrically charged, inevitably electrostatic reactions will occur between the charged accessory device wall and the emitted drug. Mutual repulsion between the charged entities pushes the drug towards the wall of the accessory device, [115–118] thus decreasing the emitted dose [119–121]. According to the GINA guidelines, [122] there are two efficient methods for neutralizing charges on the accessory device wall. The first involves washing the plastic accessory device in soapy water and letting it dry in the air: the residual soap acts as a surfactant. The second method involves priming the accessory device with puffs of the drug before inspiration. These methods are effective but they result in wasted drugs or delays, and neither is suitable in emergency cases [122]. Some disposable accessory devices are made of paper, which is antistatic and inexpensive [61].

References

1. Erzinger S, et al. Facemasks and aerosol delivery in vivo. J Aerosol Med. 2007;20(s1):S78–84.
2. Salmon B, Wilson NM, Silverman M. How much aerosol reaches the lungs of wheezy infants and toddlers? Arch Dis Child. 1990;65(4):401–3.
3. Amirav I, et al. β-agonist aerosol distribution in respiratory syncytial virus bronchiolitis in infants. J Nucl Med. 2002;43(4):487–91.
4. DiBlasi RM. Clinical controversies in aerosol therapy for infants and children. Respir Care. 2015;60(6):894–916.
5. Xi J, et al. Growth of nasal and laryngeal airways in children: implications in breathing and inhaled aerosol dynamics. Respir Care. 2014;59(2):263–73.
6. Amirav I, et al. Nasal versus oral aerosol delivery to the "lungs" in infants and toddlers. Pediatr Pulmonol. 2015;50(3):276–83.
7. Ari A, Restrepo RD. Aerosol delivery device selection for spontaneously breathing patients. Respir Care. 2012;57(4):613–26.
8. Elgendy MO, et al. Asthmatic children and MDI verbal inhalation technique counseling. Pulm Pharmacol Ther. 2020;61:101900.
9. Saeed H, et al. Impact of advanced patient counseling using training device and smartphone application on asthma control. Respir Care. 2020;65(3):326–32.
10. Myers TR. The science guiding selection of an aerosol delivery device. Respir Care. 2013;58(11):1963–73.
11. Dhand R. Aerosol delivery during mechanical ventilation: from basic techniques to new devices. J Aerosol Med Pulm Drug Deliv. 2008;21(1):45–60.
12. Ari A, Fink JB. Factors affecting bronchodilator delivery in mechanically ventilated adults. Nurs Crit Care. 2010;15(4):192–203.
13. Moustafa IO, et al. Lung deposition and systemic bioavailability of different aerosol devices with and without humidification in mechanically ventilated patients. Heart Lung. 2017;46(6):464–7.

14. Moustafa IO, et al. Clinical outcome associated with the use of different inhalation method with and without humidification in asthmatic mechanically ventilated patients. Pulm Pharmacol Ther. 2017;45:40–6.
15. Carvalho TC, McConville JT. The function and performance of aqueous aerosol devices for inhalation therapy. J Pharm Pharmacol. 2016;68(5):556–78.
16. Ari A, et al. Performance comparisons of jet and mesh nebulizers using different interfaces in simulated spontaneously breathing adults and children. J Aerosol Med Pulm Drug Deliv. 2015;28(4):281–9.
17. Ari A, Aljamhan EA, Fink J. Influence of nebulizer type position and bias flow on aerosol drug delivery in a model of adult mechanical ventilation. Respir Care. 2010;55:845–51.
18. Miller DD, et al. Aerosol delivery and modern mechanical ventilation: in vitro/in vivo evaluation. Am J Respir Crit Care Med. 2003;168(10):1205–9.
19. Hughes J, SAEZ T. Effects of nebulizer mode and position in a mechanical ventilator circuit on dose efficiency. Respir Care. 1987;32(12):1131–5.
20. Alvine GF, et al. Disposable jet nebulizers. How reliable are they? Chest J. 1992;101(2): 316–9.
21. Loffert DT, Ikle D, Nelson HS. A comparison of commercial jet nebulizers. Chest J. 1994;106(6):1788–92.
22. Hess D, et al. Medication nebulizer performance: effects of diluent volume, nebulizer flow, and nebulizer brand. Chest J. 1996;110(2):498–505.
23. Sterk P, et al. Physical properties of aerosols produced by several jet-and ultrasonic nebulizers. Bull Eur Physiopathol Respir. 1983;20(1):65–72.
24. Hess DR, Dillman C, Kacmarek RM. In vitro evaluation of aerosol bronchodilator delivery during mechanical ventilation: pressure-control vs. volume control ventilation. Intensive Care Med. 2003;29(7):1145–50.
25. O'doherty MJ, et al. Delivery of a nebulized aerosol to a lung model during mechanical ventilation. Am Rev Respir Dis. 1992;146(2):383–8.
26. Tiemersma S, et al. Vibrating membrane devices deliver aerosols more efficient than standard devices: a study in a neonatal upper airway model. J Aerosol Med Pulm Drug Deliv. 2013;26(5):280–6.
27. Arzhavitina A, Steckel H. Surface active drugs significantly alter the drug output rate from medical nebulizers. Int J Pharm. 2010;384(1):128–36.
28. Beck-Broichsitter M, et al. Impact of lyoprotectants for the stabilization of biodegradable nanoparticles on the performance of air-jet, ultrasonic, and vibrating-mesh nebulizers. Eur J Pharm Biopharm. 2012;82(2):272–80.
29. Ari A, Fink JB. Guidelines for aerosol devices in infants, children and adults: which to choose, why and how to achieve effective aerosol therapy. Expert Rev Respir Med. 2011;5(4):561–72.
30. Ari A, Restrepo RD. Aerosol delivery device selection for spontaneously breathing patients: 2012. Respir Care. 2012;57(4):613–26.
31. Watts AB, McConville JT, Williams RO III. Current therapies and technological advances in aqueous aerosol drug delivery. Drug Dev Ind Pharm. 2008;34(9):913–22.
32. Taylor KM, McCallion ON. Ultrasonic nebulisers for pulmonary drug delivery. Int J Pharm. 1997;153(1):93–104.
33. Thomas SHL, et al. Delivery of ultrasonic nebulized aerosols to a lung model during mechanical ventilation. Am Rev Respir Dis. 1993;148(4):872–7.
34. Newman S, Gee-Turner A. The Omron MicroAir vibrating mesh technology nebuliser, a 21st century approach to inhalation therapy. J Appl Therap Res. 2005;5(4):29–33.
35. Elhissi A, et al. Air-jet and vibrating-mesh nebulization of niosomes generated using a particulate-based proniosome technology. Int J Pharm. 2013;444(1):193–9.
36. Elhissi A, et al. Formulations generated from ethanol-based proliposomes for delivery via medical nebulizers. J Pharm Pharmacol. 2006;58(7):887–94.
37. Lass JS, Sant A, Knoch M. New advances in aerosolised drug delivery: vibrating membrane nebuliser technology. Expert Opin Drug Deliv. 2006;3(5):693–702.

38. Ghazanfari T, et al. The influence of fluid physicochemical properties on vibrating-mesh nebulization. Int J Pharm. 2007;339(1):103–11.
39. Zhang G, David A, Wiedmann TS. Performance of the vibrating membrane aerosol generation device: aeroneb micropump nebulizer™. J Aerosol Med. 2007;20(4):408–16.
40. Beck-Broichsitter M, et al. On the correlation of output rate and aerodynamic characteristics in vibrating-mesh-based aqueous aerosol delivery. Int J Pharm. 2014;461(1):34–7.
41. Beck-Broichsitter M, et al. Nebulization of active pharmaceutical ingredients with the eFlow® rapid: impact of formulation variables on aerodynamic characteristics. J Pharm Sci. 2014;103(8):2585–9.
42. Pitance L, et al. Delivery efficacy of a vibrating mesh nebulizer and a jet nebulizer under different configurations. J Aerosol Med Pulm Drug Deliv. 2010;23(6):389–96.
43. Skaria S, Smaldone GC, Omron NE. U22: comparison between vibrating mesh and jet nebulizer. J Aerosol Med Pulm Drug Deliv. 2010;23(3):173–80.
44. Coates AL, et al. A comparison of amount and speed of deposition between the PARI LC STAR® jet nebulizer and an investigational eFlow® nebulizer. J Aerosol Med Pulm Drug Deliv. 2011;24(3):157–63.
45. Hardaker LE, Hatley RH. In vitro characterization of the I-neb adaptive aerosol delivery (AAD) system. J Aerosol Med Pulm Drug Deliv. 2010;23(1):11–20.
46. Johnson JC, et al. Aerosol delivery of recombinant human DNase I: in vitro comparison of a vibrating-mesh nebulizer with a jet nebulizer. Respir Care. 2008;53(12):1703–8.
47. Ditcham W, et al. Lung deposition of 99mTc-radiolabeled albuterol delivered through a pressurized metered dose inhaler and spacer with facemask or mouthpiece in children with asthma. J Aerosol Med Pulm Drug Deliv. 2014;27(S1):S63–75.
48. Phillips G, Millard F. The therapeutic use of ultrasonic nebulizers in acute asthma. Respir Med. 1994;88(5):387–9.
49. Newman SP. Principles of metered-dose inhaler design. Respir Care. 2005;50(9):1177–90.
50. MacGregor T, et al. Efficiency of ipratropium bromide and albuterol deposition in the lung delivered via a soft mist inhaler or chlorofluorocarbon metered-dose inhaler. Clin Transl Sci. 2016;9(2):105–13.
51. Kwok PCL, et al. Studies of radioaerosol deposition in the respiratory tract. In: Seminars in nuclear medicine. Elsevier; 2019.
52. Terzano C. Pressurized metered dose inhalers and add-on devices. Pulm Pharmacol Ther. 2001;14(5):351–66.
53. Sheth P, Stein SW, Myrdal PB. Factors influencing aerodynamic particle size distribution of suspension pressurized metered dose inhalers. AAPS PharmSciTech. 2015;16(1):192–201.
54. Sheth P, et al. Impact of droplet evaporation rate on resulting in vitro performance parameters of pressurized metered dose inhalers. Int J Pharm. 2017;528(1–2):360–71.
55. Molina MJ, Rowland FS. Stratospheric sink for chlorofluoromethanes: chlorine atom-catalysed destruction of ozone. Nature. 1974;249(5460):810.
56. Crompton GK. How to achieve good compliance with inhaled asthma therapy. Respir Med. 2004;98:S35–40.
57. Tena AF, Clarà PC. Deposition of inhaled particles in the lungs. Arch Bronconeumol. 2012;48(7):240–6.
58. Al-Showair RAM, Pearson SB, Chrystyn H. The potential of a 2Tone trainer to help patients use their metered dose inhalers. Chest. 2007;131(6):1776–82.
59. Nicola M, et al. The impact of adding a training device to familiar counselling on inhalation technique and pulmonary function of asthmatics. Adv Ther. 2018;35(7):1049–58.
60. Elgendy MO, Abdelrahim ME, Eldin RS. Potential benefit of repeated MDI inhalation technique counselling for patients with asthma. Eur J Hosp Pharm. 2015;22(6):318–22.
61. Sanders M, Bruin R. A rationale for going back to the future: use of disposable spacers for pressurised metered dose inhalers. Pulm Med. 2015;2015(2):1–6.
62. McFadden E Jr. Improper patient techniques with metered dose inhalers: clinical consequences and solutions to misuse. J Allergy Clin Immunol. 1995;96(2):278–83.

63. van Beerendonk I, et al. Assessment of the inhalation technique in outpatients with asthma or chronic obstructive pulmonary disease using a metered-dose inhaler or dry powder device. J Asthma. 1998;35(3):273–9.
64. Bosnic-Anticevich SZ. Inhaler device handling: have we really started to address the problem? Eur Respir J. 2017;49:1700120.
65. Melani AS, et al. Inhaler mishandling remains common in real life and is associated with reduced disease control. Respir Med. 2011;105(6):930–8.
66. Lavorini F, et al. Effect of incorrect use of dry powder inhalers on management of patients with asthma and COPD. Respir Med. 2008;102(4):593–604.
67. Saji M, Alhas J, Siraj S. Study on the impact of patient counseling on the quality of life and pulmonary function of asthmatic patient. Int J Pharm Pharm Sci. 2012;4(Suppl 5):300–4.
68. Shareef J, Sajitha M, Shastry C. Impact of pharmacist provided patient counseling on quality of life in patients with asthma in a tertiary care teaching hospital. Int J Pharma Res Rev. 2014;3(2):1–10.
69. Schatz M, et al. Asthma control test: reliability, validity, and responsiveness in patients not previously followed by asthma specialists. J Allergy Clin Immunol. 2006;117(3):549–56.
70. Schatz M, et al. The minimally important difference of the Asthma Control Test. J Allergy Clin Immunol. 2009;124(4):719–723.e1.
71. Ibrahim M, Verma R, Garcia-Contreras L. Inhalation drug delivery devices: technology update. Med Devices. 2015;8:131.
72. Dal Negro RW. Dry powder inhalers and the right things to remember: a concept review. Multidiscip Respir Med. 2015;10(1):13.
73. Abdelrahim M, Assi KH, Chrystyn H. Dose emission and aerodynamic characterization of the terbutaline sulphate dose emitted from a Turbuhaler at low inhalation flow. Pharm Dev Technol. 2013;18(4):944–9.
74. Abdelrahim ME. Emitted dose and lung deposition of inhaled terbutaline from Turbuhaler at different conditions. Respir Med. 2010;104(5):682–9.
75. Ali AMA, Abdelrahim MEA. Modeling and optimization of terbutaline emitted from a dry powder inhaler and influence on systemic bioavailability using data mining technology. J Pharm Innov. 2014;9(1):38–47.
76. Chapman KR, et al. Delivery characteristics and patients' handling of two single-dose dry-powder inhalers used in COPD. Int J Chron Obstruct Pulmon Dis. 2011;6(1):353–63.
77. Newman S, Busse W. Evolution of dry powder inhaler design, formulation, and performance. Respir Med. 2002;96(5):293–304.
78. Tarsin W, Assi KH, Chrystyn H. In-vitro intra- and inter-inhaler flow rate-dependent dosage emission from a combination of budesonide and eformoterol in a dry powder inhaler. J Aerosol Med. 2004;17(1):25–32.
79. von Schantz S, et al. Evaluation of dry powder inhalers with a focus on ease of use and user preference in inhaler-naïve individuals. Int J Pharm. 2016;509(1):50–8.
80. Yun Kirby S, et al. A preference study of two placebo dry powder inhalers in adults with COPD: Ellipta® dry powder inhaler (DPI) versus DISKUS® DPI. COPD: J Chron Obstruct Pulmon Dis. 2016;13(2):167–75.
81. Hamilton M, et al. In vitro dosing performance of the ELLIPTA® dry powder inhaler using asthma and COPD patient inhalation profiles replicated with the electronic lung (eLung™). J Aerosol Med Pulm Drug Deliv. 2015;28(6):498–506.
82. Komase Y, et al. Ease-of-use preference for the ELLIPTA® dry powder inhaler over a commonly used single-dose capsule dry powder inhaler by inhalation device-naïve Japanese volunteers aged 40 years or older. Int J Chron Obstruct Pulmon Dis. 2014;9:1365.
83. Grant AC, et al. The ELLIPTA® dry powder inhaler: design, functionality, in vitro dosing performance and critical task compliance by patients and caregivers. J Aerosol Med Pulm Drug Deliv. 2015;28(6):474–85.
84. Wieshammer S, Dreyhaupt J. Dry powder inhalers: which factors determine the frequency of handling errors? Respiration. 2008;75(1):18–25.

85. Nicola M, et al. Effect of DPI's training-device on inhalation technique and clinical efficacy in asthmatics. Beni-Suef Univ J Appl Sci. 2018;7(2):178–83.
86. Elgendy MO, Abdelrahim ME, Salah Eldin R. Potential benefit of repeated MDI inhalation technique counselling for patients with asthma. Eur J Hosp Pharm. 2015.
87. Elgendy MO, Abdelrahim ME, Eldin RS. Potential benefit of repeated dry powder Inhaler's inhalation technique counseling on asthmatic patients. Pulm Ther. 2015;1(1):91–101.
88. Ari A. Drug delivery interfaces: a way to optimize inhalation therapy in spontaneously breathing children. World J Clin Pediatr. 2016;5(3):281.
89. Ari A, Fink JB. Effective bronchodilator resuscitation of children in the emergency room: device or interface? Respir Care. 2011;56(6):882–5.
90. Turpeinen M, et al. Metered dose inhaler add-on devices: is the inhaled mass of drug dependent on the size of the infant? J Aerosol Med. 1999;12(3):171–6.
91. Chavez A, McCracken A, Berlinski A. Effect of face mask dead volume, respiratory rate, and tidal volume on inhaled albuterol delivery. Pediatr Pulmonol. 2010;45(3): 224–9.
92. El Taoum KK, et al. In vitro evaluation of aerosols delivered via the nasal route. Respir Care. 2015;60(7):1015–25.
93. Kim J, et al. Hood nebulization: effects of head direction and breathing mode on particle inhalability and deposition in a 7-month-old infant model. J Aerosol Med Pulm Drug Deliv. 2014;27(3):209–18.
94. Kugelman A, et al. Hood versus mask nebulization in infants with evolving bronchopulmonary dysplasia in the neonatal intensive care unit. J Perinatol. 2006;26(1):31–6.
95. Amirav I, et al. Aerosol delivery in respiratory syncytial virus bronchiolitis: hood or face mask? J Pediatr. 2005;147(5):627–31.
96. Iles R, Lister P, Edmunds AJ. Crying significantly reduces absorption of aerosolised drug in infants. Arch Dis Child. 1999;81(2):163–5.
97. Murakami G, et al. Measurement of bronchial hyperreactivity in infants and preschool children using a new method. Ann Allergy. 1990;64(4):383–7.
98. Amirav I, et al. Feasibility of aerosol drug delivery to sleeping infants: a prospective observational study. BMJ Open. 2014;4(3):e004124.
99. Amirav I, et al. Lung aerosol deposition in suckling infants. Arch Dis Child. 2012;97(6):497–501.
100. Beggs S, et al. High-flow nasal cannula therapy for infants with bronchiolitis. Cochrane Database Syst Rev. 2014;(1):CD009609.
101. Mayfield S, et al. High-flow nasal cannula therapy for respiratory support in children. Cochrane Database Syst Rev. 2014;(3):CD009850.
102. Mikalsen IB, et al. High flow nasal cannula in children: a literature review. Scand J Trauma Resusc Emerg Med. 2016;24(1):1–12.
103. Lee JH, et al. Use of high flow nasal cannula in critically ill infants, children, and adults: a critical review of the literature. Intensive Care Med. 2013;39(2):247–57.
104. Milési C, et al. High flow nasal cannula (HFNC) versus nasal continuous positive airway pressure (nCPAP) for the initial respiratory management of acute viral bronchiolitis in young infants: a multicenter randomized controlled trial (TRAMONTANE study). Intensive Care Med. 2017;43(2):209–16.
105. Perry SA, et al. Influences of cannula size and flow rate on aerosol drug delivery through the Vapotherm humidified high-flow nasal cannula system. Pediatr Crit Care Med. 2013;14(5):e250–6.
106. Chua H, et al. The influence of age on aerosol deposition in children with cystic fibrosis. Eur Respir J. 1994;7(12):2185–91.
107. Ari A, et al. In vitro comparison of heliox and oxygen in aerosol delivery using pediatric high flow nasal cannula. Pediatr Pulmonol. 2011;46(8):795–801.
108. Anderson G, et al. Use of spacers for patients treated with pressurized metered dose inhalers: focus on the VENTOLIN™ Mini spacer. Expert Opin Drug Deliv. 2018;15(4):419–30.

109. Misik O, et al. Inhalers and nebulizers: basic principles and preliminary measurements. In: EPJ Web of Conferences. EDP Sciences; 2018.
110. Leung SSY, et al. Effect of spacers on the bipolar electrostatic charge properties of metered dose inhaler aerosols—a case study with Tilade®. J Pharm Sci. 2017;106(6):1553–9.
111. Rau JL. Practical problems with aerosol therapy in COPD. Respir Care. 2006;51(2):158–72.
112. Rahmatalla MF, et al. In vitro effect of a holding chamber on the mouth-throat deposition of QVAR® (hydrofluoroalkane-beclomethasone dipropionate). J Aerosol Med. 2002;15(4):379–85.
113. Sheth P, et al. In vitro evaluation of nonconventional accessory devices for pressurized metered-dose inhalers. Ann Allergy Asthma Immunol. 2014;113(1):55–62.
114. Goncalves TM, et al. Comparative in vitro performance of three small-volume valved holding chambers with beclomethasone/formoterol pressurized metered dose inhaler. J Aerosol Med Pulm Drug Deliv. 2013;26(4):223–7.
115. Mitchell JP, Coppolo DP, Nagel MW. Electrostatics and inhaled medications: influence on delivery via pressurized metered-dose inhalers and add-on devices. Respir Care. 2007;52(3):283–300.
116. Saini D, et al. Particle size and charge distribution analysis of pharmaceutical aerosols generated by inhalers. Pharm Dev Technol. 2007;12(1):35–41.
117. Ali M, Mazumder MK, Martonen TB. Measurements of electrodynamic effects on the deposition of MDI and DPI aerosols in a replica cast of human oral–pharyngeal–laryngeal airways. J Aerosol Med Pulm Drug Deliv. 2009;22(1):35–44.
118. Leung SSY, et al. Applicability of bipolar charge analyzer (BOLAR) in characterizing the bipolar electrostatic charge profile of commercial metered dose inhalers (MDIs). Pharm Res. 2016;33(2):283–91.
119. Barry P, O'Callaghan C. The effect of delay, multiple actuations and spacer static charge on the in vitro delivery of budesonide from the Nebuhaler. Br J Clin Pharmacol. 1995;40(1):76–8.
120. Wildhaber J, et al. Electrostatic charge on a plastic spacer device influences the delivery of salbutamol. Eur Respir J. 1996;9(9):1943–6.
121. Pierart F, et al. Washing plastic spacers in household detergent reduces electrostatic charge and greatly improves delivery. Eur Respir J. 1999;13(3):673–8.
122. (GINA), G.I.f.A. Global Strategy for Asthma Management and Prevention; 2018. https://ginasthma.org/download/832/.

Chapter 5
Transitioning Aerosol from Hospital to Home; Role of Training and Follow-Up

Contents

M. E. A. Abdelrahim et al., *Essentials of Aerosol Therapy in Critically ill Patients*,
https://doi.org/10.1007/978-3-030-85026-5_5

5.1 Challenges of Aerosol Therapy

In certain cases, such as asthma, chronic obstructive pulmonary disease (COPD), the patient is the keystone for disease prevention, and his contribution, self-management of the disease, may be greatly valuable than that of health care practitioners alone [1, 2]. The patient's ability to use different aerosol-producing devices correctly is the most significant patient-related element in controlling the aerosol therapy. Aside from this, there are biological considerations such as variations in the anatomy and physiology of the respiratory system among patients, as well as the nature and severity of the disease [3, 4].

Control of aerosol therapy is heavily influenced by the patient's age. Patient counseling and training can be facilitated or hampered by age-related physical and cognitive abilities. Elderly people and children up to the age of school need more effort from health care providers to teach them proper inhalation techniques which are related to aerosol-generating devices [5]. Using add-on devices in addition to conventional pressurized metered-dose inhalers (pMDIs) or switching to nebulizers would have better treatment results for infants and younger subjects, but this would be more expensive and time-consuming than using pMDIs alone [6]. Also, since much of the released dose is collected in the upper airways by impaction, the crying of babies results in lower aerosol accumulation in young patient's lungs [7]. A face mask can be used for aerosol delivery in children under the age of three, but if it does not match properly, the patient can inhale less of the emitted inhaled medication. However, most subjects over the age of 3 should be taught how to use the mouthpiece and the technique for taking regular inspiratory and expiratory breaths. Most subjects can learn to use spacers/valved holding chambers with a low inspiratory flow rate for at least 5 s followed by holding their breath for no more than 10 s while they are between the ages of 5 and 7. They may also be able to inhale from dry powder inhalers (DPI) with a high inspiratory rate if they are older than 5 years [8, 9].

For most chronic conditions, poor compliance is a major hindrance to successful treatment results. Missing one or more doses from the recommended dosage schedule indicates a lack of compliance with other routes of drug administration. While lack of compliance with aerosol therapy includes a lack of compliance with the correct inhalation procedure of the prescribed inhalers, as the majority of patients forget the training instructions for proper inhaler use after obtaining it from the healthcare professionals [10, 11]. As a result, in this situation involving aerosol therapy, adherence includes not only the continued use of the inhaled medication according to the dosage regimen but also the proper inhalation technique of the prescribed inhaler. Subjects receiving 14 inhaled doses per week of inhaled medicine should not miss more than three doses if they have extreme asthma or have repeated exacerbations and symptoms. Around 20% of subjects did not meet this requirement for a variety of reasons, including a drug holiday, in which the patient attempt to test the impact of discounting the inhaled medications on their wellbeing.

Other patients did not take their drugs as prescribed to prevent a specific treatment side effect, such as the cold Freon effect related to the propellant of inhaled medications [12]. Also, The most common cause of non-adherence is forgetting to take medicine.

Regarding the treatment of pulmonary disorders, patient adherence to prescription aerosol therapy is critical. Nonadherence has been linked to inadequate clinical management of the disease, increased school and work nonattendance, morbidity, unscheduled utilization of healthcare, and mortality in the past [13, 14]. A previous study found a clear connection between noncompliance with inhaled drug prescriptions and the risk of hospitalization related to exacerbations. In COPD patients, there is a clear inverse association between adherence to inhaled medications and mortality. When compared to those who did not adhere to aerosol therapy, subjects who were adherent to the therapy had 2 folds lower mortality rates [14].

Noncompliance to prescribed inhaled drugs is also linked to higher healthcare costs. In the United States, the cost of nonadherence by chronic illness patients is projected to be $300 billion a year [15]. The rate of adherence for COPD patients is greater than 50%, compared to 30–70% for asthma patients, this adherence is lower at night [16, 17]. Using an electronic monitoring system, the mean adherence rates of 122 pediatric subjects aged 7–16 years were estimated over 2 years and 3 months span. According to their results, the average adherence rate after 3 months was 76.7%, compared to 44% at the end of the study period which indicates that the adherence to medications decreases with time [18]. Prescribed inhaled drug use tends to be intermittent. A previous study that lasted for 5 years, showed that about 51% of COPD subjects received their prescription inhaled medications less than once per year [17]. A large study demonstrated the adherence rate of more than 11,000 COPD subjects who were using inhaled medications revealed that about 28% of the recruited subjects continued to use inhaled corticosteroids satisfactorily and 52% did not use all the prescribed medication but some of them [19]. While many patients recognize the value of taking their drugs as prescribed, they may still have difficulty using aerosol-generating devices correctly during their treatment. The prevalence of incorrect inhalation technique has been stated to range from 4 to 94% [20–22]. Incorrect inhalation technique could be caused by a variety of factors. Patients can be perplexed by devices that require different inhalation techniques or cannot use the aerosol-generating devices correctly. Due to a short attention span, low literacy, lack of follow-up, and insufficient time and information to learn, patients may not be able to learn how to use their inhaler correctly. Many of the problems associated with poor inhalation techniques could be resolved with patient education and training provided by healthcare practitioners. However, a shortage of clinician time and supplies, along with financial incentives for patient education, continues to be a problem that has an impact on the patient education process. Furthermore, the prescriber physicians and healthcare professionals may not fully understand the optimum mechanism and technique for using certain aerosol-generating devices [23, 24].

5.2 Factors Affecting Adherence to Aerosol Therapy

Adherence to aerosol therapy could be influence by several factors [25] that could be classified into four different categories, first is the factors related to the aerosol-generating device, second are factors related to inhaled medications, third factors related to healthcare professionals, and the last category is related to patients' factors.

5.2.1 The Aerosol Generating Devices

The optimum inhalation techniques of different aerosol-generating devices are considered complex and difficult to be applied by the patient particularly without training [11, 26]. Available aerosol-generating devices did not address the needs and capacities of patients during device development and manufacturing, resulting in several aerosol-generating devices that fail to meet the needs of many patients with pulmonary diseases. To optimize and maximize aerosol delivery to the lungs, use an inhaler that produces aerosol particles in the respirable range of less than 5 μm. The production of respirable aerosol particles is the main factor that determines the efficacy of aerosol-generating devices hence, the selection of the optimum device. While the available aerosol-generating devices are able of generating respirable aerosol particles, most patients are unable to achieve the device's necessary depth and speed of inhalation [27]. Because of their comorbidities and physical and cognitive impairments, older COPD patients have trouble using a variety of aerosol devices effectively [28], which can lead to several errors in the usage of each aerosol device. Among the aerosol generators that require a specific inhalation technique is the pMDI (Table 5.1), besides the usage steps of the pMDI, another critical issue was revealed by a previous study which showed that many subjects continue to use

Table 5.1 The correct inhalation technique of pMDI

Step 1	The patient should remove the pMDI protective cap
Step 2	The patient should shake the pMDI (canister) before using it
Step 3	The patient should exhale as far as comfortable smoothly
Step 4	The patient should put the mouthpiece of the pMDI between the teeth and cover it with lips
Step 5	The patient should ensure that the tongue does not clog the pMDI mouthpiece
Step 6	The patient should press the inhaler at the start of inhalation to emit the dose
Step 7	The patient should maintain a slow inhalation rate till filling the lungs up
Step 8	The patient should remove the pMDI from the mouth and hold the breath for 5–10 s
Step 9	The patient should wait for about 30 s before taking another aerosol dose, in case of using more than a single dose
Step 10	The patient should wash the mouth and brush the teeth
Step 11	Replace the cap of the pMDI

their pMDI after becoming empty. The reason behind this issue is the inability of patients to distinguish between empty or filled pMDI as both produce a sound of aerosol or more specifically sound of propellant passage from the pMDI nozzle [29]. As a result, a large percent of inhaler users continue to use the pMDI to deliver about 2 folds greater than it should deliver to the patient, but these extra puffs do not contain an effective medication that may lead to treatment failure and cause instability. The traditional way of knowing whether the pMDI is empty or not is the flotation technique, but there is a difference between available pMDI canisters and hence, this difference influences the flotation technique and decreases its utility [29]. This issue gave an advantage for inhalers that contain counter of the aerosol buffs or amount. Hence, aerosol-generating devices with built-in feedback notifiers become important to help patients use the devices appropriately.

For patients with obstructive pulmonary disease, DPI is an effective aerosol delivery system. It solves the pMDI coordination issue, but it necessitates the patient's ability to inhale as quickly and deeply as possible [30]. Different DPIs with varying resistance are available on the market [31]. Each has a unique method for loading the dose and delivering it, as well as a critical inhalation flow requirement [32–34]. They also vary in terms of patient preferences and the number of errors made during the handling process [32–34]. The easier a DPI is to use, the better it is for both the patient and the healthcare professional [35].

Inhaling as quickly and deeply as possible is a crucial step in dose delivery for DPIs [32–34]. Some COPD patients are unable to achieve a 30 L/min inhalation flow or a 2 L inhalation volume, preventing them from receiving the necessary dose from the DPI by inhaling as quickly and deeply as possible [21, 36].

Besides, if the DPI is loaded twice, the patient will inhale twice the required dose [37]. Patients can be exposed to unwanted side effects as a result of this.

Ellipta® is a modern multi-dose DPI with a medium resistance that has been demonstrated to be both easy to use and effective for pulmonary drug delivery [38–41]. It consists of two rolled-up blister strips containing 30 individual doses of inhaled medication that are ready for administration once the dosage is prepared [42]. Since the blisters holding the medicine are isolated and only open when the dosage is to be inhaled, the Ellipta® reduces the risk of drug interactions [42]. It was created to avoid double dosing by including a reservoir for any dose left in the blister [42]. There is no need to inhale twice from the same dose because Ellipta® has been shown to provide stable doses across a variety of patient inhalation profiles [33, 34, 40].

5.2.2 Drug-Related Factors

The frequency, type, and the number of drugs to be administrated, as well as the type of aerosol-generating device used to administer inhalable drugs, have all been linked to patient adherence to aerosol therapy. There was a connection between patient adherence and the frequency with which medication had to be taken according to previous studies [43]. Since patient adherence decreases as medication usage becomes more frequent, caregivers should consider choosing a drug that makes dosing more convenient by decreasing the amount and number of doses provided to patients, tailoring dosing to patients' schedules, and integrating medication administration into mealtimes and before bedtime. They may be able to improve patient adherence to prescription medications by doing so [44].

Combining aerosolized drugs into a single formulation simplifies the process of drug administration by reducing the number of aerosol therapy sessions required when taking prescription medications. According to a previous study, participants who used a single inhaler to deliver both fluticasone propionate and salmeterol had substantially greater adherence than the other groups which used separate inhalers [45]. These findings were confirmed through other studies which measured the level of adherence among patients who used a single inhaler to deliver both long-acting bronchodilator and corticosteroids against the control group which receives each category of medication by a separate inhaler. It was clear that subjects using both medications in a single inhaler had a better adherence rate (80%) than those used separate inhalers [46]. Besides the effect of inhaler number, another important issue that affects the adherence to aerosol therapy is the fast action of the inhaled medication. β agonists show a rapid effect that is measurable by the patients while the effect of corticosteroids is not as fast and measurable as the β agonist. The rapid effect of bronchodilators leads to the sense of good disease control by the patient. Hence, the adherence of patients is variable based on the type of inhaled medication, most patients showed higher adherence to fast relieves compared with inhaled corticosteroids [47]. Adherence to prescription corticosteroids is influenced by additional two major factors. First, patients have concluded that inhaled corticosteroids will not play a significant role in the treatment of their condition. The second reason is related to the adverse effects of corticosteroids, which may be overestimated by patients [48].

5.2.3 Healthcare Professional Related Factors

Health-care practitioners' issues begin with a poor selection of the aerosol generators and end with the inability to provide patient education about the correct inhalation technique from the device, which includes a lack of experience with certain aerosol generators, insufficient time to teach especially for those working at hospitals with high patients flow, poor or unsuitable training methods, and a lack of education materials on aerosol therapy. Unfortunately, even for those physicians with a special interest in aerosol medicine, health-care professionals' awareness and understanding of aerosol devices are poor; as a result, only a minority of health-care practitioners know how to use aerosol devices correctly [49]. For the most effective use of most inhalers, health-care practitioners must have proper training [13]. As a result, health-care providers should enhance their skills and take the advantage of any opportunity to teach and reinforce proper inhaler use across the health-care spectrum.

5.3 Factors Related to the Patient

When it comes to disease and care, each patient's ability, mood, motivation, attitudes, experience, and values, all play a role [50]. While age, socioeconomic status, marital status, and level of education all play a role in patient adherence to aerosol therapy, they are not clear predictors [51]. Another factor that could influence COPD patients' adherence to aerosol therapy is depression and this could be related to the fact that lung functions will not back to the previous normal range [52]. The financial status of the patient is a strong predictor of adherence level especially most modern inhalers are expensive. For this reason, healthcare providers should consider this factor when prescribing inhalers for those with low income [53].

There are two types of noncompliance: intended noncompliance and unintended noncompliance. Intended nonadherence could be described in the case that patients refuse to adhere to recommended medication while they recognize the value of their therapy, but they deny the diagnosis, care, or both. Because of their convictions, inability to afford drugs, fatigue, forgetfulness, a busy lifestyle, or fear of prescribed medications side effects, they do not take their prescribed medications [54]. Many patients who are intentionally non-compliant because they do not believe their condition is serious enough to warrant long-term treatment ultimately develop severe disease [55]. While other patients are worried that routine use of inhaled drugs will cause resistance, and that the drug will become ineffective in an emergency, such as during exacerbations, over time [53]. In contrast, unintentional nonadherence is caused by a lack of knowledge or confusion about the prescribed treatment, improper procedure for their prescribed aerosol-generating devices, or language barriers. As a result, they are unaware that they are not adhering to aerosol therapy and are unaware of how to properly use their aerosol-generating devices to treat pulmonary diseases.

Some patients refuse to take their inhaled medications due to a misunderstanding of their health status, the medication cost, or secondary benefits such as parental attention [55].

As symptoms improve, some people decrease the frequency of doses recommended by their physicians, while others avoid taking their drugs altogether [56]. Some patients refuse to take drugs because of side effects, and others may have unreasonable perceptions of their medications [55].

5.4 Role of Counseling in Patient Adherence

The role of patient counseling and training is very essential for optimum aerosol delivery to the patient, even if the patient has a good understanding of how to use an inhaler properly, he would always be unable to do so without clear counseling and training. Many parameters such as sleep disturbances, school absenteeism, emergency room visits, and asthma morbidity were all decreased as a result of successful patient education and training [2]. For optimum education and training for patients that are using aerosol-producing devices, the following strategies should be followed. The first point is to individualize the counseling session, each patient has a unique case that requires specific instructions, the healthcare professional should educate the patient in a one-to-one meeting. The second point is to seek the patient preference for different available aerosol generators that would be equally effective and suitable for his condition. The suitability of the device to the patient also includes the financial aspect of the patient. The third point, in the case of a patient that had used the aerosol generators before, ask patients to use their inhalers before starting the demonstration of the device usage. This point aims at the determination of the most critical mistake and misunderstanding of the patients about their aerosol generators. The fourth point is to provide practical training and demonstration of using the inhaler by the healthcare professionals in addition to verbal education, this demonstration is easier to be memorized compared with verbal training alone. Besides, recent training devices and smartphone applications are available to aid the patient in using their devices correctly. The fifth point is the proper documentation of the training session through writing a detailed label on who to use the inhaler. The sixth point is to follow up with the patient and to evaluate the inhalation technique and the disease control.

5.4.1 Counseling Sessions

Individualizing the counseling session to a single patient and encouragement to stick to prescribed drugs by open-ended questions, affirmations, reflective listening, and summary comments is more successful than a large-group counseling session. Individualized patient counseling sessions have been shown to enhance aerosol therapy adherence and clinical outcomes in previous studies [27, 57].

A lot of studies were designed to evaluate the effect of verbal counseling on the optimum use of different aerosol-generating devices such as pMDIs and DPIs [58–60]. The findings of these studies indicated the beneficial role of counseling expressed as a reduction of the number of errors related to the inhaler. The effect of patient education is not limited only to improving the usage technique of the inhaler but also the control of the disease. The asthma control test (ACT) score was significantly improved for subjects who received education sessions compared with non-educated subjects. The frequency of training sessions is an important factor that enhances the ability of the subject to use aerosol devices correctly.

The training session should include certain essential elements to ensure good patient education.

1. Provide patients with basic knowledge of their disease.
2. The patient should know the role of each medication and the importance of taking these medications as prescribed.

3. The patient should be trained on the optimum technique for using the prescribed aerosol device.
4. The patient should be trained to follow the status of the disease such as symptoms frequency and need for as-needed inhalers.

5.5 Patient Preference-Based Inhaler Selection

Patient preference is attributed to the patient's ability to perform the inhalation technique correctly and a higher level of therapy satisfaction [54, 61, 62]. As a result, using an aerosol-generating device that the patient prefers is an important part of aerosol therapy patient counseling. A patient's choice can be influenced by factors such as portability, ease of use, scale, taste, and cost of the device [63]. An aerosol-generating device is preferred by the patient based on several features such as ease of use, dose capability (single or multidose), and dose tracking [64]. Fewer steps to use the device, assurance that the dose was taken correctly, easier control of breathing maneuvers, and less resistance during inhalation were all linked to ease of use [64]. Patient satisfaction is an important factor that enhances patient adherence to aerosol therapy. Hence, choosing an inhaler that satisfies the patient's need is essential to gain improved clinical outcomes.

Patients may become confused if they are prescribed more than one form of aerosol-generating devices along with their medications due to the different usage techniques needed for each device. As a result, using the same type of aerosol generators for various inhaled drugs can help patients stick to their aerosol therapy regimen [65].

5.5.1 Inhaler Labeling

Patients are also unaware of their improper technique and do not seek further information from health-care professionals. Patient knowledge and adherence to aerosol therapy can be improved by creating customized inhaler technique labels and identifying incorrect measures on the label [66]. For each inhaler, there are critical steps that greatly affect aerosol delivery and deposition. For pMDI, a slow and deep inhalation of aerosol particles is essential to achieve higher aerosol deposition, while fast inhalation for DPI is the recommended inhalation technique. Such essential steps should be written on the label.

In aerosol therapy, written directions alone are insufficient for successful patient counseling. As a result, a successful patient counseling and training program should provide written and oral directions, as well as demonstration and training. Patients and caregivers should be able to understand the written instructions hence they should be simple and descriptive. Patients' comprehension and compliance with therapy can be improved by writing directions at or below a sixth-grade reading level and using pictures and diagrams [67]. During the counseling session, explaining each phase of the correct procedure for using an inhaler will also help resolve language barriers between the subject and the health-care provider [68]. Counseling language should not be professional to facilitate communication with the patient, professional language should be used with healthcare professionals only because of certain specific and scientific words that are not easily understood by patients. During patient counseling sessions, healthcare givers should repeat instructions and steps of using inhalers to ensure that patients understand what to do and that they could take their drugs as prescribed.

5.5.2 Aerosol Therapies Follow Up

The optimum inhalation technique education and training for certain inhalers need several counseling sessions. At each session, an evaluation of the inhalation techniques and more specifically the inhalation errors should be determined besides monitoring the clinical status and disease control of the trained patient. Follow-up faces special drawbacks represented in the absence of the patient during follow-up sessions which require more efforts by healthcare givers to communicate with their patients and remind them Following up with patients and their families is an integral part of a successful aerosol therapy counseling and training intervention. Follow-ups enable health-care providers to answer any questions patients may have, correct any errors in their inhalation technique, and ensure that patients recognize the benefits and target of the prescribed medications. Since adherence to therapy is influenced by a patient's experience and interpretation of aerosol therapy, the subsequent training sessions including follow-up are essential for optimizing aerosol therapy.

5.5.3 Evaluation of Patient Inhaler Usage Technique

Aerosol therapy for patients with pulmonary disorders is usually delivered by nebulizers, pMDIs, and DPIs. However, due to a patient's age, poor lung function, and disability, it could be difficult to use a specific aerosol-generating device; thus, patient performance must be evaluated to meet clinical targets set for disease management. A variety of tools are used to evaluate the inhalation techniques of the patients (Fig. 5.1). There are several tools and devices available for the assessment of the inhalation technique of the trained patients [61].

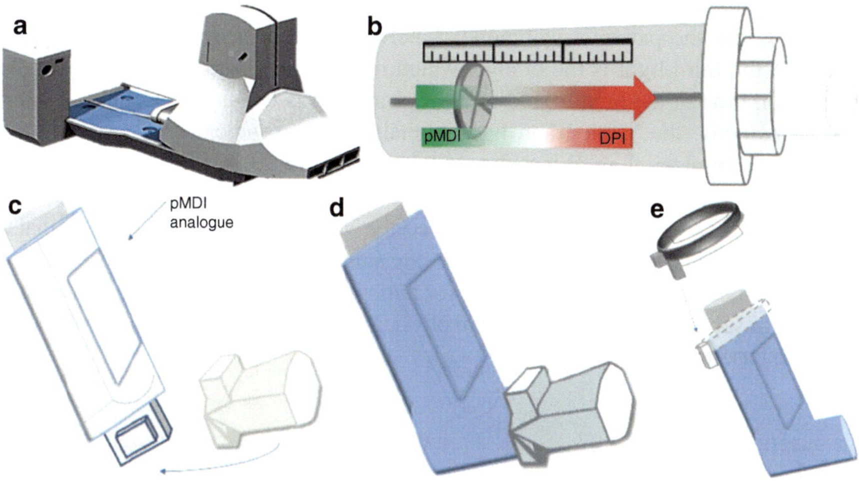

Fig. 5.1 Different types of devices used for assessment of inhalation techniques for aerosol therapy, (**a**) Mag-Flo, Dynamics (**b**) In Check DAIL, Clarke International. (**c**) Trainhaler, Clement Clarke International. (**d**) Flo-Tone, Clement Clarke International. (**e**) Clip-Tone, Clement Clarke International

5.5.4 Inhalation Manager

Inhalation manager (IM) is a computer-based measuring tool that enables quantitative testing of the inhalation capacity of patients using an inhaler. IM can assess breathing maneuvers associated with the use of different inhaler devices. Consequently, The IM is a useful tool for determining which aerosol-generating device better meets the needs and capabilities of the patient. It can also be used to train the patient on the best inhalation technique suitable for the selected inhaler [62]. It was reported by a previous study that IM is a suitable device for educating subjects on the optimum inhalation techniques. This study aimed to train randomly selected subjects how to correctly use their DPIs, two different inhalers were involved Turbuhaler and Autohaler.

5.5.5 Aerosol Inhalations Monitor (AIM)

The Vitalograph is an aerosol inhalation monitor which is an electronic pMDI and DPI trainer that measures inspiratory airflow and tracks patient hand-breath coordination during inhalation from different inhalers. A pMDI or DPI with placebo is included in the Vitalograph, which contains a responsive flow transducer that detects airflow at the start of inspiration from the included inhaler. The device gives visual light indicators, three colors are indicative of the inhalation technique status. A green light indicates that the patient's inhalation technique is right, while a red light indicates that the patient's technique is not recommended for optimum aerosol delivery, the third light is the orange, which indicates the patient did not meet the inhalation time or the breath-hold after inspiration was too short. During the training of patients, the Vitalograph has an analog needle indicator that reveals the patient's inspiratory flow. When the analog needle indicator is kept in the desired flow range, the patient receives visual feedback, which aids in attaining the best inspiratory flow [61]. An earlier study used the Vitalograph to evaluate the inhalation technique of pMDI of respiratory disease subjects over 6 weeks. It was reported that, the Vitalograph was a useful tool for patient training and education and that it resulted in substantial improvements in physical function during the follow-up compared to baseline [69].

5.5.6 *Mag-Flo Inhaler*

Mag-Flo teaches patients how to properly inhale and get the most appropriate dosage using their inhaler. The ability of patients to use a variety of DPIs such as the Accuhaler, HandiHaler Turbohaler, and Diskus could be evaluated by The Mag-Flo inhaler which is attached to a magnetic flow sensor. Using this device, the healthcare professional could educate the patient more easily also patient could be self-educated through monitoring the lighting of green color which reflects that the patient is inhaling probably from the device [63].

5.5.7 *Turbutest*

The Turbutest is a tool that is used to teach patients that use certain DPIs how to use them correctly. This tool is used specifically with Turbuhaler and Flexhaler. This device is linked to an electronic sensor that monitors and displays the patient's peak inspiratory flow, Peak inspiratory flow of more than 60 L/min is indicated by three lights, peak inspiratory flow between 40 and 60 L/min is indicated by two lights, peak inspiratory flow ranging from 30 to 40 L/min is indicated by one light, and peak inspiratory flow equal to 30 L/min is indicated by no light. In other words, the more lightning spots the better the inhalation pattern of the patient. With DPIs like the Flexhaler and Turbuhaler, two or three lights during inspiration indicate that the patient can produce adequate peak inspiratory flow. Also, the Turbutest can be used to teach patients how to prime the Flexhaler. Turbutest sensitivity with pediatric subjects was evaluated on children aged from 5 to 18 years old divided into three age groups. The sensitivity of the device was comparable among the three groups with slightly lower sensitivity in detecting the required peak inspiratory flow for pediatric subjects aged 5–6 years [70]. The Turbutest may be a useful tool for assessing and enhancing inhalation techniques in Turbuhaler DPI users.

5.5.8 2Tone Trainer

The 2Tone Trainer is a useful tool that teaches patients how to inhale at the proper inhalation speed, which improves coordination, reduces waste, and maximizes the benefits that the inhaler can provide. The rate at which patients inhale through the prescribed inhaler is important, most patients inhale from their pMDIs too quickly achieving a high inspiratory flow rate that decreases aerosol deposition in the lung. The design of the 2Tone Trainer is similar to that of the traditional pMDI but without medications. Patients who have been prescribed a pMDI could use this tool to be trained on inhaling aerosol at the optimal inhalation flow rate for better aerosol deposition. A single tone implies that the patient's inhalation flow is optimal ranging from 30 to 60 L/min, whereas two tones mean that the flow is greater than 60 L/min which is not optimum for aerosol deposition. Al-Showair et al. investigated the efficacy of the 2Tone Trainer device in preserving proper inhalation technique with a pMDI for good patient training and enhancing asthmatic outcomes. Subjects in this study were divided into three groups, the control group included subjects with optimum inhalation techniques, the second group for patients that received verbal counseling only, while the third group was for 2Tone trainer trained subjects [71]. With pMDIs, the control group had strong coordination and a slow optimum inhalation rate, while the second and third groups had poor coordination and inhalation technique at baseline. The second and third groups received verbal training on the optimum inhalation technique from pMDI in addition to the way to use the training device for the third group. Peak inspiratory flows and asthma quality-of-life questionnaire scores of the control group did not change between subsequent follow-up sessions, whereas both the second and third groups had a significant increase in asthma quality-of-life questionnaire scores [71].

5.5.9 In-Check DIAL

The In-Check DIAL is a dial-top hand-held inspiratory flow measurement tool. The resistance of different inhaler devices from the DPIs and pMDIs groups was modeled using the DIAL orifices. It allows healthcare professionals to train the patients on how to use more or less inspiratory force to achieve their optimum flow rate with a specific pMDI or DPI unit. It's amazing in terms of assessing acceptable first-time inhaler prescriptions and testing the technique patient by giving patients and healthcare providers objective and real-time response [72]. Saeed et al. measured the inspiratory flow rate for asthmatic subjects at baseline and after three training sessions on using pMDI to determine the effect of patient education and counseling on optimizing the pMDI inhalation techniques [27]. Using the In-Chick Dial showed a significant reduction in the inspired flow rate during the follow-up sessions compared with baseline, this reduction in the inhalation rate was going toward the optimum value for drawing aerosol from pMDI which is around 60 liter per minute. Another study used the device to enhance patient usage of DPI through measuring peak inspiratory flow with the In-Check DIAL in asthmatic subjects with and without DPI previous experience. Many subjects with DPI experience were unable to generate the optimum peak inspiratory flows needed with high-resistance DPIs, as measured by the In-Check DIAL [73].

5.5.10 Trainhaler and Flo-Tone

Trainhaler inhaler is a simple pMDI training device that is compatible with the traditional mouthpiece of the most available pMDI. The concept behind this instrument is to produce an alarming voice when patients reach the optimum inhalation flow rate. This device can be used to enhance the inspiratory flow rate of pMDI users to be optimum. This device could be used with a smartphone application (Trainhaler Buddy) that maximizes the benefits of the device, through recording the time of optimum inhalation rate performed by the patient. Most patients inhale with an inhalation flow above the recommended rate which results in lower lung bioavailability and higher deposition on the mouth and the upper respiratory tract of the inhaled medication [11]. This version of the training device did not account for the different resistance among the different pMDIs, hence an advanced version of the device, the Flo-Tone inhaler, has been meticulously designed to achieve additional flexibility, including the ability to suit all pMDIs and ensuring that the guidance whistle responds at the same flow rate in all pMDIs, regardless of resistance. Using this version was successful to enhance the inspiratory flow rate of the asthmatic patient through three successive visits and it was effective than traditional verbal counseling [27].

5.5.11 Clip-Tone E

Clip-Tone E is a supportive tool designed to improve the pMDI inhalation technique. The Clip-Tone device should be placed at the top of the inhaler around the canister of the pMDI, adding this tool does not change aerosol delivery from the inhaler. This device is only compatible with Evohaler devices. As the patients inhale slowly and steadily from their pMDIs, the Clip-Tone E produces a guiding whistle detected by a smartphone application which helps guide the duration of inhalation and coordination of actuation through the pMDI. When opposed to verbal counseling alone, using the Clip-tone with its smartphone application to provide visual and auditory input maintained the deep and steady inhalation over the pMDI much better. Hence, Patients are recommended to use pMDI add-on products such as Clip-tone with a smartphone application to properly administer their inhaled doses [74].

5.6 Monitoring Patient Adherence to Aerosol Therapy

Patient adherence to the prescribed aerosol therapy is a continuous process that must be monitored during disease management, but there are no standardized test or measurement methods for patients' adherence to their inhaler. Since patient adherence has a bearing on patient outcomes, clinicians should investigate it in a non-threatening and non-judgmental manner. To control adherence of the patient to the prescribed aerosol generators, a variety of approaches are used, which can be classified into direct or indirect methods, these methods vary from each other regarding the accuracy of judgment. Direct observation of patients, such as canister weighing, laboratory data, pharmacy records, and electronic monitoring, are examples of direct methods. Diaries, patient self-reports, and healthcare giver judgments are examples of indirect approaches [63].

5.7 Clinical Judgment on Therapy

Clinical judgment on aerosol therapy is the most popular approach for tracking patient adherence to the prescribed inhalers, it is simple, fast, and cheap but also the least effective method. Clinical judgment, even though it overestimates adherence of the patient to prescription inhaled medications, is still widely used in clinical practice. Furthermore, if the disease is well controlled, doctors can overlook the question of whether or not patients are taking their medications as prescribed and using the inhaler with the proper inhalation technique. Medical judgment should be used in conjunction with other approaches such as electronic tracking or pharmacy reports to improve reliability [63].

5.8 Self-Reports by Patients

Patient adherence monitoring with diary cards or patient self-reports is a simple, low-cost method that is widely used. Owing to memory bias and a desire to satisfy healthcare givers, patients could over-report their aerosol therapy adherence by using self-reports or diary cards [75]. When compared to electronic system tracking, weighing pMDI canister, and medication-dispensing data collected from pharmacies, patient self-reports show higher adherence rates that limit their usability and their value [75].

5.9 Electronic Monitoring Device

Electronic device monitoring is based on attaching a digital device to the inhaler which adds the advantage of monitoring aerosol therapy. These devices monitor the frequency of aerosol therapy administration by recording the date of using the inhaler, also, they record the actual time of inhaled drug administration. Many devices are available for this application, some of these devices can calculate the remaining doses or buffs inside the inhaler, this is particularly important for pMDI users. Among the popular monitoring devices are Smartinhaler and Chronolog DOSER (Fig. 5.2). Electronic monitoring devices are available for many inhaler designs while there are many inhalers which are not fit with any device [76].

5.10 Laboratory Measurements of Medications and Response

This method is an accurate and quantitative indicator of both adherence and good inhalation technique. The optimum inhalation technique of certain inhalers results in the highest delivered amounts of the drug to the lung, hence methods for detection of inhaled medication in biological samples could be used to determine whether the technique of the patient is optimum or not. For this quantitative measurement, the clinical pharmacokinetic methods for the determination of lung bioavailability could be used to determine the deposited amount of drug after inhalation of aerosol. Besides the analytical techniques which are expensive and are limited to certain medications and conditions, the response of the inhaled bronchodilator could be measured using spirometry. Saeed et al. measured the lung functions before and after receiving a training and educative session on the pMDI technique for three successive visits, the study reported a good bronchodilation effect for those who used the device correctly [27].

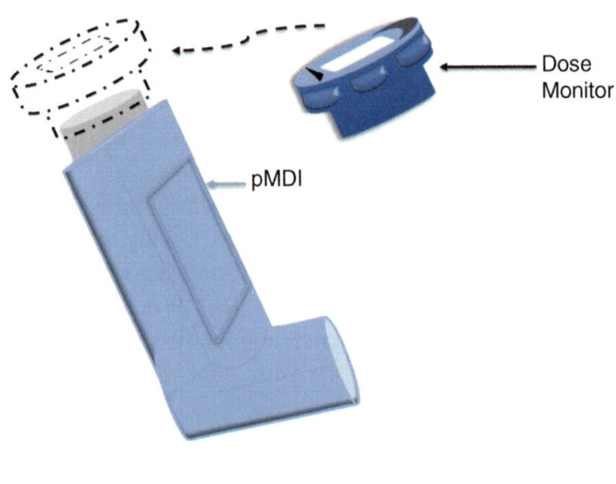

Fig. 5.2 An illustrative example of electronic monitoring devices

5.11 Pharmacy Registered Data

Another option of gathering data that refers directly to aerosol therapy adherence is collecting pharmacy records. Obtaining pharmacy registration of dispensed drugs is a low-cost, objective, and reliable method of determining patient adherence. However, these records only offer the dates of drug dispensing and there is no assurance that patients will take their drugs as prescribed by their physicians or that the device will be used correctly during drug administration. Another issue related to this method is the lack of pharmacy records since not all countries have the same regulations regarding drug dispensing and documentation, and many pharmacies do not register the name of the patient. Furthermore, the collected data could be insufficient and not accurate in case a patient takes drugs from different pharmacies. Therefore, in case the monitoring system would depend on the records registered by pharmacies, to boost the reliability of data on patient adherence, patients should be advised to get their drugs from a single pharmacy [77]. A previous study evaluated the adherence rates of pediatric subjects by collecting their drug-dispensing files from several pharmacies and informed a mean adherence rate of 61%. The investigator compared the accuracy of this method with data collected from the insurance companies and found that pharmacy data method accuracy is 92% [78].

5.12 Assessment Tools for Aerosol Therapy and Disease Control

5.12.1 Questionnaires in Asthma

A questionnaire containing a specific number of questions with a point scoring system for numerical assessment of clinical status is a good tool for the evaluation of disease control. Several available questionnaires differ in number and nature of items also in the scoring system. Questionnaires designed for evaluating asthma control can be helpful in asthma management because they allow for a structured evaluation and a fast description of a patient's asthma control. These questionnaires could be filled periodically at follow-up visits also they could be filled at home and sent by mail to the healthcare professional or to be informed through telephone [79, 80]. These questionnaires could be available as an online electronic form that is easy to be used and interpret inputs [80]. The score of the questionnaire guides the healthcare giver to change asthma medication based on predetermined cutoff points. However, poor symptom recognition may lead to an overestimation of asthma control. The ACT has a four-week recall period while the Asthma Control Questionnaire (ACQ) has a one-week recall time, which may provide a non-complete evaluation of asthma control but may not provide a detailed image of asthma control during clinic visits. As a result, frequent diaries (on daily basis) can be a more sensitive method for determining differential treatment responses than the traditional questionnaires [81]. Regarding the efficacy of both questionnaires for assessing asthma control, it was reported that both ACT and ACQ have a comparable efficacy [82]. Using questionnaires such as ACT was useful in evaluating certain training interventions on aerosol therapy for asthmatic subjects using pMDI [27]. The use of certain questionnaires requires spirometry for measuring lung functions to be a part of asthma control evaluation, hence the availability of a spirometer would guide the selection of specific questionnaires particularly for a patient who would use a daily questionnaire. Since spirometry is not included in the ACT, this test can become more practical in clinics with a large patient volume and limited resources [82]. However, both questionnaires have comparable efficacy but also, ACT is more recommended to be used with a pediatric patient because the ACQ requires further cross-validation [82].

Assessment of asthma control in pediatric subjects especially pre-school children requires specific questionnaires. Test of respiratory and asthma control in kids (TRACK) is a pediatric-specific test that consists of 5 questions and is suitable for pediatric subjects aged 1–5 years. TRACK's total score is 100 points, the higher the score the better the asthma control. Another questionnaire that could be used with pediatric asthmatics aged from 4 years is the childhood-asthma control test (C-ACT) which is characteristic by visual scale [79]. Furthermore, determination of C-ACT control of asthma can be reported not only by the parent but also by the asthmatic child itself. As parents appear to underestimate control of asthma [83], evaluation by the asthmatic child itself is more useful. The ACQ is validated for patients aged 6 years or older. Most of the available questionnaires have been designed to detect uncontrolled asthma not the controlled cases and only a few reports proposed a cut-off for well-controlled asthma [84, 85].

There is little knowledge of the potential of questionnaires for asthma control to forecast future risks, particularly for exacerbation and studies confined to adults [86, 87]. Many asthma control questionnaires have a major flaw in that children can have unexplained exacerbations after long periods of control, and exacerbations can happen in children with both good and bad short-term asthma control [88]. The only questionnaire that includes exacerbation in the scoring system is the TRACK. The coming research should concentrate on the clinical importance of asthma control questionnaires that measure exacerbations and comparing them with other questionnaires, also combining more than one questionnaire, as well as the questionnaires' ability to predict lung function decline.

The discrepancy between symptoms of certain conditions such as allergic rhinitis and flu with that of asthma may result in a non-accurate estimation of asthma control especially for questionnaires that are filled out of the clinic by the patient [89]. Combining the assessment questionnaire with measurement of lung function particularly forced expiratory volume in 1 second (FEV1) might help provide a more realistic description of the disease control status.

5.12.2 Asthma Control Questionnaire

The ACQ was the first validated questionnaire for the assessment of asthma control clinical practice which was developed by Juniper et al. [90, 91]. This questionnaire is consisting of seven questions with predetermined answered from which the patient should choose one. The ACQ covers 1 week only and should be repeated every 7 days. During these 7 days, the questionnaire assesses the nocturnal awakening, breathlessness, limitations of activity, daytime symptoms, Wheezing, frequency of short-acting bronchodilator use (rescue medication), and the value of FEV1. All the seven questions have the same scoring points that range from zero to six points for each question, the lower the score the good the asthma control. The overall score is the average score of that of the seven questions [90, 91]. This questionnaire had been validated for pediatric asthmatic patients aged between 6 and 16 years old [90]. For young children subjects of 10 years or less, they should receive a training and education session on this questionnaire to ensure the full awareness of each question. For the difference in the final score to be significant and of clinical importance, it should be at least 0.5 [84]. With a negative predictive value of 85 percent, a score of less than or equal to 0.75 suggested well-controlled asthma, and a score of greater than or equal to 1.50 indicated uncontrolled asthma with a positive predictive value of 88% [84]. Though, these cutoffs have recently been discussed, with 0.5 being suggested as a stronger cutoff point for controlled asthma and 1 or 1.25 for uncontrolled asthma [92]. There are two forms of ACQ complete and short form, the complete questionnaire consists of 20 questions while the short most common form is consisting of the previously prescribed seven questions. It was reported that the short version is similarly effective as the complete one for assessment of asthma control and it is particularly for pediatric subjects who fill the questionnaire at home [93].

5.12.3 Asthma Control Test

The ACT is a method for asthma control assessment that measures the status of the disease every 4 weeks, ACT is suitable for older pediatric subjects aged 12 years or older, while for those less than 12 years till 4 years the C-ACT should be used [94]. This questionnaire generates the asthma control score from answers to five questions on activity limitation, shortness of breath, waking up as a result of symptoms, need for extra bronchodilators, and self-evaluation of asthma control). The C-ACT is a seven-item questionnaire split into two sections that cover the previous 4 weeks for asthmatic children. The first section, which includes four questions about asthma control, limitations of activity, coughing, and nocturnal awakenings, is completed by the child using a visual scale. From 0 to 3, there are three response stages. A parent or caregiver fills out the second section, which has three questions about daytime symptoms, wheezing, and nighttime awakenings with response levels ranging from 0 to 5. While For ACT, asthmatic subjects give a rate for each of these on a scale of 1 to 5 where 1 is not controlled at all and 5 is highly controlled. The overall ACT score is the sum of all the scores to be from 5 to 25. The well-controlled cases are those with ACT score 23 or more while score less than 20 reflect the poor control of asthma, the lower the score the lower the disease control [95, 96]. The significant improvement of asthma control is restricted to three points increase in the score regarding the adult subjects while for pediatrics, two points increase is considered significant [95, 97]. ACT is an easy test that could be filled with the patient at home or through the internet without the need to visit the clinic.

5.12.4 *Asthma Therapy Assessment Questionnaire (ATAQ)*

The ATAQ is a questionnaire for children and adolescents aged from 5 to 17 years. It was created to help healthcare professionals identify pediatric subjects who are at risk of developing asthma-related complications [98]. ATAQ is consisting of 20 items which should be completed by parents, these items are categorized into four different class include self-efficacy barriers (3 items), symptom control (7 items), communication gaps (5 items), and behavior and attitude barriers (2 items) [98]. ATAQ evaluates asthma control over the previous 4 weeks through the generation of numerical scores based on giving each item either 0 or 1 point. A zero score means that the patient has no problem and the disease is controlled. The overall score ranges from 0 to 4, very poor control of asthma is indicated by score 3–4 points, while lower scores less than or equal one reflects the good asthma control [99]. Symptoms control class is scored from 0 to 7 points, 0 is reflecting the absence of problems while higher scores represent the higher level of problems related to asthma control, the highest score, 7, reflect the high possibility of asthma exacerbations [100].

5.12.5 *Test for Respiratory and Asthma Control in Kids*

The TRACK questionnaire consists of five questions, each worth 0–20 points that caregivers of pediatric asthmatic subjects or chronic respiratory symptoms must answer about nocturnal awakenings, symptoms, and physical activity limitations in the previous 4 weeks, bronchodilator use in the previous 3 months, and systemic corticosteroids use in the previous year.

TRACK is a validated parent-completed asthma control questionnaire designed for pediatric subjects under the age of 5 [43]. It was shown that this questionnaire is a valid and sensitive tool for identifying preschool children with uncontrolled respiratory symptoms [101, 102]. As opposed to consensus standards, the cutoff score of 80 points was found to be the best for distinguishing between children with controlled symptoms and those with uncontrolled asthma symptoms, with high sensitivity (83%) and precision (78%) [101]. The clinical significant change in disease status is considered in case the score increased by 10 or more points were and that suggests changes in disease management [102].

5.12.6 Questionnaires for Assessment of COPD

Two health-related quality of life questionnaires (HRQoL) for assessment of COPD subjects were recently identified and validated. The first tool is the COPD Assessment Test (CAT) that consists of eight items, each with a score ranging from 0 to 5, for an overall score of 40 points [103]. It aims to determine how COPD impacts a person's life and how the effect evolves. The CAT is easy to use and is designed to assist physicians with properly managing COPD for their patients. It is self-administered and measured by adding the scoring points of the eight evaluating items, with higher scores implying a worsening of disease's effect on HRQoL.

The second tool is The Clinical COPD Questionnaire (CCQ) which is made up of ten elements, each item score is ranging from 0 to 6, these items are classified into three class symptoms, mental, and functional domains [104]. The overall score is determined by adding the individual item scores and dividing them by the number of individual questionnaire items (10 items), yielding a total score ranging from 0 to 6, with higher scores indicating worse HRQoL [105].

Both CCQ and CAT have strong psychometric characteristics and could be completed in few minutes. The use of the CAT questionnaire is important to measure the symptom weight in COPD subjects and to aid in treatment modifications as recommended by the Global Initiative for Chronic Obstructive Lung Disease (GOLD) guidance [106].

The CAT questionnaire was developed before CCQ, however, there is no evidence that the CAT is better than the CCQ. When compared to the CCQ questionnaire, COPD patients who are undergoing pulmonary rehabilitation (PR) need more support to complete the CAT questionnaire [107]. The patient preference to a certain questionnaire is an important factor to ensure adherence to the routine filling of the questionnaire, it was reported by 60% of patients that deal with both questionnaires that the CAT is preferred than CCQ according to a previous study [108]. The CCQ questionnaire was selected by the international primary care respiratory group to be the most suitable COPD assessment tool when compared with the other eight questionnaires [109].

References

1. Thoonen B, et al. Self-management of asthma in general practice, asthma control and quality of life: a randomised controlled trial. Thorax. 2003;58(1):30–6.
2. Guevara JP, et al. Effects of educational interventions for self management of asthma in children and adolescents: systematic review and meta-analysis. BMJ. 2003;326(7402):1308–9.

3. Aydemir Y. Assessment of the factors affecting the failure to use inhaler devices before and after training. Respir Med. 2015;109(4):451–8.
4. Newman SP. Aerosol deposition considerations in inhalation therapy. Chest. 1985;88(2):152S–60S.
5. Bartolo K, et al. Predictors of correct technique in patients using pressurized metered dose inhalers. BMC Pulm Med. 2017;17(1):47.
6. Spin P, et al. A cost analysis of salbutamol administration by metered-dose inhalers with spacers versus nebulization for patients with wheeze in the pediatric emergency department: evidence from observational data in Nova Scotia. Can J Emerg Med. 2017;19(1):1–8.
7. Al-Subu AM, et al. Aerosol therapy through high flow nasal cannula in pediatric patients. Expert Rev Respir Med. 2017;11(12):945–53.
8. Fonceca AM, et al. Drug administration by inhalation in children. In: Kendig's disorders of the respiratory tract in children, 9th ed. Elsevier; 2019. p. 257–271.e3.
9. Lexmond AJ, et al. Prerequisites for a dry powder inhaler for children with cystic fibrosis. PLoS One. 2017;12(8):e0183130.
10. Ammari WG, Chrystyn H. Optimizing the inhalation flow and technique through metered dose inhalers of asthmatic adults and children attending a community pharmacy. J Asthma. 2013;50(5):505–13.
11. Nicola M, et al. The impact of adding a training device to familiar counselling on inhalation technique and pulmonary function of asthmatics. Adv Ther. 2018;35(7):1049–58.
12. Rogliani P, et al. Optimizing drug delivery in COPD: the role of inhaler devices. Respir Med. 2017;124:6–14.
13. Melani AS, et al. Inhaler mishandling remains common in real life and is associated with reduced disease control. Respir Med. 2011;105(6):930–8.
14. Vestbo J, et al. Adherence to inhaled therapy, mortality and hospital admission in COPD. Thorax. 2009;64(11):939–43.
15. DiMatteo MR. Variations in patients' adherence to medical recommendations: a quantitative review of 50 years of research. Med Care. 2004;42(3):200–9.
16. Bender BG, et al. Adherence and persistence with fluticasone propionate/salmeterol combination therapy. J Allergy Clin Immunol. 2006;118(4):899–904.
17. Haupt D, et al. Medication persistence among patients with asthma/COPD drugs. Pharm World Sci. 2008;30(5):509–14.
18. Jónasson G, Carlsen K-H, Mowinckel PJ. Asthma drug adherence in a long term clinical trial. Arch Dis Child. 2000;83(4):330–3.
19. Jung E, et al. Medication adherence and persistence in the last year of life in COPD patients. Respir Med. 2009;103(4):525–34.
20. Hardwell A, et al. Technique training does not improve the ability of most patients to use pressurised metered-dose inhalers (pMDIs). Prim Care Respir J. 2011;20(1):92–6.
21. Lavorini F, et al. Effect of incorrect use of dry powder inhalers on management of patients with asthma and COPD. Respir Med. 2008;102(4):593–604.
22. Lenney J, Innes J, Crompton GJ. Inappropriate inhaler use: assessment of use and patient preference of seven inhalation devices. Respir Med. 2000;94(5):496–500.
23. Kim S-H, et al. Inappropriate techniques used by internal medicine residents with three kinds of inhalers (a metered dose inhaler, Diskus, and Turbuhaler): changes after a single teaching session. J Asthma. 2009;46(9):944–50.
24. Self TH, et al. Inadequate skill of healthcare professionals in using asthma inhalation devices. J Asthma. 2007;44(8):593–8.
25. Rau JL. Determinants of patient adherence to an aerosol regimen. Respir Care. 2005;50(10):1346–59.
26. Elgendy MO, Abdelrahim ME, Eldin RS. Potential benefit of repeated MDI inhalation technique counselling for patients with asthma. Eur J Hosp Pharm. 2015;22(6):318–22.
27. Saeed H, et al. Impact of advanced patient counseling using a training device and smartphone application on asthma control. Respir Care. 2020;65(3):326–32.

28. Fink JB, Rubin BK. Problems with inhaler use: a call for improved clinician and patient education. Respir Care. 2005;50(10):1360–75.
29. Rubin BK, Durotoye LJC. How do patients determine that their metered-dose inhaler is empty? Chest. 2004;126(4):1134–7.
30. Ibrahim M, Verma R, Garcia-Contreras L. Inhalation drug delivery devices: technology update. Med Devices (Auckland, NZ). 2015;8:131.
31. Dal Negro RW. Dry powder inhalers and the right things to remember: a concept review. Multidiscip Respir Med. 2015;10(1):13.
32. Abdelrahim M, Assi K, Chrystyn H. Dose emission and aerodynamic characterization of the terbutaline sulphate dose emitted from a Turbuhaler at low inhalation flow. Pharm Dev Technol. 2013;18(4):944–9.
33. Ali AMA, Abdelrahim MEA. Modeling and optimization of terbutaline emitted from a dry powder inhaler and influence on systemic bioavailability using data mining technology. J Pharm Innov. 2014;9(1):38–47.
34. Abdelrahim ME. Emitted dose and lung deposition of inhaled terbutaline from Turbuhaler at different conditions. Respir Med. 2010;104(5):682–9.
35. Chapman KR, et al. Delivery characteristics and patients' handling of two single-dose dry-powder inhalers used in COPD. Int J Chron Obstruct Pulmon Dis. 2011;6(1):353–63.
36. Newman S, Busse W. Evolution of dry powder inhaler design, formulation, and performance. Respir Med. 2002;96(5):293–304.
37. Tarsin W, Assi KH, Chrystyn H. In-vitro intra- and inter-inhaler flow rate-dependent dosage emission from a combination of budesonide and eformoterol in a dry powder inhaler. J Aerosol Med. 2004;17(1):25–32.
38. von Schantz S, et al. Evaluation of dry powder inhalers with a focus on ease of use and user preference in inhaler-naïve individuals. Int J Pharm. 2016;509(1):50–8.
39. Yun Kirby S, et al. A preference study of two placebo dry powder inhalers in adults with COPD: Ellipta® dry powder inhaler (DPI) versus DISKUS® DPI. COPD: J Chron Obstruct Pulmon Dis. 2016;13(2):167–75.
40. Hamilton M, et al. In vitro dosing performance of the ELLIPTA® dry powder inhaler using asthma and COPD patient inhalation profiles replicated with the electronic lung (eLung™). J Aerosol Med Pulm Drug Deliv. 2015;28(6):498–506.
41. Komase Y, et al. Ease-of-use preference for the ELLIPTA® dry powder inhaler over a commonly used single-dose capsule dry powder inhaler by inhalation device-naïve Japanese volunteers aged 40 years or older. Int J Chron Obstruct Pulmon Dis. 2014;9:1365.
42. Grant AC, et al. The ELLIPTA® dry powder inhaler: design, functionality, in vitro dosing performance and critical task compliance by patients and caregivers. J Aerosol Med Pulm Drug Deliv. 2015;28(6):474–85.
43. Eisen SA, et al. The effect of prescribed daily dose frequency on patient medication compliance. Arch Intern Med. 1990;150(9):1881–4.
44. Claxton AJ, Cramer J, Pierce CJ. A systematic review of the associations between dose regimens and medication compliance. Clin Ther. 2001;23(8):1296–310.
45. Stoloff SW, et al. Improved refill persistence with fluticasone propionate and salmeterol in a single inhaler compared with other controller therapies. J Allergy Clin Immunol. 2004;113(2):245–51.
46. Sovani MP, et al. Poor adherence with inhaled corticosteroids for asthma: can using a single inhaler containing budesonide and formoterol help? Br J Gen Pract. 2008;58(546):37–43.
47. Bender B, et al. Adherence intervention research: what have we learned and what do we do next? J Allergy Clin Immunol. 2003;112(3):489–94.
48. Graves MM, et al. Volitional nonadherence in pediatric asthma: parental report of motivating factors. Curr Allergy Asthma Rep. 2007;7(6):427–32.
49. Ari A, Restrepo RD. Aerosol delivery device selection for spontaneously breathing patients: 2012. Respir Care. 2012;57(4):613–26.

50. DiMatteo MR, Haskard KB, Williams SL. Health beliefs, disease severity, and patient adherence: a meta-analysis. Med Care, 45. 2007:521–8.
51. Serra-Batlles J, et al. Patient perception and acceptability of multidose dry powder inhalers: a randomized crossover comparison of Diskus/Accuhaler with Turbuhaler. J Aerosol Med. 2002;15(1):59–64.
52. Fan VS, et al. Costs of pulmonary rehabilitation and predictors of adherence in the National Emphysema Treatment Trial. COPD. 2008;5(2):105–16.
53. Le TT, et al. Do asthma medication beliefs mediate the relationship between minority status and adherence to therapy? J Asthma. 2008;45(1):33–7.
54. Schulte M, et al. Handling of and preferences for available dry powder inhaler systems by patients with asthma and COPD. J Aerosol Med Pulm Drug Deliv. 2008;21(4):321–8.
55. Rubin BK. What does it mean when a patient says,"my asthma medication is not working?". Chest. 2004;126(3):972–81.
56. Menckeberg TT, et al. Patients' understanding of the reasons for starting and discontinuing inhaled corticosteroids. Br J Clin Pharmacol. 2008;66(2):255–60.
57. Eakin MN, Rand CS. Improving patient adherence with asthma self-management practices: what works? Ann Allery Asthma Immunol. 2012;109(2):90–2.
58. Saeed H, et al. Effect of human error, inhalation flow, and inhalation volume on dose delivery from Ellipta® dry-powder inhaler. J Pharm Innov. 2019;14(3):239–44.
59. Elgendy MO, et al. Asthmatic children and MDI verbal inhalation technique counseling. Pulm Pharmacol Ther. 2020;61:101900.
60. Elgendy MO, Abdelrahim ME, Eldin RS. Potential benefit of repeated dry powder inhaler's inhalation technique counseling on asthmatic patients. Pulm Ther. 2015;1(1):91–101.
61. Lavorini F, et al. The ADMIT series-issues in inhalation therapy. 6. Training tools for inhalation devices. Prim Care Respir J. 2010;19(4):335–41.
62. Kamin WE, et al. The inhalation manager: a new computer-based device to assess inhalation technique and drug delivery to the patient. J Aerosol Med. 2003;16(1):21–9.
63. Ari AJ. Patient education and adherence to aerosol therapy. Respir Care. 2015;60(6):941–57.
64. Molimard M, Colthorpe P. Inhaler devices for chronic obstructive pulmonary disease: insights from patients and healthcare practitioners. J Aerosol Med Pulm Drug Deliv. 2015;28(3):219–28.
65. Ari A, Fink JB. Guidelines for aerosol devices in infants, children and adults: which to choose, why and how to achieve effective aerosol therapy. Expert Rev Respir Med. 2011;5(4):561–72.
66. Basheti IA, et al. Evaluation of a novel educational strategy, including inhaler-based reminder labels, to improve asthma inhaler technique. Patient Educ Couns. 2008;72(1):26–33.
67. Safeer RS, Keenan JJ. Health literacy: the gap between physicians and patients. Am Fam Physician. 2005;72(3):463–8.
68. Goodyer L, et al. Inhaler technique in Turkish people with poor English: a case of information discrimination? Pharm World Sci. 2006;28(2):107–14.
69. Skaer T, et al. Metered-dose inhaler technique and quality of life with airways disease: assessing the value of the Vitalograph in educational intervention. J Int Med Res. 1996;24(4):369–75.
70. Manuyakorn W, et al. Sensitivity of Turbutester and Accuhaler tester in asthmatic children and adolescents. Pediatr Int. 2010;52(1):118–25.
71. Al-Showair RA, Pearson SB, Chrystyn HJC. The potential of a 2Tone Trainer to help patients use their metered-dose inhalers. Chest. 2007;131(6):1776–82.
72. Azouza W, Chrystyn HJ. Clarifying the dilemmas about inhalation techniques for dry powder inhalers: integrating science with clinical practice. Prim Care Respir J. 2012;21(2):208–13.
73. Amirav I, Newhouse MT, Mansour YJ. Measurement of peak inspiratory flow with in-check dial device to simulate low-resistance (Diskus) and high-resistance (Turbohaler) dry powder inhalers in children with asthma. Pediatr Pulmonol. 2005;39(5):447–51.
74. Wael W, et al. The effect of clip-tone® and its smartphone application on optimization of metered-dose inhaler inhalation technique. Eur Respir Soc. 2020;56:4157.

75. Bender B, et al. Measurement of children's asthma medication adherence by self report, mother report, canister weight, and doser CT. Ann Allergy Asthma Immunol. 2000;85(5):416–21.
76. Chan AHY, et al. Using electronic monitoring devices to measure inhaler adherence: a practical guide for clinicians. J Allergy Clin Immunol Pract. 2015;3(3):335–349.e5.
77. McQuaid EL, et al. Medication adherence in pediatric asthma: reasoning, responsibility, and behavior. J Pediatr Psychol. 2003;28(5):323–33.
78. Sherman J, et al. Telephoning the patient's pharmacy to assess adherence with asthma medications by measuring refill rate for prescriptions. J Pediatr. 2000;136(4):532–6.
79. Schatz M, et al. Validity of the Asthma Control Test™ completed at home. Am J Manag Care. 2007;13(12):661.
80. Peters SP, et al. Real-world Evaluation of Asthma Control and Treatment (REACT): findings from a national Web-based survey. J Allergy Clin Immunol. 2007;119(6):1454–61.
81. Okupa AY, et al. Daily diaries vs retrospective questionnaires to assess asthma control and therapeutic responses in asthma clinical trials: is participant burden worth the effort? Chest. 2013;143(4):993–9.
82. Jia CE, et al. The Asthma Control Test and Asthma Control Questionnaire for assessing asthma control: systematic review and meta-analysis. J Allergy Clin Immunol. 2013;131(3):695–703.
83. Pijnenburg MW, et al. Monitoring asthma in children. Eur Respir J. 2015;45(4):906–25.
84. Juniper EF, et al. Identifying 'well-controlled'and 'not well-controlled' asthma using the Asthma Control Questionnaire. Respir Med. 2006;100(4):616–21.
85. Álvarez-Gutiérrez FJ, et al. Relationship of the Asthma Control Test (ACT) with lung function, levels of exhaled nitric oxide and control according to the Global Initiative for Asthma (GINA). Arch Bronconeumol. 2010;46(7):370–7.
86. Meltzer EO, et al. Use of the Asthma Control Questionnaire to predict future risk of asthma exacerbation. J Allergy Clin Immunol. 2011;127(1):167–72.
87. Ko FW, et al. Evaluation of the asthma control test: a reliable determinant of disease stability and a predictor of future exacerbations. Respirology. 2012;17(2):370–8.
88. Forno E, et al. Risk factors and predictive clinical scores for asthma exacerbations in childhood. Chest. 2010;138(5):1156–65.
89. Voorend-van Bergen S, et al. Asthma control questionnaires in the management of asthma in children: a review. Pediatr Pulmonol. 2015;50(2):202–8.
90. Juniper EF, et al. Asthma Control Questionnaire in children: validation, measurement properties, interpretation. Eur Respir J. 2010;36(6):1410–6.
91. Juniper E, et al. Development and validation of a questionnaire to measure asthma control. Eur Respir J. 1999;14(4):902–7.
92. Olaguibel JM, et al. Measurement of asthma control according to Global Initiative for Asthma guidelines: a comparison with the Asthma Control Questionnaire. Respir Res. 2012;13(1):1–10.
93. McCallister JW, et al. Sex differences in asthma symptom profiles and control in the American Lung Association Asthma Clinical Research Centers. Respir Med. 2013;107(10):1491–500.
94. Liu AH, et al. Development and cross-sectional validation of the Childhood Asthma Control Test. J Allergy Clin Immunol. 2007;119(4):817–25.
95. Schatz M, et al. Asthma Control Test: reliability, validity, and responsiveness in patients not previously followed by asthma specialists. J Allergy Clin Immunol. 2006;117(3):549–56.
96. Nathan RA, et al. Development of the asthma control test: a survey for assessing asthma control. J Allergy Clin Immunol. 2004;113(1):59–65.
97. Schatz M, et al. The minimally important difference of the Asthma Control Test. J Allergy Clin Immunol. 2009;124(4):719–723.e1.
98. Skinner EA, et al. The asthma therapy assessment questionnaire (ATAQ) for children and adolescents. Dis Manag. 2004;7(4):305–13.
99. Cloutier MM, et al. Asthma outcomes: composite scores of asthma control. J Allergy Clin Immunol. 2012;129(3):S24–33.

100. Diette GB, et al. Using the pediatric asthma therapy assessment questionnaire to measure asthma control and healthcare utilization in children. Patient. 2009;2(4):233–41.
101. Murphy KR, et al. Test for respiratory and asthma control in kids (TRACK): a caregiver-completed questionnaire for preschool-aged children. J Allergy Clin Immunol. 2009;123(4):833–839.e9.
102. Zeiger RS, et al. Test for Respiratory and Asthma Control in Kids (TRACK): clinically meaningful changes in score. J Allergy Clin Immunol. 2011;128(5):983–8.
103. Jones P, et al. Development and first validation of the COPD Assessment Test. Eur Respir J. 2009;34(3):648–54.
104. Van der Molen T, et al. Development, validity and responsiveness of the Clinical COPD Questionnaire. Health Qual Life Outcomes. 2003;1(1):1–10.
105. Kon SS, et al. The Clinical COPD Questionnaire: response to pulmonary rehabilitation and minimal clinically important difference. Thorax. 2014;69(9):793–8.
106. Rabe KF, et al. Global strategy for the diagnosis, management, and prevention of chronic obstructive pulmonary disease: GOLD executive summary. Am J Respir Crit Care Med. 2007;176(6):532–55.
107. Ringbaek T, Martinez G, Lange PJ. A comparison of the assessment of quality of life with CAT, CCQ, and SGRQ in COPD patients participating in pulmonary rehabilitation. COPD. 2012;9(1):12–5.
108. Tsiligianni IG, et al. Assessing health status in COPD. A head-to-head comparison between the COPD assessment test (CAT) and the clinical COPD questionnaire (CCQ). BMC Pulm Med. 2012;12(1):1–9.
109. Cave AJ, et al. Assessment of COPD wellness tools for use in primary care: an IPCRG initiative. Int J Chron Obstruct Pulmon Dis. 2012;7:447.
110. Toumas-Shehata M, et al. Exploring the role of quantitative feedback in inhaler technique education: a cluster-randomised, two-arm, parallel-group, repeated-measures study. NPJ Prim Care Respir Med. 2014;24(1):1–6.

Chapter 6
The Aerosol Generators Available for Critically Ill Patient

Contents

6.1 Introduction

Although there are several treatments for pulmonary diseases, which may be given orally or via injection, it is unlikely that these will be as effective as inhaled bronchodilators or anti-inflammatory drugs. Hence, inhaled therapy is likely to predominate for pulmonary diseases including critically ill patients. Their rapid onset, low doses, higher pulmonary deposition and lower systemic effects are its main advantages [1, 2]. Aerosol therapy is probably better given during breaks in mechanical ventilation. This may also facilitate coughing and the clearing of respiratory secretions. If discontinuing mechanical ventilation results in patient distress, it should be continued and the aerosol generator get attached to the circuit [3]. In this situation, the inhaled medication, given during non-invasive ventilation (NIV) or high flow

M. E. A. Abdelrahim et al., *Essentials of Aerosol Therapy in Critically ill Patients*,
https://doi.org/10.1007/978-3-030-85026-5_6

nasal cannula (HFNC), offers better and quicker clinical effects than with unassisted breathing. This is strongly appreciated for NIV-dependent critically ill patients, compared to taking the patient off the ventilator and delivering during spontaneous unassisted breathing, due to their urgent need for respiratory aid as well as regular prescribed inhaled medications for many days [4–6]. Many aerosol generators are commercially available for treatment of critically ill patients. Some of them have been adapted for clinical use during mechanical ventilation. However, others has not demonstrated their efficacy in clinical settings and needs further research [7]. Clinicians and therapists must be aware of the individual characteristics of different inhalers applied for pulmonary or systemic diseases and the major regulations of choosing the appropriate inhaler device to maximize clinical benefits and minimize possible side effects.

6.2 Discussion and Analysis of Main Topics

From a clinical perspective, an appropriate inhaler device should satisfy the patient and physician criteria especially successful delivery of the therapeutic agent to the target site within the lungs and the ease of use of the device to provide consistent clinical control. However, from a pharmaceutical perspective, an ideal inhaler-device should be; environmentally friendly (no propellant), easy to manufacture, provide uniform dosing of active ingredient, protected against contamination with a long shelf life [8]. The principal categories of aerosol generators used for inhalation therapy are nebulizers, pressurized metered dose inhalers (pMDIs), dry powder inhalers (DPIs) and soft mist inhalers (SMIs). Only pMDIs and nebulizers have been adapted for clinical use during mechanical ventilation. While it is feasible to employ DPIs during mechanical ventilation (see below), their efficacy has not been demonstrated in clinical settings [7]. Similarly, inhaled drug dose efficiency and optimal connection of an SMI to a ventilation circuit remain unknown [9].

6.2.1 Nebulizers

Nebulizers convert either a solution or a micronized suspension into an aerosol suitable for inhalation so they are frequently used for drugs that cannot be conveniently formulated into a pMDI or a DPI. Moreover, they have the potential to deliver relatively large therapeutic doses to the patient, for that reason they are ideal when the therapeutic dose is too large for delivery using any of the alternative aerosol generators [10, 11].

Respirable solutions are concentrated solutions that contain preservatives and antioxidants which sometime cause bronchospasm. For that reason, they must be diluted before administration. The standard practice is to use small-unit dose iso-tonic solutions (Respules) free from preservatives and antioxidants for dilution. Nebulizers differs according to mechanism of energy generated; high velocity air stream dispersion (air-jet nebulizers “JNs”), ultrasonic energy dispersion (ultrasonic nebulizers “USNs”) and vibration energy dispersion (vibrating mesh nebulizers “VMNs”) [11, 12].

6.2.1.1 Air-Jet Nebulizer (JNs)

JNs use compressed air or oxygen from a compressed gas cylinder either through a hospital air-line or electrical compressor to convert a liquid respirable solution into a suitable mist for inhalation [13]. High velocity gas passed through a narrow Venturi nozzle, typically 0.3–0.7 mm in diameter, either co-axially (Inspiron Mini-neb) or tangentially (concentric Nebulizers, e.g. Turret, Respirgard II). An area of negative pressure results in drowning liquid from a fluid reservoir up a feed tube where a proportion of the resultant aerosol leaves the nebulizer chamber and directly carried in the airstream as shown in Fig. 6.1. The aerosol leaving the nebulizer is diluted by atmospheric air and inhaled through a face-mask or mouth-piece. However, the remaining, large, non-respirable droplets impact on baffles or the walls of the nebulizer chamber and are recycled into the reservoir fluid. Therefore, the particle size of aerosol is significantly modified within the nebulizer by the ‘filtering’ effect of the baffles in the JN and due to droplet aggregation, solvent evaporation and condensation. Moreover, they have a tendency to concentrate the respirable solution [10, 15].

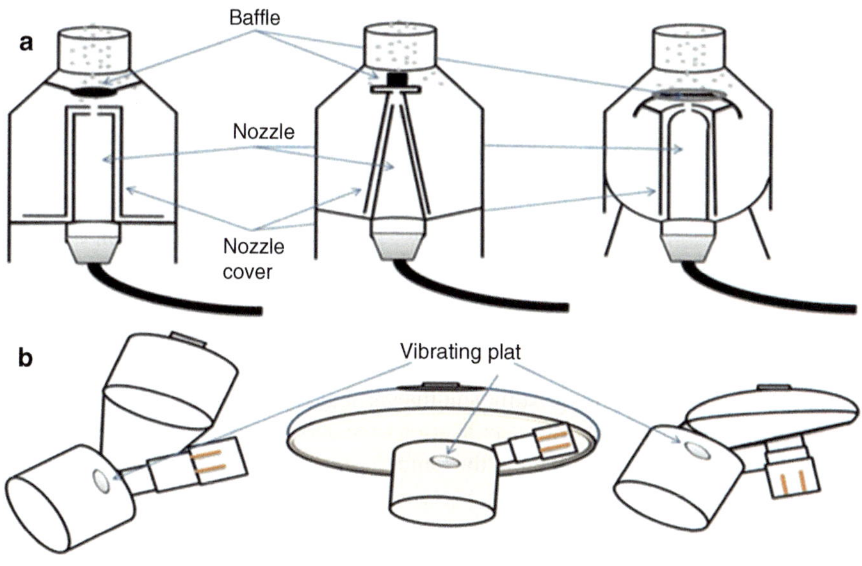

Fig. 6.1 Different types of nebulizers; (**a**) different designs of JN, (**b**) different types of VMNs [14]

Traditional JNs are accompanied by high aerosol wastage caused by continuous operation since the expiratory phase of breathing constitutes approximately two-third of the breathing cycle [10], a large proportion of the total emitted dose is lost, in addition to upward movement of aerosol leaving a large residual volume of respirable solution with high drug concentration (solute) [16]. It was reported that >50% of the aerosol is retained in JNs and tubing with lower pulmonary deposition which suggest inefficiency of JNs [17, 18]. Reported methods to improve JNs efficiency includes; diluting the nebulized solution but that increases nebulization time [19–22], applying intermittent nebulization over continuous delivery, using breath-enhanced or breath-actuated JNs or using reservoirs that conserve aerosols during expiration phase like Circulaire® II hybrid [21–23]. Moreover, it was proven that the gas flow rate of JN is a major determinant of the aerosol particle size [19, 24]. A laser diffraction analysis of four JNs showed that when the flow rate was increased from 4 to 8 L min^{-1}, a 50% reduction in the MMAD with a linear increase in the fine particle dose (FPD) (particles less than 5 μm) was observed [25]. Actually, increasing the flow rate increases the shearing forces to which the surfaces of droplets are exposed, resulting in smaller droplets and smaller particle size with a better lung deposition. Moreover, viscosity and surface tension of respirable solution might be expected to affect the nebulizer performance and aerosol characteristics, since energy is required to overcome viscous forces for creating a new surface. Atomization theory suggests that the mean diameter of aerosol droplets will decrease as viscosity decreases [26]. It was proven that the low viscosity solutions offered less resistance to the essential aerosol disintegration process, thereby producing smaller droplets and higher aerosol output [12].

JNs are recommended for suspensions such as corticosteroid formulations, e.g. Pulmicort Respules, AstraZeneca [10], and recombinant human deoxyribonuclease [27]. The activity and structural integrity of the enzyme was maintained, when JNs were employed, unlike USN which caused denaturation of the protein due to the elevated temperatures. However, studies with lactate dehydrogenase have suggested that there was an irreversible time-dependant loss of enzyme activity with JNs due to long nebulization time [28].

6.2.1.2 Ultrasonic Nebulizers (USNs)

USNs use a transducer of a piezo-electric crystal to produce high frequency sound waves in the nebulizing unit to produce vertical capillaries of liquid. When the amplitude of energy applied is sufficient the vertical capillaries break up to provide an aerosol. USNs have a shorter nebulization time and greater particle size than that of JNs [29, 30]. They cause a rise in the temperature of the nebulised solution so not suitable for thermo-labile drugs, e.g. proteins and can't be used with viscous respirable solutions. They are less used than JNs despite their compactness which makes them easy to be carried [11, 31, 32].

6.2.1.3 Vibrating Mesh Nebulizer (VMNs)

Conventional nebulizers lack portability due to the need of an electrical or compressed gas source, have low efficiency and variability in performance [33]. VMNs can overcome many of the drawbacks of conventional nebulizers. VMNs have much greater aerosol output efficiency, fraction of fine particles (FPF), precision and consistency of pulmonary drug delivery than conventional JNs or USNs. These devices are relatively quiet, portable, time-saving with minimal residual volume after nebulization [16, 23, 34–37]. For that reason diluting the respiratory solution with either water or saline will not increase the drug delivery from VMNs due to their minimal residual volumes [20–22]. These nebulizers nebulise solutions at a rate of 0.3–0.6 $mL.min^{-1}$. The nebulization time is shorter than conventional nebulizers [38]. Their main disadvantage is the substantially higher cost than other nebulizers [39, 40]. Aerogen Pro VMN was proven to have a three to five fold higher efficiency for delivering aerosol to the lungs than conventional JN or USN [41, 42]. Hence, similar clinical effects could be obtained through VMNs with lower doses compared to conventional nebulizers. It is recommended to adjust the dose if changing nebulizer type to avoid possible toxicity [43].

VMNs are powered by an alternating current or a rechargeable battery pack. They apply a vibrating mesh or plate with multiple apertures to generate an aerosol. The aperture plate has about 1000 tapered holes that are electroformed in a sheet. The wider portion of the hole is toward the medication, and the narrower end is toward the atmosphere. The medication is placed in a reservoir above (e.g. Aerogen Pro, Aerogen Solo) or against (e.g. e-flow) the domed aperture plate (Fig. 6.1). When electric current is applied, the ceramic vibrational element expands and contracts, causing the domed aperture plate to move upward and downward by a few micrometers, which creates a micro-pump action that extrudes medication through the apertures to produce an aerosol [34]. The energy required for nebulisation is applied to the vibrational element rather than to the nebulised solution, hence the increase in temperature of the solution during operation is very low causing negligible risk of denaturing proteins and of reducing the activity of enzymes or antibiotics during nebulization [44–47]. When suspensions are nebulized, blockage of the apertures with drug particles can occur. Therefore, they must be cleaned regularly [48].

During mechanical ventilation, VMNs had proved superiority over conventional nebulizers [14]. They could be applied to generate aerosol continuously, or it can be adapted to generate aerosol only during inspiration which offer much better aerosol delivery and minimal leakage [49]. Furthermore, placing VMNs within the ventilation circuit is not affecting its setting unlike JNs [50, 51]. A study compared Aerogen Pro and two JNs, MistyNeb (Allegiance Healthcare Corp, McGaw Park, Ill) and Vix One (Westmed, Mexico), for delivery of 2.5 mg of salbutamol sulphate to a simulated pediatric patient during mechanical ventilation with high frequency oscillation. Aerogen Pro delivered significantly higher salbutamol amount (582 ± 89 μg) to the end of the endotracheal tube than MistyNeb (201 ± 87 μg) or Vix One (197 ± 50 μg) at p 5 cmH_2O and required adjustment of ventilator flow settings during operation to maintain ventilator parameters with initiation and discontinuation of nebulization. Opening the medication reservoir to refill the Aerogen Pro did not result in any change of the ventilator parameters. In contrast, both of the JNs required interruption of ventilation in order to refill [52].

6.2.2 *Pressurized Metered Dose Inhalers (pMDIs)*

pMDIs are the standard aerosol generator for the treatment of pulmonary diseases since they provide reliable, reproducible, effort-independent dosing, high protection from environmental humidity or bacterial infection and at the same time they are the most portable and the least expensive aerosol generators available [53–57]. A pMDI consists of a canister with a metering valve containing a drug in suspension/solution with surfactants, lubricants and a propellant under pressure (Fig. 6.2). The canister is lodged upside down in a plastic support called the actuator. By pressing the bottom of the canister, a pre-metered drug dose is released. When the canister is depressed, liquid propellant containing the drug substance is forced into the actuator where flashing occurs. The resulting gas under high pressure forces the propellant together with the excipients and the drug substance as particles or droplets of drug solution exit through the actuator orifice, thus creating the aerosol cloud. These emerge at a very high speed. The aerosol cloud consists of a so-called heterodisperse aerosol consisting of a variety of particle sizes from approximately 1 to 35 μm. The large particles have considerable inertia resulting in their deposition on the tongue and in the oropharynx. It was reported that from 100 μg salbutamol in the Ventolin (chlorofluorocarbons (CFC) formulation) leaving the actuator orifice,

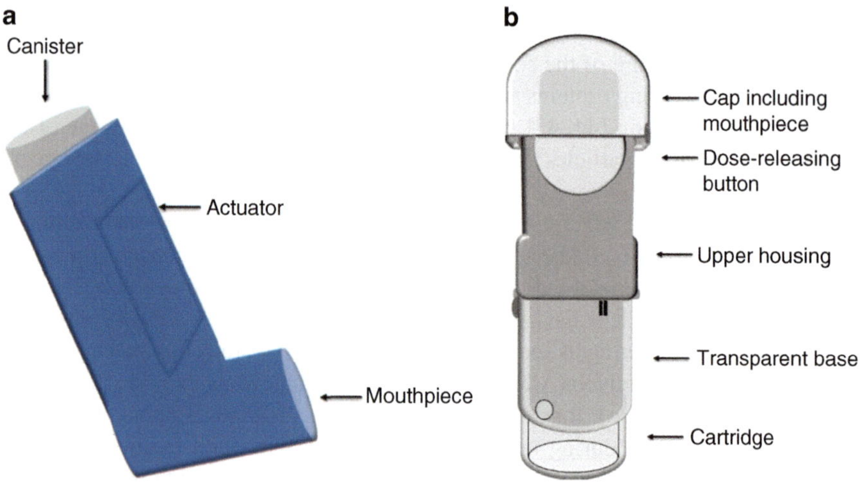

Fig. 6.2 Portable inhaler devices (**a**) pressurized metered dose inhalers (pMDIs) and (**b**) soft mist inhaler (SMI)

approximately 10 μg remains in the actuator and mouthpiece, 75–80 μg is deposited in the mouth and throat and only about 10–15 μg reaches the lungs [58]. It was reported that an average of 8.8% of the nominal dose was deposited in the lungs (3.0% in the alveoli and 5.8% on the conducting airways) and 80% in the mouth. The remainder of the dose was either expired [1.0%] or deposited in the aerosol actuator (9.8%) [58]. It was reported that 2 mg salbutamol was delivered by pMDI with a spacer as do 5 mg through JN and 3 mg through VMN [43]. Therefore, pMDI delivery system is considered quite inefficient, but this dose distribution was sufficient to provide maximum bronchodilation in stable mild–moderate asthmatics [59].

For effective particle deposition in the lower airways, the aerodynamic diameter of particles should be <5 μm. However, particularly for patients with obstructive lung disease, particle size should ideally be within the 2–3 μm range [60–62]. Particle size delivered by pMDIs is influenced by a variety of factors [63], including:

1. Pressure inside the canister.
2. Physical and chemical properties of the propellant and additives.
3. Drug used, its concentration and the delivered volume.
4. Metering valve and delivery outlet design.
5. Mouthpiece and delivery outlet cleanness.
6. Propellant evaporation time.
7. Distance to travel from the delivery outlet.

Therefore, the major limitation of the conventional "press and breathe" pMDIs is that coordination between actuation and inhalation is highly required to minimize oro-pharyngeal deposition and subsequent systemic side effects [64, 65]. Similarly, during NIV, dose actuation through pMDI must be at the beginning of the inspiration phase to enhance the performance of pMDIs use [63]. A number of studies have shown that about 25% of patients who have been taught how to use pMDIs in a chest clinic [66], and 75% of elderly patients [67] may not perform the inhalation manoeuvre very efficiently. A recent study of asthmatics revealed that only 7.5% performed the correct technique [68]. Their performance was improved by using spacers and applying new technologies which reduced the delivery speed such as breath-actuated pMDIs (BA-pMDIs) as the Autohaler (Teva, UK) and the Easi-Breathe (Teva, UK), breath-coordinated pMDIs (BC-pMDIs) and spray-velocity modifiers like Neohaler and Tempo [63, 69, 70]. In addition to the critical role of patient training with the use of a training aid device, like 2Tone Trainer, which looks like a pMDI but without a canister in addition to verbal counselling to help training and maintaining a slow inhalation flow [68, 71]. At present, there is no evidence that a breath actuated pMDI helps to overcome the 'cold Freon' effect, as the spray is fired direct into the oro-pharynx just like a standard pMDI.

Moreover, pMDIs were firstly formulated using CFC propellants which have environmental concerns, causing the destruction of the atmospheric ozone layer [72], and causing cold freon effect (early breath cut off caused by a cold sensation provoked by CFC in the pharynx) [63, 73]. Therefore, pharmaceutical companies have reformulated pMDIs with hydrofluoroalkans (HFAs) propellants which are

2000 times more potent greenhouse gases than CFCs but do not damage the ozone layer [74]. Modern pMDI devices contain non-ozone depleting propellants like HFA, which emit aerosol with more ultrafine particles and lower velocity than CFC-pMDIs; (53%) from a HFA beclometasone dipropionate (BDP) compared to (4%) with a CFC BDP, leading to a significant improvement in lung deposition and clinical efficacy [64, 75]. The Main problems associated with pMDIs use includes [8]:

- Canister not shaken well before delivery
- Cap not removed
- Patient breathe in before or after delivery
- Patient breathe in through the nose
- Patient breathe out before inhalation is complete
- Patient delivers multiple doses during the same breathe
- Not coordinating drug actuation with inhalation
- Too fast inhalation flow
- Inhalation is interrupted by 'Freon effect' (early breath cut off caused by a cold sensation provoked by CFC in the pharynx)

6.2.2.1 Add-on Devices (Spacers)

Spacers/ad-on devices are extension tubes attached to the pMDI mouthpiece. They reduce both the aerosol velocity, particle size and decrease the need for patient co-ordination between actuation and inhalation of the aerosol. They have a size selective function, retaining large particles, reducing drug deposition in the oropharynx, the systemic bioavailability of the inhaled drug and the 'cold-Freon effect' [76, 77]. Different spacers can bind to JNs and VMNs as well. Their main disadvantages are that they are bulky, and difficult to carry around; in addition, the valves sometimes stick or become otherwise faulty [63, 78]. The spacers are classified into three categories, simple tube spacer, holding chambers spacers and reverse-flow spacers. The simple tube spacer is an extension to the inhaler mouthpiece. Valved holding chambers usually contain a one-way valve in the mouthpiece. They can reduce drug loss associated with poor hand-breath co-ordination. A reverse-flow spacer is a device in which the spray is fired away from the patient into a bag or chamber, from which the patient then inhales [77, 79].

Many spacers were developed and adapted for use during mechanical ventilation. The standard T-piece of pMDI, pMDI Tee Adapter, is characterized by a small internal volume which cause early particle deposition and condensation on its inner walls due to early stopping of generated particles from pMDI canister which is estimated after 45 mm, despite that it remains the standard piece used with pMDI during NIV [43, 80]. This drawback also exists with the VMNs T-piece due to the similarity between both pMDI port and the VMNs T-piece in the downward movement of generated aerosol. While JN T-piece shows a different behavior due to the upward movement of aerosol particles so any condensed aerosol within JN T-piece has a chance to be returned to the nebulizer reservoir and to be nebulized again [16].

Several types of spacers were developed to overcome the main drawback of the standard T-piece and improve the propellant evaporation including; AeroChamber Mini [MC], AeroChamber Vent [VC], AeroChamber MV [AC], Combihaler and Minimhal, to be used with both single-limb and dual-limb NIV circuits [76, 81]. Combihaler and Minimhal are newly developed spacers with inlets to both pMDI and VMN which allow delivering preliminary pMDI puffs for initial bronchodilation to enhance subsequent pulmonary deposition of nebulized drugs. Minimhal have a smaller volume than Combihaler [81–83].

There are many factors that could affect aerosol delivery through a spacer. Firstly, spacer volume; spacers range from small-volume e.g. Aerochamber, Optimiser and Inhalet to large-volume spacer e.g. Nebuhaler, Volumatic and Fisonair. An in-vitro study compared the pMDI alone to the pMDI plus a large-volume holding chamber (Volumatic) (GlaxoSmithKline, Ware, UK). They estimated the aerodynamic characteristics of fluticasone propionate, flunisolide and beclomethasone dipropionate, at inhalation flows of 30 L min^{-1}. A significant reduction of the MMAD and increase of the FPD was obtained for all three drugs with the pMDI plus Volumatic spacer [84]. Evaluating a small volume spacer, Optimiser, for use with the Easi-Breathe inhaler showed that oro-pharyngeal deposition was reduced by 80% by the use of the spacer. The Optimiser spacer removes most of the non-respirable drug, without compromising FPD delivered from the Easi-Breathe inhaler [85]. Small-volume spacers are more portable than large-volume spacers but they can cause earlier particle deposition and condensation on its inner walls due to the early stopping of the generated aerosol unlike large-volume ones [43, 80]. Using a large-volume spacer increases the lung dose in adults by approximately 50% in dual-limb ventilation circuit as it could retain higher fraction of aerosol for subsequent breathing in this closed circuit. Combihaler as a large volume spacer proved superiority when compared to T-piece (small volume spacer) with VMN in a dual-limb ventilation circuit but not in single-limb ventilation [86, 87]. However, in single-limb ventilation circuit which is an open-circuit with an open expiration port, this conservative effect of large spacer was diminished. Unfortunately, the large volume design of Combihaler does not suit the aerosol therapy within a single limb NIV circuit and its large dead volume forces the patient to rebreathe the exhaled air kept in the spacer [86, 87].

Additionally, spacer material; most of spacers are constructed of plastic material and so the surfaces can accumulate static charge unless specially treated. Drug delivery from a spacer could be improved by placing an antistatic lining on the inner walls of the spacer [88]. It has been found that washing a plastic spacer in detergent without subsequent rinsing in tap water and then allowing it to air dry [89, 90], priming by using the spacer several times [91] or using a spacer made of metal [92] can decrease the electrostatic charges on the spacer surface and help increase drug output from plastic spacers. On the other hand, rubbing the spacer with a cloth increases the electrostatic charge. In a metal spacer the aerosol half-life is about 30 s compared with about 10 s in a plastic spacer; a shorter half-life increases the need for co-ordination between actuation and inhalation. Therefore non-electrostatic metal spacers ensure delivery of significantly higher doses than plastic spacers [93].

Not only spacer volume and material could affect aerosol delivery but also spacer design. Certain spacers (Volumatic, Nebuhaler) are designed to fit only a single type of pMDI, whereas others can be used with all types (AeroChamber). The most suitable kind of spacer must be chosen. Nebuhaler, an example of a large volume spacer, its shape was intended to replicate the shape of the aerosol cloud emitted from pMDI. Early versions of Nebuhaler were described as the pear-shaped extension tube [94]. Some devices can be used to deliver aerosols from pMDIs to intubated or tracheotomised patients [95], others could be used during mechanical ventilation [96, 97].

Finally, inhalation from the spacer must be slow. Multiple actuations should be avoided because this will reduce drug output from the spacer. Each actuation must be followed by at least 30 s to allow propellant evaporation and consistent dose deposition [98]. It had been found that, taking multiple tidal breaths from a large-volume spacer is more practical than taking single deep breath, and this result in a satisfactory bronchodilator response [99]. During an acute asthma exacerbation, a high dose (10–15 puffs) of short-acting β_2-agonist pMDI via a large-volume spacer was found to be an effective alternative to nebulizer [95, 100, 101]. Cost-analysis studies showed that treatment with either pMDIs plus spacers or nebulizers produce equivalent responses during acute exacerbation, but pMDI plus spacer use was associated with shorter periods of hospitalization [102].

6.2.3 *Dry Powder Inhalers (DPIs)*

Dry powder inhalers can be divided into two main groups, single dose and multi-dose inhalers, based on their functional elements (powder container, metering system, disintegration principle and the mouthpiece). Multi-dose inhalers are divided in two different designs: the reservoir systems and the multiple unit-dose inhalers [65]. The early DPIs were all unit-dose systems. Firstly, single-dose inhalers which utilize pre-metered doses dispensed into hard gelatine capsules. The capsule cap and body must be separated before inhalation (Rotacaps for Rotahaler) or the capsule has to be pierced at both ends (Capsules for Aerolizer (Novartis Pharma, GmbH, Germany), Handihaler (Boehringer Ingelheim, Germany) and Breezhaler (Novartis Pharma, GmbH, Germany)). However, regarding multiple unit-dose inhalers, they were introduced starting with Diskhaler (GlaxoWellcome, UK) in which single doses are filled, by the manufacturer, into suitable dose compartments (Rotadisk). The dose is released by piercing the upper and the lower surfaces of a blister before inhalation [71]. Then, The Diskus/Accuhaler (GlaxoSmithKline, UK) was launched. It contains 60 discrete dispensed doses packed on a long strip which is coiled within the inhaler. Similarly, many other multi-unit DPIs inhalers were then well-developed with simpler technique such as Ellipta (GlaxoWellcome, UK). Finally, the reservoir systems includes the powder formulation stored in a reservoir containing 100–200 equal doses from which a single dose is dispensed with a special dose-metering unit. They require careful manipulation of the device during dose preparation. Turbuhaler (AstraZeneca, UK) as an example was introduced to deliver 500 μg per dose of terbutaline sulphate devoid of carrier, and then it was used for other drugs [8]. The mouthpiece may be used to control the resistance to airflow of the inhaler device and the direction of the aerosol cloud in the mouth and throat, in order to reduce drug deposition in the oro-pharyngeal cavities [103]. Newer reservoir DPIs have been introduced with the advantage of giving a fairly consistent emitted dose irrespective of the inhalation technique used by patients of all age groups e.g. Clickhaler (ML Laboratories PLC; St. Albans, UK), Pulvinal (Chiesi, Farmaceutici, Italy) and Easyhaler (Orion Corporation, Finland) [104]. Moreover, Novolizer (Viatris, Germany) was introduced with special characteristics together with the feedback mechanisms which overcome inherent problems of DPIs [74, 105]. It is a reservoir DPI with a refillable cartridge system. The dose has to be inhaled at a flow >35 $L.min^{-1}$. No dose is released when the patient inhalation flow is less than 35 $L.min^{-1}$ [106], but it has a medium to low resistance which permits a relatively high PIFR [69.0 ± 18.0 L min^{-1}] to be easily achieved through the device making it particularly valuable for inhalation therapy in asthmatic children [105, 107].

The total emitted dose (TED) and fine particle fraction (FPF) released by DPIs have been shown to vary considerably and be affected by differences in inspiratory flow [108]. The inhalation profile may affect both the dose emitted and particle size distribution [109]. A study was conducted to compare Easyhaler, Turbohaler and Diskus concluded that TED and FPF showed less flow dependency with Easyhaler and Diskus than with Turbohaler [110]. Another study have tested the aerodynamic characteristics of the emitted aerosol from both Seretide Diskus (salmeterol xinafoate 50 μg; fluticasone propionate 500 μg) and Symbicort Turbohaler (formoterol 6 μg; budesonide 200 μg). They found that the dose characteristics of Turbohaler were more dependent on the patient's inhalation flow [111]. Therefore, patients cannot use all DPIs equally well [112]. Changing an inhalation device can have adverse effects on both the safety and efficacy of an inhaled drug. Hence, DPIs should not be regarded as interchangeable [113, 114].

The main limitation of DPIs is that a sufficient peak inspiratory flow rate (PIFR) is required by the patients to obtain the optimal therapeutic dose which vary according to inhaler resistance; [ranging from 30 $L.min^{-1}$ for high resistance to 65 $L.min^{-1}$ for low resistance] [115, 116]. The PIFR achieved by a patient through a DPI depends upon the specific resistance of the device and the patient inspiratory capability for a set of inspiratory effort. The lower the specific resistance in the DPI the higher will be the PIFR [117]. Therefore, resistance to airflow is one of the design parameters for DPIs that could be used to control the inspiratory flow profile and optimize particle deposition in the airways [118].

Patients with reduced inspiratory capacity may not get the full benefit from the DPI [110, 119, 120]. Drug delivery across the Diskus® resistance was reported to be 92 ± 9% at flow rates ≥60 $L.min^{-1}$ if compared to 76 ± 12% at 30 $L.min^{-1}$ [110]. Also, a pilot in-vivo study with 10 subjects showed that a pulmonary drug deposition of 27% was achieved through Turbohaler® at faster flow rates (60 $L.min^{-1}$) if compared to 15% deposition at slower flow rates (35 $L.min^{-1}$) [119]. Many other studies have reported an association between suboptimal PIFR and increased risk of acute exacerbations of COPD and readmissions [121, 122]. Loh et al. was the first study to show that suboptimal PIFR had significant effect on clinical outcomes. The suboptimal group had fewer days to both all causes of admission (65.5 vs. 101 days, $p = 0.009$) and COPD readmission (63.5 vs. 144 days, $p = 0.002$) if compared to the optimal group. In their study analysis, PIFR was the only significant variable associated with readmission [121]. Optimal PIFR is therefore a major requirement of successful inhaler use. PIFR should be routinely measured if prescribing DPIs is being considered, especially in COPD females [115]. Patients with COPD have been reported to have a lower inhalation flow than adult asthmatics when they use DPI. Also, the more severe the airway obstruction the lower was the inhalation flow through a variety of DPIs [123]. Also it was recommended that Turbohaler was not suitable for pre-school children due to the low flow achieved by this group [124].

Some of the recent DPIs incorporate an additional energy source to supplement airflow to the inspiratory force of the patient, in order to aerosolize the drug particles into the inhaled air stream, but not quite used yet and will have the patient co-ordination problems. Future generations of DPIs focus on both the inhaler device and the powder formulation properties. They enable optimum therapeutic benefits through effective respiratory deposition. The continued expansion on the development of DPIs that improve drug delivery deep in lung allow innovative powder formulations to target many drugs in different diseases like cystic fibrosis, lung cancers, influenza and diabetes [125–127].

DPIs could be employed in-line in ventilator circuits, either by employing the ventilator's inspiratory airflow to generate an aerosol or by first producing an aerosol from the DPI and then entraining the drug particles in the airflow from the ventilator. Everard and colleagues modified the Turbohaler for use in a ventilator circuit [128]. These investigators removed the outer covering of the Turbohaler and enclosed the inner cylinder containing the spiral disaggregation channels in a chamber. Once the device was loaded, air flowing through the chamber carried the aerosol beyond the endotracheal tube (ETT). The system employed by Everard and colleagues was reported to deliver approximately 20% of the nominal dose to a filter placed at the distal end of the ETT. That are comparable to those achieved with pMDIs and spacers [129]. Moreover, Everard and colleagues employed a dry ventilator circuit, because humidity is well known to reduce drug delivery from DPIs [130]. Drug losses are likely to be higher when a DPI is employed in a ventilator circuit. Because mechanically ventilated patients routinely receive warm and humidified gas, the feasibility of administering dry powders in a humid environment was a big challenge. Therefore, current in-line DPIs either perform poorly, are difficult to operate, and/or require large volumes (~1 L) of air which encourage further research. A new low-air volume (LV) DPIs were produced recently with an acceptable high-quality aerosol with only 10 mL of dispersion air per actuation and were easy to load and operate (Fig. 6.3). Best case performance included a device emitted dose of approximately 85% (of loaded dose) and device emitted MMAD of 1.77 μm. Maximum emitted dose through the low flow nasal cannula (LFNC) system and small diameter (4 mm) nasal cannula was approximately 65% (of the loaded dose)

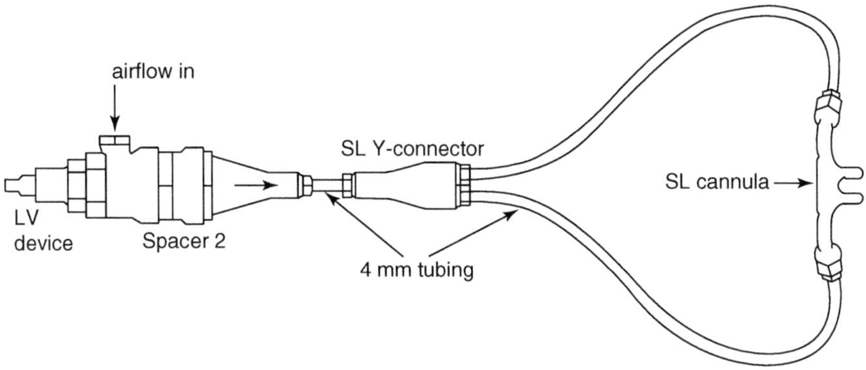

Fig. 6.3 Schematic drawing showing the overall layout of the in-line DPI delivery system with each component labeled [131].

and device emitted MMAD of 1.93 μm. Potential applications of this device include the delivery of high dose inhaled medications such as surfactants, antibiotics, mucolytics, and anti-inflammatories. This performance should enable application in high and low flow mechanical ventilation systems with high efficiency lung delivery to both infants and children [132].

6.2.4 *Soft Mist Inhalers (SMIs)*

SMIs are novel, multidose, propellant-free, hand-held, liquid inhalers that represent a new category of inhaler devices. They deliver aerosol cloud that are slower moving and last 4–10 times longer than aerosols from pMDIs. Aerosol cloud generated by SMI has at least twice higher FPF (particles smaller than 5.8 μm) than both pMDIs and DPIs [133, 134]. That would allow a higher proportion of the TED to be delivered to the lungs and less to the oro-pharynx [135, 136].

There is currently only one commercially available SMI, the Respimat® Soft Mist™ Inhaler (Boehringer Ingelheim, Germany). It is a hand-held inhaler with a hinged cap. Medication is stored as a solution in the drug cartridge, an aluminum cylinder containing a double-walled, plastic, collapsible bag that contracts as the solution is used. Twisting the base of the device 180° compresses a spring and provides mechanical power to aerosolize the dose of drug and also transfers a metered dose of drug (usually 10–15 μL) from the drug cartridge through a capillary tube to the pump cylinder. When the dose-release button is activated, the energy from the compressed spring forces the drug through a nozzle system called the "uniblock" using a technique derived from microchip technology (Fig. 6.2). Respimat® was firstly marketed with 120 actuations and a dose indicator. This indicator does not count individual doses but gives an estimate of doses remaining. After 120 actuations have been delivered, a locking mechanism is activated to prevent further use by preventing twisting of the base [137]. The dose can be administered to the patient with the inhaler held in any position [135].

Many scintigraphic studies showed that SMIs deliver a higher proportion of TED to the lungs than with pMDIs with/without spacer in healthy subjects [136, 138], and COPD patients [139]. More recent studies proved that Respimat® showed deeper lung deposition of ICS if compared to Turbohaler® DPI or CFC-pMDI in mild to moderate asthmatic subjects. Mean whole lung deposition of drug from the Respimat® SMI was found to be 51.6% of the metered dose ($p < 0.001$) if compared to 28.5% and 17.8% with Turbohaler® DPI fast (60 L/min) and slow (30 L/min) inhalation flow rates, respectively or 8.9% from the Becloforte® pMDI. Moreover, the deposition pattern within the lungs was more peripheral for Respimat® SMI than for Turbohaler® DPI [134, 135]. It could be attributed to slow movement of the mist at the push of a button in Respimat®, with no need to the force of patient's inhalation like DPI. Moreover, the combination of smaller particle size, lower velocity and longer duration of the aerosol cloud improved coordination of inhalation with actuation, enhanced lung deposition and decreased oro-pharyngeal deposition if compared to pMDIs [135, 139]. These main findings allow reducing the dose in the SMI to half, or even one quarter, of the nominal dose of the pMDI with comparable efficacy and safety as proven by many clinical trials in asthmatics [140–145], and COPD patients [146]. A continuing challenge with this inhaler, however, is the expense of treatment if compared to other commercially available inhalers which is affecting affordability by the patient [135].

Inhaled drug dose efficiency and optimal connection of an SMI to a ventilation circuit remain unknown. Clinicians try to connect SMI to the ventilator circuit in various creative ways. Currently, an in-line adapter for the SMI is commercially available to provide an access port in the ventilator circuit that facilitates the administration of medication from the SMI as prescribed to mechanically ventilated adult patients [147]. The efficiency of administering SMI with this in-line adapter has not been reported. A current study hypothesized that, with the long aerosol release time of the SMI, the release of aerosol during expiration of the ventilator system may increase the delivered dose compared to release during inspiration. They compared in-line adapter with different adapters via endotracheal tube with a range of actuation timing during mechanical ventilation or by manual resuscitation [9]. They found that the in-line adapter yielded the greatest delivered dose only with expiratory synchronization. A T-adapter without valve connected to the SMI resulted in an unacceptable leak volume during ventilation therefore it should not be used. Finally, SMI administration during mechanical ventilation should be avoided until more efficient adapters are available based on low dose efficiency of the current available connections. They reported that drug delivery of the SMI in an intubated lung model was greatly reduced if compared to that in a spontaneous breathing model. Further research on the relationship among delivered drug dose/ therapeutic effects and the optimal method of delivery to patients with NIV or tracheostomized patients with spontaneous breathing is desired [9].

6.3 Conclusion

Different aerosol generators greatly vary in their efficiency of aerosol delivery to critically ill patients. Only pMDIs and nebulizers have been adapted for clinical use during mechanical ventilation. pMDI with a spacer have higher efficiency of aerosol output than VMN which have a three–five fold higher efficiency for delivering aerosol to the lungs than conventional JN or USN. On the other hand DPI and SMI have not yet proven their efficiency when applied within ventilation circuit. A new low-air volume DPI was currently introduced, to be included in the ventilation circuit, with an acceptable high-quality aerosol However, SMI administration during mechanical ventilation should be avoided until more efficient adapters are available and further research must be encouraged in this field. For non-ventilated patients, SMI is the highest efficient aerosol generator, providing higher and deeper aerosol output than CFC- pMDIs with/without spacer and DPIs. It could overcome most of their limitations. If prescribing DPIs is being considered, patient PIFR should be routinely measured to choose the matched DPI resistance for optimal therapeutic effect. Finally, changing the type of aerosol generator necessitates dose adjustment to avoid possible toxicity or sub-therapeutic doses.

Key Major Recommendations

1. It is recommended to adjust the dose if changing type of aerosol generator to avoid possible toxicity or sub-therapeutic doses.
2. It was proven that diluting the respiratory solution with either water or saline will increase the drug delivery from JNs even with longer treatment time, unlike VMNs due to their minimal residual volumes.
3. pMDI plus spacer use is a better alternative to nebulizer use and is associated with shorter periods of hospitalization.
4. PIFR should be routinely measured if prescribing DPIs is being considered, especially in COPD females. Moreover, DPIs should not be regarded as interchangeable.
5. SMI administration during mechanical ventilation should be avoided until more efficient adapters are available based on low dose efficiency of the current available connections.

References

1. Larsson S, Svedmyr N. Bronchodilating effect and side effects of Beta2-adrenoceptor stimulants by different modes of administration (tablets, metered aerosol, and combinations thereof) a study with salbutamol in asthmatics. Am Rev Respir Dis. 1977;116(5):861–9.
2. Darquenne C. Aerosol deposition in health and disease. J Aerosol Med Pulm Drug Deliv. 2012;25(3):140–7.
3. Mukhopadhyay A, et al. Effects of inhalational bronchodilator treatment during noninvasive ventilation in severe chronic obstructive pulmonary disease exacerbations. J Crit Care. 2009;24(3):474.e1–5.

4. Michotte J-B, et al. In vitro comparison of five nebulizers during noninvasive ventilation: analysis of inhaled and lost doses. J Aerosol Med Pulm Drug Deliv. 2014;27(6):430–40.
5. Duarte AG. Inhaled bronchodilator administration during mechanical ventilation. Respir Care. 2004;49(6):623–34.
6. Madney YM, et al. The influence of changing interfaces on aerosol delivery within high flow oxygen setting in adults: an in-vitro study. J Drug Deliv Sci Technol. 2020;55:101365.
7. Dhand R. Inhalation therapy with metered-dose inhalers and dry powder inhalers in mechanically ventilated patients. Respir Care. 2005;50(10):1331–45.
8. Abdelrahim M. Relative bioavailability of terbutaline to the lungs following inhalation using different methods. niversity of Bradford; 2009.
9. Fang T-P, et al. Optimal connection for tiotropium SMI delivery through mechanical ventilation: an in vitro study. Pharmaceutics. 2020;12(3):291.
10. McCallion O, et al. Jet nebulisers for pulmonary drug delivery. Int J Pharm. 1996;130(1):1–11.
11. Taylor KM, McCallion ON. Ultrasonic nebulisers for pulmonary drug delivery. Int J Pharm. 1997;153(1):93–104.
12. Mc Callion O, Patel M. Viscosity effects on nebulisation of aqueous solutions. Int J Pharm. 1996;130(2):245–9.
13. Abdelrahman MA, et al. Effect of holding chamber as an add-on device on aerosol delivery and fugitive aerosol from different jet nebulizers. J Pharm Innov. 2019:1–7.
14. Saeed H, et al. Effect of nebulizer designs on aerosol delivery during non-invasive mechanical ventilation: a modeling study of in vitro data. Pulmon Ther. 2017;3(1):233–41.
15. Dhand R, Tobin MJ. Inhaled bronchodilator therapy in mechanically ventilated patients. Am J Respir Crit Care Med. 1997;156(1):3–10.
16. Waldrep J, Dhand R. Advanced nebulizer designs employing vibrating mesh/aperture plate technologies for aerosol generation. Curr Drug Deliv. 2008;5(2):114–9.
17. Dhand R. Aerosol delivery during mechanical ventilation: from basic techniques to new devices. J Aerosol Med Pulm Drug Deliv. 2008;21(1):45–60.
18. Bosco AP, Rhem RG, Dolovich MB. In vitro estimations of in vivo jet nebulizer efficiency using actual and simulated tidal breathing patterns. J Aerosol Med. 2005;18(4):427–38.
19. Vecellio L, et al. Disposable versus reusable jet nebulizers for cystic fibrosis treatment with tobramycin. J Cyst Fibros. 2011;10(2):86–92.
20. Saeed H, et al. Effects of nebulizer fill volume on the efficacy and safety of the bronchodilator. J Drug Deliv Sci Technol. 2020;56:101508.
21. Saeed H, et al. Effects of fill volume and humidification on aerosol delivery during single-limb noninvasive ventilation. Respir Care. 2018;63(11):1370–8.
22. Saeed H, et al. Fill volume, humidification and heat effects on aerosol delivery and fugitive emissions during noninvasive ventilation. J Drug Deliv Sci Technol. 2017;39:372–8.
23. Ari A. Jet, ultrasonic, and mesh nebulizers: an evaluation of nebulizers for better clinical outcomes. Eurasian J Pulmonol. 2014;16:1–7.
24. Rau JL, Hess D. A guide to aerosol delivery devices for respiratory therapists. AARC Times; 2009. p. 53.
25. Clay M, et al. Factors influencing the size distribution of aerosols from jet nebulisers. Thorax. 1983;38(10):755–9.
26. Mercer TT. Production and characterization of aerosols. Arch Intern Med. 1973;131(1):39–50.
27. Cipolla D, et al. Assessment cf aerosol delivery systems 2 for recombinant human deoxyribonuclease. STP Pharm Sci. 1994;4(1):5062.
28. Niven RW, Brain JD. Some functional aspects of air-jet nebulizers. Int J Pharm. 1994;104(1):73–85.
29. Arzhavitina A, Steckel H. Surface active drugs significantly alter the drug output rate from medical nebulizers. Int J Pharm. 2010;384(1):128–36.
30. Miller DD, et al. Aerosol delivery and modern mechanical ventilation: in vitro/in vivo evaluation. Am J Respir Crit Care Med. 2003;168(10):1205–9.

31. Ari A, Fink JB. Guidelines for aerosol devices in infants, children and adults: which to choose, why and how to achieve effective aerosol therapy. Expert Rev Respir Med. 2011;5(4):561–72.
32. Ari A, Restrepo RD. Aerosol delivery device selection for spontaneously breathing patients: 2012. Respir Care. 2012;57(4):613–26.
33. Smith E, Denyer J, Kendrick A. Comparison of twenty three nebulizer/compressor combinations for domiciliary use. Eur Respir J. 1995;8(7):1214–21.
34. Dhand R. Nebulizers that use a vibrating mesh or plate with multiple apertures to generate aerosol. Respir Care. 2002;47(12):1406–16; discussion 1416–8.
35. Dhand R. New nebuliser technology-aerosol generation by using a vibrating mesh or plate with multiple apertures. Business briefing: long-term health care strategies; 2003. p. 1–4.
36. Watts AB, McConville JT, Williams RO III. Current therapies and technological advances in aqueous aerosol drug delivery. Drug Dev Ind Pharm. 2008;34(9):913–22.
37. Ari A, et al. Influence of nebulizer type, position, and bias flow on aerosol drug delivery in simulated pediatric and adult lung models during mechanical ventilation. Respir Care. 2010;55(7):845–51.
38. Fink J, et al. In vitro characteristics of the aeroneb portable nebulizer system. J Aerosol Med. 2001;14(3):1–11.
39. Ghazanfari T, et al. The influence of fluid physicochemical properties on vibrating-mesh nebulization. Int J Pharm. 2007;339(1):103–11.
40. Zhang G, David A, Wiedmann TS. Performance of the vibrating membrane aerosol generation device: Aeroneb Micropump Nebulizer™. J Aerosol Med. 2007;20(4):408–16.
41. Fink JB, Barraza P, Bisgaard J. Aerosol delivery during mechanical ventilation with high frequency oscillation: an in-vitro evaluation. Chest. 2001;120(4).
42. Fink J, Schmidt D. In vitro comparison of nebulizers for aero-sol delivery during mechanical ventilation. Am J Respir Crit Care Med. 2002;165:A375.
43. Hassan A, et al. In-vitro/in-vivo comparison of inhaled salbutamol dose delivered by jet nebulizer, vibrating mesh nebulizer and metered dose inhaler with spacer during non-invasive ventilation. Exp Lung Res. 2017;43(1):19–28.
44. Pitance L, et al. Delivery efficacy of a vibrating mesh nebulizer and a jet nebulizer under different configurations. J Aerosol Med Pulm Drug Deliv. 2010;23(6):389–96.
45. Ari A, Aljamhan EA, Fink J. Influence of nebulizer type position and bias flow on aerosol drug delivery in a model of adult mechanical ventilation. Respir Care. 2010;55:845–51.
46. Skaria S, Smaldone GC. Omron NE U22: comparison between vibrating mesh and jet nebulizer. J Aerosol Med Pulm Drug Deliv. 2010;23(3):173–80.
47. Coates AL, et al. A comparison of amount and speed of deposition between the PARI LC STAR® jet nebulizer and an investigational eFlow® nebulizer. J Aerosol Med Pulm Drug Deliv. 2011;24(3):157–63.
48. Fink J, Schmidt D, Power J. Comparison of a nebulizer using a novel aerosol generator with a standard ultrasonic nebulizer designed for use during mechanical ventilation. In: American Thoracic Society 97th International Conference. San Francisco, CA. 2001.
49. Ari A, Fink JB. Factors affecting bronchodilator delivery in mechanically ventilated adults. Nurs Crit Care. 2010;15(4):192–203.
50. Hardaker LE, Hatley RH. In vitro characterization of the I-neb Adaptive Aerosol Delivery (AAD) System. J Aerosol Med Pulmon Drug Deliv. 2010;23(S1):S11–20.
51. Johnson JC, et al. Aerosol delivery of recombinant human DNase I: in vitro comparison of a vibrating-mesh nebulizer with a jet nebulizer. Respir Care. 2008;53(12):1703–8.
52. Fink JB, Barraza P, Bisgaard J. Aerosol delivery during mechanical ventilation with high frequency oscillation: an in-vitro evaluation. Chest. 2001;120:277S.
53. Elgendy MO, et al. Asthmatic children and MDI verbal inhalation technique counseling. Pulm Pharmacol Ther. 2020;61:101900.
54. Saeed H, et al. Impact of advanced patient counseling using a training device and smartphone application on asthma control. Respir Care. 2020;65(3):326–32.

55. Nicola M, et al. The impact of adding a training device to familiar counselling on inhalation technique and pulmonary function of asthmatics. Adv Ther. 2018;35(7):1049–58.
56. Elgendy MO, Abdelrahim ME, Eldin RS. Potential benefit of repeated MDI inhalation technique counselling for patients with asthma. Eur J Hosp Pharm. 2015;22(6):318–22.
57. Azouz WAA. Novel methodology to characterise how asthma and chronic obstructive pulmonary disease patients use their inhalers and methods to improve their inhaler technique objective assessment of how patients use inhalers. University of Huddersfield; 2012.
58. Newman SP, et al. Deposition of pressurised aerosols in the human respiratory tract. Thorax. 1981;36(1):52–5.
59. Ruffin R, Kenworthy M, Newhouse M. Response of asthmatic patients to fenoterol inhalation: a method of quantifying the airway bronchodilator dose. Clin Pharmacol Therap. 1978;23(3):338–45.
60. Zanen P, Go LT, Lammers J-WJ. The optimal particle size for β-adrenergic aerosols in mild asthmatics. Int J Pharm. 1994;107(3):211–7.
61. Zanen P, Go LT, Lammers J. Optimal particle size for beta 2 agonist and anticholinergic aerosols in patients with severe airflow obstruction. Thorax. 1996;51(10):977–80.
62. Bisgaard H. What dose fraction represents the respirable dose? Respir Med. 1997;91:20–1.
63. Terzano C. Pressurized metered dose inhalers and add-on devices. Pulmon Pharmacol Therap. 2001;14(5):351–66.
64. Newman SP. Principles of metered-dose inhaler design. Respir Care. 2005;50(9):1177–90.
65. Harb HS, et al. Real-life assessment of chronic obstructive pulmonary disease patient performance with different inhalers. Int J Clin Pract. 2020;75:e13905.
66. Crompton G. Problems patients have using pressurized aerosol inhalers. Eur J Respir Dis Suppl. 1982;119:101.
67. Allen SC, Prior A. What determines whether an elderly patient can use a metered dose inhaler correctly? Br J Dis Chest. 1986;80:45–9.
68. Al-Showair RA, Pearson SB, Chrystyn H. The potential of a 2Tone trainer to help patients use their metered-dose inhalers. Chest. 2007;131(6):1776–82.
69. Newman SP, et al. Improvement of drug delivery with a breath actuated pressurised aerosol for patients with poor inhaler technique. Thorax. 1991;46(10):712–6.
70. Murphy KR, et al. Therapeutic equivalence of budesonide/formoterol delivered via breath-actuated inhaler vs pMDI. Respir Med. 2015;109(2):170–9.
71. Harb HS, et al. First-time handling of different inhalers by chronic obstructive lung disease patients. Exp Lung Res. 2020;46(7):258–69.
72. Molina MJ, Rowland FS. Stratospheric sink for chlorofluoromethanes: chlorine atom-catalysed destruction of ozone. Nature. 1974;249(5460):810–2.
73. Said AS, Harding LP, Chrystyn H. Urinary pharmacokinetic methodology to determine the relative lung bioavailability of inhaled beclometasone dipropionate. Br J Clin Pharmacol. 2012;74(3):456–64.
74. Crompton GK. How to achieve good compliance with inhaled asthma therapy. Respir Med. 2004;98:S35–40.
75. Leach CL, et al. Influence of particle size and patient dosing technique on lung deposition of HFA-beclomethasone from a metered dose inhaler. J Aerosol Med. 2005;18(4):379–85.
76. Harb HS, et al. Update efficacy of aerosol therapy with noninvasive ventilator approach (non-invasive ventilation and nasal high flow). J Drug Deliv Sci Technol. 2020;59:101922.
77. Newman SP. Spacer devices for metered dose inhalers. Clin Pharmacokinet. 2004;43(6):349–60.
78. Aswania O, Chrystyn H. Relative lung bioavailability of generic sodium cromoglycate inhalers used with and without a spacer device. Pulm Pharmacol Ther. 2001;14(2):129–33.
79. Newman SP, Newhouse MT. Effect of add-on devices for aerosol drug delivery: deposition studies and clinical aspects. J Aerosol Med. 1996;9(1):55–70.
80. Boukhettala N, et al. In vitro performance of spacers for aerosol delivery during adult mechanical ventilation. J Aerosol Med Pulm Drug Deliv. 2015;28(2):130–6.

81. Eckes M, Porée T. Influence of the position on the in vitro performances of a new spacer for pediatric use in a mechanical ventilation circuit. In: Pediatric pulmonology. Hoboken: Wiley; 2019.
82. Madney YM, et al. Aerosol delivery through an adult high-flow nasal cannula circuit using low-flow oxygen. Respir Care. 2019;64(4):453–61.
83. Madney YM, et al. Nebulizers and spacers for aerosol delivery through adult nasal cannula at low oxygen flow rate: an in-vitro study. J Drug Deliv Sci Technol. 2017;39:260–5.
84. Terzano C, Mannino F. Probability of particle and salbutamol deposition in the respiratory tract: comparison between MDI and autohaler. Monaldi Arch Chest Dis. 1996;51(3):236–42.
85. Hardy J, et al. A small volume spacer for use with a breath-operated pressurised metered dose inhaler. Int J Pharm. 1996;142(1):129–33.
86. Harb HS, et al. Is Combihaler usable for aerosol delivery in single limb non-invasive mechanical ventilation? J Drug Deliv Sci Technol. 2017;40:28–34.
87. Harb HS, et al. Performance of large spacer versus nebulizer T-piece in single-limb noninvasive ventilation. Respir Care. 2018;63(11):1360–9.
88. O'callaghan C, et al. Improvement in sodium cromoglycate delivery from a spacer device by use of an antistatic lining, immediate inhalation, and avoiding multiple actuations of drug. Thorax. 1993;48(6):603–6.
89. Wildhaber JH, et al. High-percentage lung delivery in children from detergent-treated spacers. Pediatr Pulmonol. 2000;29(5):389–93.
90. Pierart F, et al. Washing plastic spacers in household detergent reduces electrostatic charge and greatly improves delivery. Eur Respir J. 1999;13(3):673–8.
91. Bisgaard H, et al. A non-electrostatic spacer for aerosol delivery. Arch Dis Child. 1995;73(3):226–30.
92. Bisgaard H. A metal aerosol holding chamber devised for young children with asthma. Eur Respir J. 1995;8(5):856–60.
93. Bisgaard H. Delivery of inhaled medication to children. J Asthma. 1997;34(6):443–67.
94. Barry PW, O'Callaghan C. The influence of inhaler selection on efficacy of asthma therapies. Adv Drug Deliv Rev. 2003;55(7):879–923.
95. Cates C. Spacers and nebulisers for the delivery of beta-agonists in non-life-threatening acute asthma. Respir Med. 2003;97(7):762–9.
96. Dhand R, Tobin M. Bronchodilator delivery with metered-dose inhalers in mechanically-ventilated patients. Eur Respir J. 1996;9(3):585–95.
97. Manthous CA, et al. Treatment of bronchospasm by metered-dose inhaler albuterol in mechanically ventilated patients. Chest. 1995;107(1):210–3.
98. Barry P, o'Callaghan C. Multiple actuations of salbutamol MDI into a spacer device reduce the amount of drug recovered in the respirable range. Eur Respir J. 1994;7(9):1707–9.
99. Castro-Rodriguez JA, Rodrigo GJ. β-Agonists through metered-dose inhaler with valved holding chamber versus nebulizer for acute exacerbation of wheezing or asthma in children under 5 years of age: a systematic review with meta-analysis. J Pediatr. 2004;145(2):172–7.
100. Cates CJ, et al. Holding chambers versus nebulisers for beta-agonist treatment of acute asthma. Cochrane Database Syst Rev. 2003;(2).
101. Duarte AG, Momii K, Bidani A. Bronchodilator therapy with metered-dose inhaler and spacer versus nebulizer in mechanically ventilated patients: comparison of magnitude and duration of response. Respir Care. 2000;45(7):817–23.
102. Chou KJ, Cunningham SJ, Grain EF. Metered-dose inhalers with spacers vs nebulizers for pediatric asthma. Arch Pediatr Adolesc Med. 1995;149(2):201–5.
103. De Boer A, et al. Inhalation characteristics and their effects on in vitro drug delivery from dry powder inhalers: part 3: the effect of flow increase rate (FIR) on the in vitro drug release from the Pulmicort 200 Turbuhaler. Int J Pharm. 1997;153(1):67–77.
104. Chrystyn H. Closer to an 'Ideal Inhaler' with the Easyhaler®. Clin Drug Investig. 2006;26(4):175–83.

105. Vogelberg C, et al. Clinical evaluation of the peak inspiratory flow generated by asthmatic children through the Novolizer®. Respir Med. 2004;98(10):924–31.
106. Kohler D. The Novolizer®: overcoming inherent problems of dry powder inhalers. Respir Med. 2004;98:S17–21.
107. Richter K. Successful use of DPI systems in asthmatic patients—key parameters. Respir Med. 2004;98:S22–7.
108. Chrystyn H. The DiskusTM: a review of its position among dry powder inhaler devices. Int J Clin Pract. 2007;61(6):1022–36.
109. Miller N, et al. Aerodynamic sizing with simulated inhalation profiles: total dose capture and measurement. In: Respiratory drug delivery VII. Raleigh, NC: Serentec Press; 2000. p. 191–6.
110. Palander A, et al. In vitro comparison of three salbutamol-containing multidose dry powder inhalers. Clin Drug Investig. 2000;20(1):25–33.
111. Tarsin WY, et al. Emitted dose estimates from Seretide® Diskus® and Symbicort® Turbuhaler® following inhalation by severe asthmatics. Int J Pharm. 2006;316(1–2):131–7.
112. Gustafsson P, et al. Can patients use all dry powder inhalers equally well? Int J Clin Pract. 2005;59:13–8.
113. Chrystyn H. Do patients show the same level of adherence with all dry powder inhalers? Int J Clin Pract. 2005;59:19–25.
114. Williams AE, Chrystyn H. Survey of pharmacists' attitudes towards interchangeable use of dry powder inhalers. Pharm World Sci. 2007;29(3):221–7.
115. Harb HS, et al. Prevalence and predictors of suboptimal peak inspiratory flow rate in COPD patients. Eur J Pharm Sci. 2020;147:105298.
116. Ghosh S, Ohar JA, Drummond MB. Peak inspiratory flow rate in chronic obstructive pulmonary disease: implications for dry powder inhalers. J Aerosol Med Pulm Drug Deliv. 2017;30(6):381–7.
117. Clark A, Hollingworth A. The relationship between powder inhaler resistance and peak inspiratory conditions in healthy volunteers—implications for in vitro testing. J Aerosol Med. 1993;6(2):99–110.
118. De Koning J, et al. Effect of an external resistance to airflow on the inspiratory flow curve. Int J Pharm. 2002;234(1–2):257–66.
119. Borgstrom L, et al. Lung deposition of budesonide inhaled via Turbuhaler: a comparison with terbutaline sulphate in normal subjects. Eur Respir J. 1994;7(1):69–73.
120. Mahler DA, et al. Comparison of dry powder versus nebulized beta-agonist in patients with COPD who have suboptimal peak inspiratory flow rate. J Aerosol Med Pulm Drug Deliv. 2014;27(2):103–9.
121. Loh CH, et al. Suboptimal inspiratory flow rates are associated with chronic obstructive pulmonary disease and all-cause readmissions. Ann Am Thorac Soc. 2017;14(8):1305–11.
122. van der Palen J. Peak inspiratory flow through Diskus and Turbuhaler, measured by means of a peak inspiratory flow meter (In-Check DIAL®). Respir Med. 2003;97(3):285–9.
123. Tarsin W, et al. Inter-individual variability of peak inhalation rate through different inhalers by asthmatic children and adults and those with COPD. Eur Respir J. 2001;18(Suppl 33):P900.
124. Pedersen S, Mortensen S. Use of different inhalation devices in children. Lung. 1990;168(1):653–7.
125. Hill M. Characteristics of an active multiple dose dry powder inhaler. Respir Drug Deliv. 1994;4:109–16.
126. Brown B, et al. A piezo-electronic inhaler for local & systemic applications. Drug Deliv Technol. 2004;4(8):90–3.
127. Young PM, et al. The development of a novel high-dose pressurized aerosol dry-powder device (PADD) for the delivery of pumactant for inhalation therapy. J Aerosol Med. 2004;17(2):123–8.

128. Everard ML, Devadason SG, Le Souef PN. In vitro assessment of drug delivery through an endotracheal tube using a dry powder inhaler delivery system. Thorax. 1996;51(1):75–7.
129. Mitchell JP, et al. The delivery of chlorofluorocarbon-propelled versus hydrofluoroalkane-propelled beclomethasone dipropionate aerosol to the mechanically ventilated patient: a laboratory study. Respir Care. 2003;48(11):1025–32.
130. Jashnani RN, Byron PR, Dalby RN. Testing of dry powder aerosol formulations in different environmental conditions. Int J Pharm. 1995;113(1):123–30.
131. Farkas D, Hindle M, Longest PW. Application of an inline dry powder inhaler to deliver high dose pharmaceutical aerosols during low flow nasal cannula therapy. Int J Pharm. 2018;546(1–2):1–9.
132. Farkas D, Hindle M, Longest PW. Development of an inline dry powder inhaler that requires low air volume. J Aerosol Med Pulm Drug Deliv. 2018;31(4):255–65.
133. Hochrainer D, et al. Comparison of the aerosol velocity and spray duration of Respimat® Soft Mist™ inhaler and pressurized metered dose inhalers. J Aerosol Med. 2005;18(3): 273–82.
134. Pitcairn G, et al. Deposition of corticosteroid aerosol in the human lung by Respimat® Soft Mist™ inhaler compared to deposition by metered dose inhaler or by Turbuhaler® dry powder inhaler. J Aerosol Med. 2005;18(3):264–72.
135. Anderson P. Use of Respimat® soft Mist™ inhaler in COPD patients. Int J Chron Obstruct Pulmon Dis. 2006;1(3):251.
136. Steed K, et al. Lung and oropharyngeal depositions of fenoterol hydrobromide delivered from the prototype III hand-held multidose Respimat nebuliser. Eur J Pharm Sci. 1997;5(2):55–61.
137. Dalby R, Spallek M, Voshaar T. A review of the development of Respimat® Soft Mist™ inhaler. Int J Pharm. 2004;283(1–2):1–9.
138. Newman SP, et al. Lung deposition of fenoterol and flunisolide delivered using a novel device for inhaled medicines: comparison of RESPIMAT with conventional metered-dose inhalers with and without spacer devices. Chest. 1998;113(4):957–63.
139. Brand P, et al. Higher lung deposition with Respimat® Soft Mist™ inhaler than HFA-MDI in COPD patients with poor technique. Int J Chron Obstruct Pulmon Dis. 2008; 3(4):763.
140. Kässner F, Hodder R, Bateman ED. A review of ipratropium bromide/fenoterol hydrobromide (Berodual®) delivered via Respimat® Soft Mist™ inhaler in patients with asthma and chronic obstructive pulmonary disease. Drugs. 2004;64(15):1671–82.
141. Vincken W. Clinical efficacy and safety of the combination of ipratropium bromide and fenoterol inhaled via the Respimat© Soft Mist™ inhaler for relief of airflow obstruction. Expert Rev Respir Med. 2008;2(1):11–26.
142. Kunkel G, et al. Respimat®(a new soft mist inhaler) delivering fenoterol plus ipratropium bromide provides equivalent bronchodilation at half the cumulative dose compared with a conventional metered dose inhaler in asthmatic patients. Respiration. 2000;67(3):306–14.
143. von Berg A, et al. Efficacy and safety of ipratropium bromide plus fenoterol inhaled via Respimat® Soft Mist™ inhaler vs. a conventional metered dose inhaler plus spacer in children with asthma. Pediatr Pulmonol. 2004;37(3):264–72.
144. Vincken W, Dewberry H, Moonen D. Fenoterol delivery by Respimat® soft mist inhaler versus CFC metered dose inhaler: cumulative dose-response study in asthma patients. J Asthma. 2003;40(6):721–30.
145. van Noord JA, et al. Delivery of Fenoterol via Respimat®, a novel 'Soft Mist' Inhaler. Respiration. 2000;67(6):672–8.
146. Iacono P, et al. Improved delivery of ipratropium bromide using Respimat®(a new soft mist inhaler) compared with a conventional metered dose inhaler: cumulative dose response study in patients with COPD. Respir Med. 2000;94(5):490–5.
147. FDA. RTC 26-C In-line Aerosol Adapter. 2017. https://www.accessdata.fda.gov/cdrh_docs/pdf16/K162753.pdf.

Chapter 7
Mechanisms of Aerosol Lung Deposition

Contents

7.1 Principles of Aerosol Delivery

The main principle of aerosol therapy is that the response of the inhaled medications depends on the percent of drug that could pass through the upper airways deep into the lungs. Delivery of aerosol particles to the lung depends mainly on certain factors or key elements like the velocity of the produced aerosol particles and their particle size [1, 2].

Aerosol particles with a size of more than 5 μg mainly deposit in the upper airways and cannot pass to the lung or in other words they are not inhalable particles.

M. E. A. Abdelrahim et al., *Essentials of Aerosol Therapy in Critically ill Patients*,
https://doi.org/10.1007/978-3-030-85026-5_7

The aerosol particle size is expressed as a mass median aerodynamic diameter (MMAD) [3].

The percentage of the deposited aerosol particle in the lung also depends on the patient's inhalation flow rate. Slow inhalation will results in higher aerosol particle deposition in the lungs [4]. Inhaling aerosol particles through the nose will also result in a lower amount that could be deposited in the lower airways compared to inhaling through the mouth [5].

Aerosol in the range between 1 and 7 μg could distribute and deposit in the respiratory system by different manners as fine particles mainly distribute peripherally while the larger aerosol particles would deposit centrally in the conducting tubes [6–8]. The pattern of particle deposition also could be affected by the breath-holding, inhalation rate, and geometry of the airways [9].

Aerosol-producing devices currently available in the market produce a wide range of aerosol particle sizes, in the respirable range. So the particles will be deposited and distributed in different regions of the lung and that could enhance the therapeutic response of the inhaled medications [10, 11].

7.2 Physical Principles that Control Aerosol Delivery and Deposition

Numerous factors control the delivery and distribution of aerosol particles in the respiratory system some of them are related to the patient like inhalation flow rate, age, breathing pattern, the anatomy of the respiratory system, and adherence to the therapy. Also, factors that control aerosol distribution could be related to the device or the drug formulation like particle size and velocity, viscosity of the drug, hygroscopic properties, and the type of formulation.

7.2.1 Particle Size

A key element and essential factor that affects aerosol delivery is the particle size of the emitted drug [12]. Aerosol particles deposition depend on its size so particle with size greater than 5 μg will deposit in the upper airways (oropharynx), while particles less than 3 μg will pass deep to the lower airways. Hence, the smaller the particle size the more the targeting of aerosol delivery to the lower and small airways [13]. The greater the size of the aerosol droplet the larger the volume of medication that will be carried in these droplets. The large aerosol particles greater than 10 μg that will be deposited in the upper airways (oropharynges) will result in less effective therapy by decreasing the percentage of lung deposited amount.

Aerosol particles produced from aerosol-producing devices have different sizes which are called poly-disperse droplets. Aerodynamic characteristics of aerosol droplets could be determined by MMAD and geometric standard deviation (GSD) [14]. MMAD describes the aerodynamic diameter of emitted aerosol when 50% of the emitted aerosol has particle mass less than the given value for MMAD. GSD describes the distribution of aerosol particles. The small MMAD less than 5 is very essential for delivering inhaled corticosteroids, as the greater the MMAD of emitted corticosteroids the greater the amount that will deposit in the oropharynx causing adverse effects like oral thrush (candidiasis) [15–17].

7.2.2 Inertial Impaction

The velocity and mass of aerosol particles determine the momentum in which the movement of particles through the airstream is dependent. Inertia will drive the aerosol particle to move continuously depending on the velocity of it. The direction of the airflow may be changed in some areas like the oropharynx or airway bifurcations however, not all particles will change the direction of movement. The large particle with a size higher than 5 μg will continue the movement till deposition in the first drawback in their way [18]. Large aerosol particles deposit mainly in the upper airways (oropharynx) due to the high velocity of the air stream produced by the patient [19, 20].

7.2.3 Gravitational Sedimentation

The settling of aerosol particles or any particles is controlled by gravity. The air in which the drug particles travel has a resistance when it balances with the gravity, aerosol particles will deposit with a steady velocity. So, breath-holding after aerosol inhalation is needed to allow the aerosol particles to settle down. Breath-holding more than 10 s after aerosol inspiration has no additional benefits on aerosol deposition [21, 22].

Large aerosol particles will deposit in the upper airways or airway bifurcations, as a result, the smaller droplets will pass deep to the lower airways by the action of gravity. Inertial impaction is the main way by which large particles impact the oropharynx while gravitational sedimentation is the cause of smaller aerosol particles less than 3 μm deposition. Sedimentation has a greater effect on particles greater than 0.5 μg [23, 24].

7.2.4 Brownian Motion and Diffusion

Brownian motion affects mainly the very small particles less than 0.1 μg, in which the aerosol particles move according to the gas in which they are suspended. Aerosol particles less than 0.5 μg are less affected by the diffusion power. In general, particles ranged from 0.1 to 1 microgram are slowly affected by sedimentation and diffusion as mechanisms of deposition [12, 25].

7.2.5 Electrostatic Attraction

The attraction of two particles that are charged might lead to their deposition also this electrostatic charge may lead to the deposition of aerosol particles to the charged mucosa which is a disadvantage of the electrostatic charges. Not only the electrostatic charges could be presented in the biological system and the medication, but also in the add-on devices like spacers which used with pMDIs, but no sufficient investigations were carried in this area [26].

7.2.6 Variables Related to the Patient

The patient is the cornerstone for the success of disease control and his role (self-management of the disease) could be more beneficial than that of the health care professionals in some conditions like asthma [27, 28]. The most important patient-related factor in aerosol therapy is the patient's ability to use aerosol-producing devices correctly. Besides this factor, there are biological factors like anatomy and physiology differences of the respiratory system between patients and the severity of the disease [29, 30].

The age of the patient plays an important role in aerosol therapy control. Age-related physical and cognitive skills could facilitate or complicate the process of patient training or counseling. Elderly and children till the age of the school take more effort from health care professionals to educate them on the correct inhalation technique [31]. Infants and younger children would achieve higher therapeutic outcomes by using add-on devices plus the traditional pMDIs or shifting to nebulizers but this will be more costly and take more time compared to pMDI [32]. Also crying of infants will result in lower deposition of aerosol in the lung because most of the emitted dose will be deposited in the upper airways by impaction [33]. At an age of fewer than 3 years, a facial mask should be used for aerosol delivery, but if it was not fitting well, the patient will inhale less amount of the drug. But regarding age more than 3 years, most subjects could be learned how to use the mouthpiece and the technique by which they could take frequent inspiratory and expiratory breaths. At the age of 5–7 years, most subjects can learn how to use spacers with a low inspiratory flow rate for at least 5 s followed by holding their breath for not more than 10 s. Also at the age of more than 5 years, they could be able to inhale from DPI with a fast inspiratory rate [26, 34].

Poor compliance is a big drawback in the way to achieve good therapeutic outcomes for most chronic disorders. Lack of compliance for other routes of drug administration expressed by missing one or more doses from the prescribed dose regimen. Lack of compliance for aerosol therapy contains an additional element which is the compliance for correct inhalation technique of the prescribed devices, as the majority of patients forget the training instruction for the correct use of the device after receiving it from the healthcare professionals [35, 36]. So the adherence in this condition related to aerosol therapy is not only the continuous use of the drug according to the dose regimen, but also adherence to the correct Inhalation technique. Adherence to the medications for severe asthmatic patients or those who have frequent exacerbations and symptoms (patients taking 14 inhaled doses per week (twice daily) of inhaled medication), means that they should not miss more than three doses. About 20% of patients did not reach this criterion due to several reasons like a drug holiday, which means that the patients try to test the result of discounting the medication and its effect on their health. Other patients did not adhere to their medications to avoid a certain side effect of the treatment like the cold Freon effect of the inhaled medications [37]. Forgetting to take medication is still the major cause of poor adherence.

7.2.7 Deposition in the Oropharyngeal Regions

Recent studies on realistic upper airway replicas and Computational fluid dynamic (CFD) simulation, lead to considerable progress related to the understanding of the aerosol transport and deposition processes in the oropharyngeal regions. 50% of the complete opening [38]. Airway replica studies from *Magnetic resonance imaging* (MRI) scans have provided reproducible deposition evidence that can be used to evaluate the process of in-vivo aerosol particles deposition. The impaction parameter showed a monotonic increase in deposition results, suggesting that impaction is the most common deposition mechanism in the oropharyngeal airway. The deposition performance falls within the same range as the in vivo deposition results. The dominant deposition mechanism, according to these studies, is inertial impaction by the curved streamline of the main flow in the oropharyngeal area at the back of the oral cavity, and deposition triggered by a constriction in the larynx [39]. When the idealized replica is coated to avoid particle bounce, aerosol deposition in the idealized replica is in near agreement with those in the Lovelace Respiratory Research Institute realistic mouth–throat replica for liquid and solid aerosol [40]. The deposition in the USP induction port was also much smaller, according to the same report.

7.3 Oral Deposition for the Dry Powder Inhalers (DPIs)

The oropharyngeal depositions of inhaled particles emitted from DPIs were 60% to 70% higher than that expected using the oral deposition model in the human lung deposition model, according to data obtained with gamma scintigraphy of several DPIs [41]. The mouthpiece design of some DPIs was speculated to be the true cause of the high oropharyngeal aerosol deposition. A previous study focused on the deposition of monodisperse aerosol at flow rates ranging from 5 to 90 liter per minute using two DPIs (Turbuhaler and Diskus), a metered-dose inhaler (pMDI) with a holding chamber, two nebulizers, and a straight tube with a 17-mm diameter [42]. In an idealized mouth and throat testing model, the oropharyngeal deposition was measured. The oropharyngeal aerosol deposition of two nebulizers using a combination of pMDI and holding chamber was identical to the straight tube deposition. The two DPIs, on the other hand, had substantially higher aerosol particles deposition than the straight tube, up to 14 folds higher.

7.3.1 Lung Clearance Mechanisms

After the aerosol particles have been deposited in the lungs, aerosolized medications are either cleared from the lungs, absorbed into the systemic circulation, or degraded through drug metabolism. There is a two-layer mucus blanket over the ciliated epithelium which extends from the trachea to the terminal bronchioles: a high viscosity gel layer above a low-viscosity periciliary or sol layer. The mucus secreted from the airway epithelial goblet cells and submucosal glands is forming the two-layer mucus blanket. The rate of mucus movement depends on the airway region and is defined by the number of ciliated cells and their beat frequency in the normal lung. Movement is relied on factors affecting ciliary functioning and the mucus quality and quantity and is slower in the small airways than in the trachea [43, 44]. Insoluble drug particles are deposited in the high viscosity gel layer and then moved by the mucus upward movement caused by the cilia metachronous beating to the pharynx and finally to the gastrointestinal tract. Mucociliary clearance removes the major amount of drug particles that are deposited in the conducting airways and the rest are absorbed into the circulatory or lymphatic system through the airway epithelium. The intact airway epithelial cells, the optimal sol layer depth and chemical composition, normal ciliary structure and activity, and the mucus rheology in the physiological range are factors that should be available to ensure normal mucociliary clearance. Several lung diseases as bronchiectasis, immotile cilia syndrome, asthma, and cystic fibrosis (CF) decrease the mucociliary clearance of aerosolized drugs, and the cough clears the secretions from the lung [2, 45, 46]. The ciliary function in bronchiectasis and immotile cilia syndrome may be non-existent or impaired. The ciliary function and structure in CF affect their ability to clear the mucus efficiently [47].

Soluble drug particles removed by mucociliary clearance as well as the absorptive mechanisms at the conducting airways and its transport is been more resistant by pulmonary epithelium than the endothelium or the interstitium [47]. Lipophilic molecules cross simply by passive transport through the airway epithelium. Lipophobic molecules pass by extracellular pathways, like tight junctions, or through active transport by endocytosis and exocytosis [48] particles are absorbed from the submucosal region, into the bronchial circulation, systemic circulation, or lymphatic system. The main phagocytic cells for the lung are the alveolar macrophages which defense against the drug particles trapped in the alveolar region that also can be absorbed into the systemic circulation.

It was proven that there is a converse relationship between the permeability of alveoli and molecular weight [47]. In the in-vivo study, peak serum DDAVP levels (1-des amino-8-d-arginine vasopressin) that have low molecular weight (1.1 kDa) is observed at 1 h after directly administration by intratracheal instillation, but of albumin that has a high molecular weight (67 kDa) observed from (16 to 25 h) after directly administration by intratracheal instillation. So, the rate of absorption from the alveoli depends on the size of protein, but various proteins cleared more rapidly from the lung than predicted for their size which is indicative of receptor-mediated endocytosis. As in human growth hormone that has (22 kDa m wt), the peak serum levels occurred at 0.5–4 h after direct administration by intratracheal instillation [49].

It isn't clear to know about the effect of the drug-metabolizing activities of the lung on the pharmacokinetics and pharmacodynamics of an inhaled drugs. The conducting airways and alveoli in the lung contain all metabolizing enzymes (such as Phase 1 cytochrome-450 (CYP450) enzymes, flavin-containing monooxygenases (FMO), aldehyde dehydrogenase, NADPH-CYP450 reductase, and monoamine oxidase (MAO)) as in the liver but with a lesser extent, CYP450 enzymes are lower 5–20 times in the lung than in the liver [50]. Esterase is in higher concentrations in alveolar macrophages than in alveolar type I and II cells, it hydrolyses beclomethasone dipropionate to its beclomethasone and monopropionate. The monooxygenase system metabolizes steroids, lipophilic xenobiotics, and fatty acids. The lung is a poor site for sulphation. So, proteins and peptides are hydrolyzed in the lung by neutral endopeptidase and cathepsin H. More than 95% of proteins as insulin, are absorbed completely from the lung, So the metabolism of most proteins in the alveoli is not the main mechanism of clearance [49]. It is a blur to know the extent of metabolized proteins and peptidases, but Vasoactive intestinal polypeptide (VIP) is supposed to be finally degraded form through the passage across the pulmonary epithelium and into the blood circulation [49]. Various sources for the proteases, that hydrolyze the proteins and peptides, are like the alveolar macrophages and other inflammatory cells, as neutrophils. The higher level of proteases at the inflamed site of the lung impairs the efficacy of the aerosolized proteins and peptidases [51]. Therefore, to decrease the proteins' metabolism and improve their pulmonary absorption, co-administration with protease inhibitors as sodium glycocholate and bacitracin is necessary [52].

7.3.2 *The Optimal Site for Aerosol Therapy Deposition for Management of Lung Diseases*

The efficacy of inhaled drugs depends on two factors (the dose deposited and its distribution in the lung) but the effect of the drug distribution in the lung is still unclear. The effect of the drug might be impaired if the inhaled drug is administrated within suboptimal dose or to a site in the lung away from targeted disease or receptor. It is demonstrated that after administration of a small dose of inhaled histamine that deposited mainly in the central airways, it made an efficacy as 11 times the dose of inhaled histamine that deposited diffusely in the lung, indicating that the histamine receptors distributed predominantly in the central airways which affecting on drug response [53]. However, in the lung, other receptors are distributed irregularly as salbutamol (β2-agonist), and ipratropium bromide (M3 antagonist). As β receptors are mainly deposited in the alveolar wall but also, they are located in the airway smooth muscle with unknown significant effect. Two adrenergic receptors are present in high density in the airway epithelium from the wide bronchi to the terminal bronchioles, according to autoradiographic studies. The number of -receptors in airway smooth muscle is lower in the bronchioles than in the bronchi [54]. As well, submucosal glands and airway ganglia have a high density of M3 receptors and they are located in a moderate density in airway smooth muscles, alveolar walls, and nerves in intrapulmonary bronchi [55]. So, the drugs should be delivered to their target site according to the distribution of their receptors in the lung. For example, to ensure the therapeutic efficacy of salbutamol, it should be delivered to the medium and small airways in the lung, but ipratropium bromide should be delivered to the conducting airways. While anti-inflammatory aerosol therapy is distributed through the whole lung to produce the most beneficial efficacy, inflammatory cells, like eosinophils, macrophages, lymphocytes, and dendritic cells are distributed in the airways and at the alveolar tissue in asthma [56].

Also, it was demonstrated that to produce an identical bronchodilation effect of ipratropium bromide, it should be administrated at 3.3 μm or 7.7 μm aerosol, while the therapeutic efficacy of ipratropium bromide is greater when it administrated with 3.3 μm aerosol, suggesting that due to deliver drug aerosol to the site of their receptors in the lung which increase its efficacy [57]. So, the particle size of aerosol therapy affects its deposition in the lung and can increase the therapeutic efficacy of the drug. A study in asthmatic patients informed that when 250 μg terbutaline was administrated by a metered-dose inhaler (MDI) with three different particle sizes (10–15 μm, 5–10 μm and <5 μm), they produced a different therapeutic effect [58]. The smallest particle size of terbutaline (<5 μm) produced the best increase in specific airway conductance (saw), forced expiratory volume in 1 s (FEV1), and flow at 50% of vital capacity (V50), so the bronchodilation effect of smaller particle size of aerosols was more effective than that produced by a larger one, as in the narrowing airway, the smaller particle size has the best deposition and retention in the lung. Another study applied in asthmatic patients with mild to moderate case, demonstrated that when salbutamol aerosols administrated with three monodisperses (mass median aerodynamic diameter (MMAD) of 5 μm, 2.8 μm, 1.5 μm), It was founded that the aerosol with 2.8 μm particle size caused the greater bronchodilation effect than the other two aerosols [59]. The findings of the studies reported that the smallest particle size is better than the large particle size (5 μm) aerosol, as it penetrates more deeply into the lung than the larger particle size and thus, will produce more dilation effect in the small airways than the effect produced by larger particles, that filtered out in the upper airways. But the 2.8 μm aerosol produces more bronchodilation effect than the 1.5-μm aerosol, as the smallest aerosol is peripherally deposited and there is not a smooth muscle in the alveolar region and thus will produce less effect. So the ideal particle size for anticholinergic or β2 agonist aerosols to get the greatest bronchodilation effect is about 3 μm in asthmatic patients who have severe airflow obstruction (FEV1 $< 40\%$) [60].

To ensure the best therapeutic efficacy of antibiotics, it should be targeted to the site of infection to be treated in the respiratory tract. So, in pneumonia, effective antibiotic therapy should be distributed through the lungs. As in pneumonia shows a mixture of purulent tracheobronchitis and alveolar infection. *Pneumocystis carinii* that cause the most common life-threatening infection pneumonia between HIV patients, present predominately in the alveolar spaces and the apical region in case of relapse after treatment with inhaled pentamidine (1-μm MMAD) that happened due to the poorer apical deposition of the antibiotic [61]. The aerosol is more deposited in the lower lung than the upper lung because of the intrapleural pressure regional changes when standing or sitting in an upright position. The poorer apical deposition of 4 μm aerodynamic diameter aerosol is shown in an experiment by 2:1 ratio between the lower and upper lobes after analysis of the aerosol deposition sites in the normal lung at the upright position [62]. So, to reduce this gradient and increase the antibiotic deposition in the upper lung regions, aerosolized pentamidine should be administrated by patients in the supine position and thus will decrease the risk of relapse in the apical lobes of the lung [61].

The optimum inhaled antibiotic therapy's site of deposition in patients with chronic lung infection with Pseudomonas aeruginosa will be a uniform distribution in the conducting airways because infection initiates in the smaller airways then bronchioles and moves towards the larger airways and located in the airway lumen with a partial invasion of the lung parenchyma [63]. But the regions of highest infection, contain a large amount of mucus at the bronchi and bronchioles that may prevent deposition of aerosols in sites distal to the airway obstruction, and so it will reduce the clinical efficacy of the inhaled antibiotic [64].

7.4 Optimal Site of Aerosol Therapy Deposition for Management of Systemic Diseases

Pulmonary drug delivery is restricted to local therapy in the lung or nose because the accessible inhalation devices deposit in the lungs 10–15% of the released dose. The topical effect of steroids and bronchodilators is achieved by administrated a suitable lung dose using inhalation devices. But larger doses of the drug are required for the treatment of the systemic disease and achieving systemically therapeutic drug levels. Lately, progression in aerosol and formulation technologies is an aid in using pulmonary drug delivery as a route of administration for the treatment of the systemic disease as it has more advantages than oral, intravenous, transdermal, buccal, vaginal, nasal, or ocular routes of administration. This progression aids in producing small particles of aerosols that are deposited in the alveolar region in the lungs by large doses, so they allow more efficient systemic absorption.

The available administration routes of protein are intravenous, intramuscular, or subcutaneous injection. It cannot be absorbed into the blood circulation after oral administration as it digested before absorption, and also cannot be administered transdermally or intranasally because it cannot pass naturally via the skin or nasal membrane due to its large size. Insulin that has 5.7 kDa molecular weight and 2.2 nm in diameter, its peaks appear rapidly in the blood (15–60 min) after inhalation [65]. So, inhaled macromolecules that have low molecular weight (<40 kDa) and (<5–6 nm in diameter) are absorbed and appear in the blood rapidly. But albumin and α1-antitrypsin that have 68 kDa m.wt and 45–51 kDa m.wt respectively, are absorbed slowly and their peaks appear in the blood at 20 h and between 12 and 48 h, respectively [66]. Therefore, macromolecules that have a high molecular weight of more than 40 kDa and diameter >5–6 nm are absorbed slowly after inhalation and take many hours to appear in the blood.

The inhaled drugs overcome many barriers primarily as surface lining fluid, lung surfactant, epithelium, interstitium and basement membrane, and the endothelium, and then they are available to be absorbed into the bloodstream. The mechanism of the drug absorption is still unclear, but it has assumed that the drugs pass through the cell in different ways as large transitory pores in the epithelium which produced by apoptosis or cell injury, paracellular transport between trijunctions or junctions, or adsorptive or receptor-mediated (absorptive transcytosis) [49]. And its absorption is regulated with a thin alveolar–vascular permeable barrier. Pulmonary drug delivery promotes greater bioavailability of the deposited macromolecule in the lung (10–200 times) than gastrointestinal and nasal values, and also provide effective drug delivery to the blood circulation because the entire cardiac output passes through the lung only and the lung contains about (200–600 million) alveoli and a large surface area of epithelium with a single thin (0.2–0.7 μm thickness) cellular layer [67]. These large surface areas, thin cellular layer, antiprotease defense mechanism, and slow surface clearance allow an efficient gas change via passive transport and deliver the drug into the bloodstream efficiently [68].

References

1. Deng Q, et al. Particle deposition in the human lung: health implications of particulate matter from different sources. Environ Res. 2019;169:237–45.
2. Rossman CM, et al. Nasal ciliary ultrastructure and function in patients with primary ciliary dyskinesia compared with that in normal subjects and in subjects with various respiratory diseases. Am Rev Respir Dis. 1984;129(1):161–7.
3. Jabbal S, Poli G, Lipworth B. Does size really matter?: relationship of particle size to lung deposition and exhaled fraction. J Allergy Clin Immunol. 2017;139(6):2013–2014.e1.
4. Haidl P, et al. Inhalation device requirements for patients' inhalation maneuvers. Respir Med. 2016;118:65–75.

5. Amirav I, et al. Nasal versus oral aerosol delivery to the "lungs" in infants and toddlers. Pediatr Pulmonol. 2015;50(3):276–83.
6. Fang C-P, et al. Effect of lung airway branching pattern and gas composition on particle deposition in bronchial airways: III. Experimental studies with radioactively tagged aerosol in human and canine lungs. Exp Lung Res. 1993;19(3):377–96.
7. Esch JL, Spektor DM, Lippmann M. Effect of lung airway branching pattern and gas composition on particle deposition. II. Experimental studies in human and canine lungs. Exp Lung Res. 1988;14(3):321–48.
8. Perinel S, et al. Micron-sized and submicron-sized aerosol deposition in a new ex vivo preclinical model. Respir Res. 2016;17(1):78.
9. Kadota K, et al. Effects of inhalation procedure on particle behavior and deposition in the airways analyzed by numerical simulation. J Taiwan Inst Chem Eng. 2018;90:44–50.
10. Finlay W, et al. Validating deposition models in disease: what is needed? J Aerosol Med. 2000;13(4):381–5.
11. FARR SJ. The physico-chemical basis of radiolabelling metered dose inhalers with 99mTc. J Aerosol Med. 1996;9(s1):S27–36.
12. Cheng YS. Mechanisms of pharmaceutical aerosol deposition in the respiratory tract. AAPS PharmSciTech. 2014;15(3):630–40.
13. Dolovich M. Physical principles underlying aerosol therapy. J Aerosol Med. 1989;2(2):171–86.
14. Sheth P, Stein SW, Myrdal PB. Factors influencing aerodynamic particle size distribution of suspension pressurized metered dose inhalers. AAPS PharmSciTech. 2015;16(1):192–201.
15. Dekhuijzen PR, et al. Incidence of oral thrush in patients with COPD prescribed inhaled corticosteroids: effect of drug, dose, and device. Respir Med. 2016;120:54–63.
16. Matera MG, et al. Safety of inhaled corticosteroids for treating chronic obstructive pulmonary disease. Expert Opin Drug Saf. 2015;14(4):533–41.
17. Postma DS, et al. Asthma-related outcomes in patients initiating extrafine ciclesonide or fine-particle inhaled corticosteroids. Allergy, Asthma Immunol Res. 2017;9(2):116–25.
18. Lourenço RV, Cotromanes E. Clinical aerosols: I. Characterization of aerosols and their diagnostic uses. Arch Intern Med. 1982;142(12):2163–72.
19. Chen X, et al. Numerical investigation of particle deposition in a triple bifurcation airway due to gravitational sedimentation and inertial impaction. Powder Technol. 2018;323:284–93.
20. Sera T, et al. Numerical simulation of airflow and microparticle deposition in a synchrotron micro-CT-based pulmonary acinus model. Comput Methods Biomech Biomed Engin. 2015;18(13):1427–35.
21. Gonda I. Targeting by deposition, in Pharmaceutical Inhalation Aerosol Technology. 2nd ed. Boca Raton: CRC Press; 2016. p. 84–104.
22. Inthavong K, et al. Micron particle deposition in a tracheobronchial airway model under different breathing conditions. Med Eng Phys. 2010;32(10):1198–212.
23. Talaat K, Xi J. Computational modeling of aerosol transport, dispersion, and deposition in rhythmically expanding and contracting terminal alveoli. J Aerosol Sci. 2017;112:19–33.
24. Nicolaou L. Inertial and gravitational effects on aerosol deposition in the conducting airways. J Aerosol Sci. 2018;120:32–51.
25. Koullapis P, et al. Regional aerosol deposition in the human airways: the SimInhale benchmark case and a critical assessment of in silico methods. Eur J Pharm Sci. 2018;113:77–94.
26. Fonceca AM, et al. Drug administration by inhalation in children. In: Kendig's disorders of the respiratory tract in children, 9th ed. Elsevier; 2019. p. 257–271.e3.
27. Thoonen B, et al. Self-management of asthma in general practice, asthma control and quality of life: a randomised controlled trial. Thorax. 2003;58(1):30–6.
28. Guevara JP, et al. Effects of educational interventions for self management of asthma in children and adolescents: systematic review and meta-analysis. BMJ. 2003;326(7402):1308–9.
29. Aydemir Y. Assessment of the factors affecting the failure to use inhaler devices before and after training. Respir Med. 2015;109(4):451–8.

30. Newman SP. Aerosol deposition considerations in inhalation therapy. Chest. 1985;88(2):152S–60S.
31. Bartolo K, et al. Predictors of correct technique in patients using pressurized metered dose inhalers. BMC Pulm Med. 2017;17(1):47.
32. Spin P, et al. A cost analysis of salbutamol administration by metered-dose inhalers with spacers versus nebulization for patients with wheeze in the pediatric emergency department: evidence from observational data in Nova Scotia. Can J Emerg Med. 2017;19(1):1–8.
33. Al-Subu AM, et al. Aerosol therapy through high flow nasal cannula in pediatric patients. Expert Rev Respir Med. 2017;11(12):945–53.
34. Lexmond AJ, et al. Prerequisites for a dry powder inhaler for children with cystic fibrosis. PLoS One. 2017;12(8):e0183130.
35. Ammari WG, Chrystyn H. Optimizing the inhalation flow and technique through metered dose inhalers of asthmatic adults and children attending a community pharmacy. J Asthma. 2013;50(5):505–13.
36. Nicola M, et al. The impact of adding a training device to familiar counselling on inhalation technique and pulmonary function of asthmatics. Adv Ther. 2018;35(7):1049–58.
37. Rogliani P, et al. Optimizing drug delivery in COPD: the role of inhaler devices. Respir Med. 2017;124:6–14.
38. Cheng KH, et al. Measurements of airway dimensions and calculation of mass transfer characteristics of the human oral passage. 1997.
39. Xi J, Longest PW. Transport and deposition of micro-aerosols in realistic and simplified models of the oral airway. Ann Biomed Eng. 2007;35(4):560–81.
40. Zhou Y, Sun J, Cheng Y-S. Comparison of deposition in the USP and physical mouth–throat models with solid and liquid particles. J Aerosol Med Pulm Drug Deliv. 2011;24(6):277–84.
41. Clark A, Newman S, Dasovich N. Mouth and oropharyngeal deposition of pharmaceutical aerosols. J Aerosol med. 1998;11(s1):S-116–21.
42. DeHaan WH, Finlay WH. In vitro monodisperse aerosol deposition in a mouth and throat with six different inhalation devices. J Aerosol Med. 2001;14(3):361–7.
43. Brain J, Blanchard J. Aerosols in medicine: principles, diagnosis and therapy. New York: Elsevier Science Publishers; 1993.
44. Smaldone G, et al. Interpretation of "24 hour lung retention" in studies of mucociliary clearance. J Aerosol Med. 1988;1(1):11–20.
45. Houtmeyers E, et al. Regulation of mucociliary clearance in health and disease. Eur Respir J. 1999;13(5):1177–88.
46. Isawa T, et al. Mucociliary clearance and transport in bronchiectasis: global and regional assessment. J Nucl Med. 1990;31(5):543–8.
47. Effros RM. Measurements of pulmonary epithelial permeability in vivo. Am Rev Respir Dis. 1983;127:S59–65.
48. Summers Q. Inhaled drugs and the lung. Clin Exp Allergy. 1991;21(3):259–68.
49. Folkesson H, et al. Alveolar epithelial clearance of protein. J Appl Physiol. 1996;80(5):1431–45.
50. Upton RN, Doolette DJ. Kinetic aspects of drug disposition in the lungs. Clin Exp Pharmacol Physiol. 1999;26(5–6):381–91.
51. Bhat M, et al. Drug metabolism and enzyme kinetics in the lung. Lung Biol Health Dis. 2007;221:147.
52. Yamamoto A, Umemori S, Muranishi S. Absorption enhancement of intrapulmonary administered insulin by various absorption enhancers and protease inhibitors in rats. J Pharm Pharmacol. 1994;46(1):14–8.
53. Ruffin R, et al. The effects of preferential deposition of histamine in the human airway. Am Rev Respir Dis. 1978;117(3):485–92.
54. Carstairs J, Nimmo A, Barnes PJ. Autoradiographic visualization of beta-adrenoceptor subtypes in human lung. Am Rev Respir Dis. 1985;132(3):541–7.
55. Mak J, Barnes PJ. Autoradiographic visualization of muscarinic receptor subtypes in human and Guinea pig lung. Am Rev Respir Dis. 1990;141(6):1559–68.

56. Carroll N, Cooke C, James A. The distribution of eosinophils and lymphocytes in the large and small airways of asthmatics. Eur Respir J. 1997;10(2):292–300.
57. Johnson MA, et al. Delivery of albuterol and ipratropium bromide from two nebulizer systems in chronic stable asthma: efficacy and pulmonary deposition. Chest. 1989;96(1):6–10.
58. Rees P, Clark T, Moren F. The importance of particle size in response to inhaled bronchodilators. Eur J Respir Dis. 1982;119:73–8.
59. Zanen P, Go LT, Lammers J-WJ. The optimal particle size for β-adrenergic aerosols in mild asthmatics. Int J Pharm. 1994;107(3):211–7.
60. Zanen P, Go LT, Lammers J. Optimal particle size for beta 2 agonist and anticholinergic aerosols in patients with severe airflow obstruction. Thorax. 1996;51(10):977–80.
61. Baskin MI, Abd AG, Ilowite JS. Regional deposition of aerosolized pentamidine: effects of body position and breathing pattern. Ann Intern Med. 1990;113(9):677–83.
62. Gerrity T, Garrard C, Yeates D. Theoretic analysis of sites of aerosol deposition in the human lung. Chest. 1981;80(6 Suppl):898–901.
63. Tena AF, Clarà PC. Deposition of inhaled particles in the lungs. Arch Bronconeumol. 2012;48(7):240–6.
64. Anderson PJ, et al. Effect of cystic fibrosis on inhaled aerosol boluses 1–3. Am Rev Respir Dis. 1989;140:1317–24.
65. Mastrandrea LD. Inhaled insulin: overview of a novel route of insulin administration. Vasc Health Risk Manag. 2010;6:47.
66. Byron PR, PATTON JS. Drug delivery via the respiratory tract. J Aerosol Med. 1994;7(1):49–75.
67. Hickey AJ, Mansour HM. Inhalation aerosols: physical and biological basis for therapy, vol. 1. Boca Raton: CRC Press; 2019.
68. Patton JS. Mechanisms of macromolecule absorption by the lungs. Adv Drug Deliv Rev. 1996;19(1):3–36.

Chapter 8
Factors Affecting Aerosol Deposition in Critically Ill Patient

Contents

8.1 Introduction

The inhaled therapies are rapidly expanding for treating systemic as well as pulmonary disorders. The lung is a major route by which inhaled therapies could reach the systemic circulation especially for drugs with a relatively poor systemic bioavailability through the gastrointestinal tract (GIT) (e.g., beclomethasone, only about 20% of drug reaches the systemic circulation through GIT) [1]. Also, many inhaled medications are commonly administered to critically ill patients undergoing mechanical ventilation for treating various pulmonary disorders such as short and long-acting bronchodilators (B agonists and anticholinergics), inhaled corticosteroids (ICS), antibiotics, antibacterial, antiviral, antifungal, mucolytic, prostaglandins, proteins and surfactant [2, 3]. Several factors affect aerosol delivery during mechanical ventilation. These factors can be classified into five main categories: ventilator-related factors, circuit-related factors, device-related factors, drug-related factors, and patient-related factors (Table 8.1) [3]. The lack of knowledge of these

M. E. A. Abdelrahim et al., *Essentials of Aerosol Therapy in Critically ill Patients*,
https://doi.org/10.1007/978-3-030-85026-5_8

Table 8.1 Factors affecting aerosol delivery in mechanically ventilated patients [3]

Type of factors	Factors
Ventilator-related	Ventilation mode Respiratory rate Tidal volume Duty cycle Breath-triggering mechanism Inspiratory wave-form
Circuit-related	Humidity of gas Density of gas Endotracheal tube size
Device-related	*pMDIs:* Type of spacer/adapter Position of the spacer in the circuit Type of pMDI Timing of pMDI actuation
	Nebulizers: Type of nebulizer Position of the nebulizer in the circuit Mode of nebulization Gas-flow Fill volume Nebulization duration
Drug-related	Aerosol particle size The target site for delivery Formulation Dose Onset and duration of action
Patient-related	Type of lung disease Severity of disease Presence of dynamic hyperinflation Patient-ventilator synchrony

factors leads to suboptimal practice during treatment of mechanically ventilated patients caused by a significant loss of aerosol in the ventilator circuits and artificial airways which decreases the efficiency of pulmonary drug delivery of aerosol [3]. A clear understanding and attention to these factors are very important in optimizing the efficiency of aerosol delivery to critically ill patients [4, 5].

8.2 Discussion and Analysis of Main Topics

In the past, the efficiency of aerosol delivery was impaired by extensive drug deposition within the ventilator-circuit and artificial airway owing to many factors such as circuit humidity [6]. It was repeatedly reported that the efficiency of aerosol delivery was significantly lower in mechanically ventilated patients if compared to ambulatory patients [7, 8]. For routine aerosol therapy in mechanically ventilated patients, higher doses are needed than that employed in ambulatory patients to compensate for the extensive drug deposition in the ventilator circuit. Improvement in techniques of aerosol delivery and development of newer aerosol generators enhanced the efficiency of aerosol delivery in mechanically ventilated patients to a level that matches and may even exceed that reported in spontaneously breathing ambulatory patients [9]. Now, administering inhaled therapies to mechanically ventilated patients has a firmly established scientific basis. Knowledge and understanding of principles of aerosol delivery in those patients have evolved rapidly [10, 11]. Successful aerosol therapy during mechanical ventilation depends on optimal drug deposition at the intended sites within the lung. Optimizing drug delivery to the lung in the mechanically ventilated patient requires consideration of a host of factors that significantly influence aerosol drug delivery [12].

8.2.1 Ventilator-Related Factors

First of all, characteristics of the ventilator breath significantly influence aerosol drug delivery. Spontaneous modes have been proven to be more comfortable and effective than controlled modes (either volume-controlled (VC) or pressure-controlled (PC)) in optimizing aerosol drug delivery during mechanical ventilation. That was attributed to the fact that during spontaneous modes the patient can modify both the timing and size of each breath, which in turn encourage synchrony with the ventilator [4]. For example, a study compared continuous positive air pressure (CPAP) with controlled ventilation modes at equivalent tidal volume (Vt). It was concluded that CPAP increased aerosol drug delivery by up to 30% compared to controlled modes [13]. Therefore, spontaneous modes of breathing should be recommended, if tolerable by the patient. When spontaneous modes are non-tolerable, controlled modes could be then considered. The main advantage of VC ventilation is the high stability of Vt with changing lung mechanics. However, PC ventilation could provide more stable ventilatory support than VC if there is a significant and variable leak like that in non-invasive ventilation (NIV) [14]. The nebulizer efficiency during NIV was found to be lower in PC mode if compared to VC mode in patients with low compliance and low resistance. However, pressurized metered-dose inhaler (pMDI) efficiency was similar with both controlled modalities [15].

Moreover, Vt of $\geq$500 mL (in an adult) emphasizes that the dead space is cleared of aerosol, which enhances aerosol drug delivery to the lower respiratory tract [13]. Low Vt decreases aerosol drug delivery to the lower respiratory tract. Also, longer inspiratory time and slower inspiratory flow enhance aerosol drug delivery in both ambulatory [16] and mechanically ventilated patients [13]. Drug delivery is linearly correlated with a longer duty cycle (ratio of inspiratory time to total breathing cycle time) with both pMDIs and nebulizers [13, 17]. With duty cycles of 0.3 or greater, pMDI drug delivery was significantly better with a slower inspiratory flow (40 L/min) if compared with a faster inspiratory flow (80 L/min) [17]. It is recommended to use an inspiratory flow of 30–50 L/min if tolerated [4]. Higher inspiratory flow increases turbulence and inertial impaction; thereby reduces aerosol drug delivery. Moreover, aerosol drug delivery is better when the pMDI is synchronized with a simulated spontaneous breath than with a controlled breath of similar Vt. During spontaneous breaths, the amount of aerosol drug delivered increased with higher Vt (an effect that was not observed with other mechanical ventilation modes) [13].

The use of a breath-triggering mechanism (bias flow) with a nebulizer could dilute the aerosol and increase the washout of the aerosol into the expiratory limb between breaths. Therefore, it was recommended to use a lower bias flow of ≤2 L/min with nebulizers [4]. However, the bias flow could not significantly influence aerosol drug delivery from a pMDI [13]. The additional gas flow of the nebulizer could interfere with the ventilator's ability to sense the onset of the patient's inspiration. Also, the type of ventilator used affects the efficiency of aerosol drug delivery with a nebulizer [18, 19]. Matching the ventilator with the nebulizer is required to better control the aerosol drug delivery in mechanically ventilated patients.

The influence of the inspiratory flow pattern (the inspiratory waveform) on aerosol drug delivery was recently studied. The inspiratory waveform during PC ventilation mode differs from that of VC ventilation mode. Also, the lung mechanics affect both the duration of inspiratory flow and inspiratory flow pattern during PC ventilation mode. Square waveform delivers less aerosol than a decreasing ramp or sinusoidal waveform. The aerosol drug delivery efficiency of the air-jet nebulizer (JN) was reported to be affected by the inspiratory flow pattern, inspiratory time, lung mechanics and was significantly lower during PC ventilation mode if compared to that during VC ventilation mode ($p = 0.03$). In contrast, the efficiency of aerosol drug delivery from a pMDI was not affected by any of these factors and remained remarkably consistent [15].

8.2.2 *Circuit-Related Factors*

Firstly, patient interfaces pose a significant barrier to effective aerosol drug delivery. Endotracheal tube (ETT) and tracheostomy are the interfaces used for invasive mechanical ventilation [20]. However, NIV circuits include more variable interfaces including; nasal masks, oro-nasal masks, total face masks, helmets, nasal pillows, and mouthpieces with or without the oral mask [128].

All NIV interfaces show common unintentional leaks between the skin and the interface [21]. The selection of patient interface must depend on patient tolerance and preference [22]. Oro-nasal masks and nasal masks are the most common interfaces for NIV [5]. The Tight-fitting of the interface is the most important factor determining the success of aerosol therapy. On the other hand, overfitting of the interface may cause skin breakdown [23, 24].

In infant and pediatric invasive mechanical ventilation, there was a significant aerosol impaction on the endotracheal tube (ETT) (ETT internal diameter of 3–6 mm) [25, 26]. However, in adult invasive mechanical ventilation, there was no difference in nebulizer efficiency with ETT of internal diameter 7 mm versus an internal diameter of 9 mm [27]. Drug losses within the ETT could be reduced by placing the aerosol generator at a distance from the ETT instead of being proximal to it [6]. In vitro studies show minimal drug deposition within ETTs with JNs, however, significant ETT deposition of aerosol occurs with ultrasonic nebulizers (USNs) [28]. When a pMDI with spacer is employed, the presence of humidity in the circuit enhanced aerosol deposition in the ETT by approximately three fold [10, 13, 17]. Aerosol deposition in tracheostomy tubes has not been well studied in as much detail as ETT. One study found that approximately 10% of the nominal dose from a nebulizer was deposited in the tracheostomy tube of mechanically ventilated patients with a majority of aerosol deposition (approximately 7%) occurred during exhalation [29]. But in vitro studies are unable to accurately determine aerosol deposition during exhalation, so that such studies could significantly underestimate the actual aerosol loss in the artificial airway [3].

Additionally, the gas in the ventilator circuit is usually heated and humidified to prevent the dryness of the airway mucosa. Humidification leads to a higher aerosol deposition in the ventilator circuit [17] and decreases aerosol drug delivery to the lower respiratory tract from both pMDIs and nebulizers by ≥40% if compared with a dry circuit [10, 18, 30]. On the other hand, bypassing the humidifier is not recommended in mechanically ventilated patients. The impact of humidity on aerosol drug delivery can be overcome by delivering higher drug doses with careful attention to the administration technique [31–33]. Also, dry-circuit conditions could be employed for delivery of very expensive and critical drugs (e.g., antibiotics and prostaglandins) but in this case, drug administration should be achieved within a short period (<10–15 min) to minimize the effects of dry gas on the airway mucosa.

Heat and moisture exchangers (HMEs) are passive humidification systems that transfer part of the heat and moisture from the exhaled breath to the next inspired breath. They are often employed to provide humidification of inspired air during mechanical ventilation [34]. The filter in the HME is a barrier to efficient aerosol drug delivery and the device must be removed from the circuit during aerosol delivery. Also, placement of nebulizers between the HME and patient airway may overload the HME and increase work of breathing, it must be avoided [4]. The Circuvent (DHD Health Care Corp. Wampsville, New York) allows aerosol drug delivery without removing the HME from the circuit by turning a dial on the device, a piece of tubing bypasses the HME. After aerosol generation is completed, the dial is turned back to allow inspiratory airflow to pass through the HME [3].

Moreover, the Inhalation of a low-density gas such as helium-oxygen (heliox) 80/20 or 70/30 mixture, which is less dense than air or oxygen, improves aerosol drug delivery in both pediatric and adult models of mechanical ventilation [35, 36]. Similarly, studies in ambulatory patients have shown higher aerosol retention in the lungs when patients breathed heliox instead of air [37, 38]. Heliox creates the persistence of laminar flows in the airways improving aerosol deposition by decreasing particle-impaction losses. With pMDIs, there was a 50% increase in the amount of aerosol delivered to the lower respiratory tract with the use of heliox if compared to air or oxygen [36]. In contrast, JN operation with heliox reduced both the drug output and respirable mass, requiring two fold higher flows, which may alter ventilator parameters [36, 39]. A practical method to enhance aerosol drug delivery from a JN during mechanical ventilation is to operate the nebulizer with oxygen at a flow rate of 6–8 L/min and to entrain the aerosol generated into a ventilator-circuit containing heliox [36]. Moreover, VMNs and USNs generate aerosol without being affected by heliox [4].

Finally, many ventilator circuits incorporate a right-angle elbow adapter between the ETT and the 'Y' adapter which connects the inspiratory and expiratory limb of the circuit. Using a right-angle elbow adapter decreases aerosol drug delivery from a pMDI on a humidified ventilator circuit but not on a non-humidified circuit. It was reported that the removal of the right-angle elbow adapter enhanced the aerosol drug delivery from a pMDI on a humidified ventilator circuit but not on a non-humidified circuit. It is unclear whether the efficiency gained by removing the elbow is not lost further down the airway [17]..

8.2.3 Device-Related Factors

Both nebulizers and pMDIs are used to deliver inhaled therapies to mechanically ventilated patients. The majority of drug particles in pMDI and nebulizer aerosols are in the range of 1–5 μm. Larger aerosol particles are trapped in the ventilator circuit and patient interface. pMDIs are chiefly used to deliver B adrenergic and anticholinergic bronchodilators and corticosteroids. Nebulizers have been used to deliver antibiotics, mucolytics, prostaglandins, and surfactants in addition to bronchodilators and corticosteroids [12].

Firstly, the position of the aerosol generator in the ventilator circuit significantly affects its efficiency in delivering drugs to the lower respiratory tract. It varies according to the type of ventilation circuit; in a single-limb circuit, the aerosol generator is commonly placed between the patient interface and the expiration port more proximal to the patient. In the dual-limb circuit, the JN was more efficient when placed closer to the ventilator, however, other aerosol generators like the vibrating mesh nebulizer (VMN), USN, and pMDI, that do not add flow into the ventilator circuit, were more efficient when placed 6 inches from the Y adapter than when it is placed close to the ventilator [4, 5]. Placing the JN at a distance from the ETT offers higher efficiency than placing it between the patient Y-piece and the ETT [27, 40] because the ventilator circuit serves as a spacer for aerosol to accumulate between inspirations. Adding a reservoir between the nebulizer and ETT also modestly enhances the efficiency of aerosol drug delivery [41]. One preliminary investigation found that placing a JN proximal to the humidifier (between the ventilator and the humidifier) significantly enhanced the efficiency of aerosol drug delivery in a heated, humidified ventilator circuit [42].

Moreover, the efficiency of aerosol generation differs markedly among different aerosol generators [27, 43]. Hassan et al. observed that a 2 mg salbutamol delivered by pMDI with a spacer was equal to 3 mg delivered by VMN and 5 mg delivered by JN [44]. Commercially available pMDIs are designed for use with ambulatory patients. For a pMDI to be employed in a ventilator circuit, the canister must be removed from the actuator and connected to the ventilator circuit with a different adapter. Several types of commercially available adapters are used to connect the pMDI canister to the ventilator circuit [45]. When a pMDI canister is uncoupled from its original actuator and employed with a different actuator (the various circuit adapters), it becomes part of a different device that has different aerosol characteristics and performance. For example, using the canister of a chlorofluorocarbon (CFC) propellant pMDI in the actuator of a hydrofluoroalkane (HFA) propellant pMDI (or vice versa) would change the aerosol properties and aerosol drug delivery [17].

Similarly, the type of pMDI propellant formulation [46], and the drug formulation can also affect aerosol drug delivery [45]. Adapters that are used to connect a pMDI to ventilator circuit include elbow adapters, inline devices (unidirectional or bidirectional), and chamber or reservoir adapters [47]. An elbow adapter connects to the ETT, whereas the inline and chamber adapters are placed in the inspiratory limb of the ventilator circuit. With a chamber spacer, the pMDI aerosol has an opportunity to slow, and propellant evaporation decreases the size of the aerosol particles. Both of those phenomena reduce aerosol drug loss caused by inertial impaction on the walls of the ventilator circuit and ETT. In contrast, when a pMDI is employed with an adapter connected directly to the ETT, considerable aerosol loss occurs within the ETT, which may result in negligible therapeutic effects, even after administration of up to 100 pMDI doses [48]. Several investigators have shown that employing a chamber spacer with a pMDI in a ventilator circuit results in four- to six-fold greater aerosol drug delivery than either an elbow adapter or a unidirectional inline spacer [49–52]. A bidirectional inline spacer increases the volume of air into which the aerosol is actuated and correspondingly produces a 1.5–2.5 fold increase in aerosol drug delivery, compared with a unidirectional inline spacer [45]. The efficiency of aerosol drug delivery with a pMDI and bidirectional inline spacer was reported to be comparable with that achieved with chamber spacers [45]. A pMDI with a chamber spacer connected to the circuit at approximately 6 inches from the ETT provides efficient aerosol drug delivery to mechanically ventilated patients [33]. Moreover, careful attention to optimal inhaler technique is essential during mechanical ventilation [4]. When using pMDI, it is important to wait at 15 s or greater intervals between actuations to allow proper propellant evaporation. Also, the drug in the pMDI formulations is separated when standing. Therefore, it is recommended to shake the inhaler before each actuation [53]. Not shaking a pMDI canister reduces total and respirable dose up to 35% [4, 54]. Also, the actuation of a pMDI must be synchronized with the precise onset of inspiratory airflow from the ventilator [50].

Factors that affect nebulizer efficiency are, nebulizer type, operating pressure and/or flow, diluent volume, and the duration of treatment. VMNs are specifically designed for use in a ventilator circuit. It has higher aerosol delivery efficiency than conventional JN [55], and in contrast to USN, the VMN does not increase the temperature of the solution during nebulization [56]. As with JN, aerosol drug delivery from a USN is significantly reduced by humidity in the ventilator circuit [42].VMNs is a good alternative for aerosol drug delivery in mechanically ventilated patients because aerosol deposition with USNs and VMNs is more than 10% without the addition of low-dense gas into the ventilator circuit [2]. Also, the greater the dead volume, the less amount of drug is nebulized. JNs do not aerosolize below a dead volume of 1–2.5 mL. VMN nebulizers have smaller residual volumes than JN or USNs. Previous studies showed that >50% of the nebulized drug was retained in JNs and tubing with lower aerosol drug delivery to lungs which proves the inefficiency of such types of nebulizers [57, 58]. When the standard JN is used under normal heated humidification conditions, aerosol deposition varies between 1 and 3%. This can be increased to 15% if the ventilator settings and other factors are optimized. Attempts to improve the aerosol delivery of JNs were successively conducted by diluting the nebulized solution by either water or saline with a longer nebulization time (a fill volume of 4–5 mL is preferred) and encouraging the intermittent nebulization of respiratory solution over continuous delivery [59, 60]. If they are run continuously, the flow rate should be set at 6–8 L/min and the ventilator parameters such as Vt and pressure should be adjusted accordingly [2]. Intermittent operation of the nebulizer that is synchronized with inspiratory airflow from the ventilator is more efficient for aerosol drug delivery, compared with a continuous aerosol generation [18]. That aids in minimizes aerosol wastage during the exhalation phase of the breathing cycle [3]. Moreover, the higher the gas pressure and/or flow to the nebulizer, the smaller the particle size generated [43, 61]. Table 8.2 summarizes possible recommendations to optimize aerosol delivery in mechanically ventilated patients [4, 5].

8.2.4 Drug-Related Factors

The efficiency of aerosolized therapies is dependent upon the effective dose (amount deposited in the lung) and its distribution. If a drug aerosol is delivered at a suboptimal dose or to a different part of the lung other than that of the target disease or receptor, the effectiveness of therapy is significantly reduced [62]. Muscarinic receptors are mostly located in the medium and large airways, although muscarinic antagonist effects also occur in the small airways. The Beta receptors and corticosteroid receptors are distributed throughout the airways [63]. Large, medium, and small airways (generations from 8 to 23 with internal diameter < 2 mm) are significantly affected in asthma and chronic obstructive pulmonary disease (COPD). Therefore, aerosol drug delivery throughout the airways is desirable [64]. Airway smooth muscle, which is affected by bronchodilators, is denser in medium and larger airways than that in the terminal and respiratory bronchioles [1]. The optimal site of deposition of aerosolized antibiotics in the respiratory tract depends on the infection being treated. Many types of pneumonia represent a mixture of tracheobronchitis and alveolar infection for which a successful therapy requires the antibiotic to be evenly distributed throughout the lungs. However, those confined to the alveolar region would probably benefit from a greater peripheral aerosol penetration

Table 8.2 Possible recommendations to optimize aerosol delivery in mechanically ventilated patients [4, 5]

Factors	Recommendations
Mode of ventilation	– Prefer VC ventilation mode when using a nebulizer in patients with low compliance and low resistance, if possible – Use spontaneous modes, if tolerable by patients
Vt	– Set Vt greater than the volume of tubing and ETT between the nebulizer and the patient. For adults, it should be set to ≥500 mL, if appropriate for the patient
Inspiratory time and duty cycle	– Increase inspiratory time while minimizing the degree of iPEEP. A duty cycle of 0.3 or greater is recommended
Inspiratory flow	– Use an inspiratory flow of 30–50 L/min, if tolerated
Breath-triggering mechanism (bias flow)	– Use lower bias flow ≤2 L/min with nebulizers – Synchronize the actuations with inspiration when using pMDIs
Inspiratory waveform	– Choose sinusoidal or decreasing ramp waveforms
Patient interface	– Oro-nasal masks and nasal masks are the best interfaces for NIV (consider tight-fitting) – For invasive ventilation, place the largest diameter ETT that the patient can safely tolerate and keep it clear of secretions
Heat /humidity	– Remove the HME before aerosol generation and place it back into the circuit after the treatment – Apply the Circuvent during aerosol generation – Do not place nebulizers between the HME and patient airway – Increase the dose, as needed for clinical response – Do not remove the heated humidifier from the circuit, except for expensive drugs (short term <10–15 min)
The density of inhaled gas	– Use heliox 80:20 or 70:30 for optimal delivery of aerosols through the ventilator circuit – Do not dilute less than 50:50 for effect – Use a lower flow of oxygen to power JN. If you do use heliox, increase the flow rate by two fold – Use VMN, USN, or pMDI with spacer when using heliox
Right-angle elbow adapter	– Remove the right-angle elbow adapter, when using a humidified ventilator circuit
Position of aerosol generator in the circuit	– In a single-limb circuit, the aerosol generator is commonly placed more proximal to the patient – In a dual-limb circuit, place the JN closer to the ventilator – Place the pMDI, VMN, and USNs in the inspiratory limb 6 inches from the Y adapter
pMDI-related factors	– Synchronize pMDI actuations with inspiration. Actuate at 15 s or greater intervals – Use chamber spacers with the pMDIs for aerosol administration to mechanically ventilated patients – Bidirectional inline adapters are a better option than unidirectional low-volume spacers – Shake the pMDI before the first actuation of each dose (up to eight puffs) administered

(continued)

Table 8.2 (continued)

Factors	Recommendations
Nebulizer-related factors	– Choose the VMN, USN, or pMDI with spacer for aerosol drug delivery in mechanically ventilated patients – Run the JN intermittently, if the ventilator has that option – Set the flow rate at 6–8 L/min or as recommended by the manufacturer and adjust the ventilator parameters (Vt and pressure), if you run the JN continuously – Use the VMN nebulizer when possible – In the absence of the VMN nebulizer, use a fill volume of 4–5 mLl unless the JN is specifically designed for a smaller fill volume – Use USN or VMN for aerosol delivery, when possible – Set the flow rate at 6–8 L/min or as recommended by the manufacturer and adjust the ventilator parameters (Vt and pressure), if you run the JN continuously

VC volume-controlled, *Vt* tidal volume, *ETT* endotracheal tube, *iPEEP* intrinsic positive end-expiratory pressure, *pMDI* pressurized metered-dose inhaler, *NIV* non-invasive ventilation, *HME* heat and moisture exchanger, *JN* air-jet nebulizer, *VMN* vibrating mesh nebulizer, *USN* ultrasonic nebulizer

and deposition. Targeting the aerosolized medications to their intended sites within airways can be accomplished by altering the aerosol particle size and/or the inspiratory flow rate [62].

Aerosol particle size is the first determinant of aerosol deposition in the lungs. Three processes affect aerosol drug deposition: inertial impaction, sedimentation, and diffusion. Inertial impaction and sedimentation of aerosols are the dominant mechanisms of deposition of most inhaled medications [62]. Depending on the characteristics of the aerosol, device, and patient, a part of the drug is swallowed and absorbed into the systemic circulation and/or is excreted through the GIT. Larger particles tend to early deposit by inertial impaction in the oropharynx and large conducting airways particularly at airway bifurcations and areas of obstruction, whereas smaller particles tend to deposit in the small conducting and distal airways, including the alveoli and terminal bronchioles. Sedimentation of aerosolized particles depends on gravity, residence time in the airway (breath-hold time), airway dimensions, and patient position. The inhaled drugs most likely to reach the airways, and thus exert local clinical effects, are aerosol particles in the fine-particle fraction (FPF) of 1–5 μm. It was concluded that deposition of particles 3–7 μm occurs largely in the conducting airways, whereas particles <2–3 μm can reach the alveoli, particularly those <1 μm. Particles <0.5–1 μm undergo Brownian motion, settle very slowly, and maybe re-exhaled or may diffuse into the pulmonary capillaries after impaction [1, 62]. Each deposition process occurs rapidly, allowing the drug to exert its effects within minutes before entering the systemic circulation. The FPF varies widely among inhalers, with 12–35% for dry powder inhaler (DPI), 10–50% for pMDI, and 30–50% for the soft mist inhaler (SMI) [63, 65].

Not only is the lung deposition of an aerosol affected by particle size, but also the clinical effectiveness of the aerosol. It was shown that the bronchodilation response to cumulative doses of salbutamol delivered either as a 3.3 μm or 7.7 μm aerosol was significantly higher with the finer (3.3 μm) aerosol, suggesting that targeting drug aerosol to its receptor location in the lung significantly influence its effectiveness [66]. Rees et al. reported a varying clinical effect of 250 mg of aerosolized terbutaline given by a pMDI either as <5 μm, 5–10 μm, or 10–15 μm in asthmatics. The highest improvement of forced expiratory volume in 1 s (FEV1), specific airway conductance (sGaw) and flow at 50% of vital capacity (V50) was reported with <5 μm aerosol, suggesting that smaller particle size was considerably more effective than larger particle size in producing bronchodilation owing to best penetration and retention in the lungs [67]. Also, a study examined the effect of equal doses of salbutamol and ipratropium bromide of three different particle size aerosols (1.5 μm, 2.8 μm, and 5 μm) on the lung functions. Their findings suggest that smaller particle size penetrate more deeply into the lung and exert more bronchodilation of the small airways than larger particles but the 1.5 μm aerosol induced significantly less bronchodilation than the 2.8 μm aerosol, suggesting that particle size of 1.5 μm may be deposited too peripherally to be effective since smooth muscle is not present in the alveolar region. Therefore, the optimal particle size for B2 agonist or anticholinergic aerosols was proven to be about 3 μm [68, 69].

Inhaled drugs are either cleared from the lungs, absorbed into the systemic circulation, or metabolized [62]. Clearance of drugs from the lungs is affected by pharmacokinetic properties including half-life (t1/2), and physicochemical properties, such as lipophilicity/hydrophilicity, solubility, molecular weight, protein-binding, and charge. Hydrophilic molecules cross the airway epithelium via extracellular pathways and lipophilic molecules by passive transport. Lipophilic inhaled medications promote slow clearance from the lungs and thus exert a long effect. Drug particles with a low dissolution rate that reaches the alveolar space are phagocytized by alveolar macrophages or absorbed into the pulmonary circulation. Non-absorbed particles that are deposited in the airways are cleared by mucociliary clearance and cough. Some inhaled medications undergo metabolism in the lungs, such as ICS; beclomethasone dipropionate, whose metabolites diffuse into the bloodstream [62, 70].

Moreover, drug formulation plays an important role in producing an optimal aerosol therapy. Not only is it important to have a pharmacologically active drug, but it must also be efficiently delivered to the lungs, to the appropriate site of action, and remain in the lungs for a reasonable time until the desired pharmacological effect occurs. A drug designed to treat a systemic disease, such as insulin for diabetes, must be deeply deposited in the lung periphery to ensure maximum systemic bioavailability. For gene therapy or antibiotic treatment in cystic fibrosis (CF), prolonged residence in the lungs may be required to obtain the optimal therapeutic effect of the drug. Thus, a formulation that is retained in the lungs for the desired length of time and could overcome the clearance mechanisms of the lung may be necessary such as using liposomes and biodegradable polymer microspheres as pulmonary drug delivery vehicles for sustained release therapy. Moreover, formulating dry powders for inhalation involves either precipitation, micronization via jet milling, freeze-drying, or spray-drying using various excipients, such as lipids and polymers, or carrier systems like lactose. Each one has its unique advantages as well as disadvantages, the choice between them depends on the therapeutic agent being formulated [71].

8.2.5 Patient-Related Factors

Even with strict adherence to optimal ventilator parameters, adequate circuit conditions, optimal inhaler technique, and position and efficient drug formulation with optimal particle size, the patient himself has a direct effect on the efficiency of aerosol deposition and distribution in the lung owing to many factors including; lung diseases, airway geometry, humidity and clearance mechanisms. These patient-related factors can directly affect the extent of aerosol deposition and therefore influence the therapeutic effectiveness of inhaled therapies [62].

Unfortunately, bronchoconstriction, airway obstruction, and inflammation can alter the pulmonary deposition of aerosol. An obstruction decreases the cross-sectional area of the lung. That increases air velocity and turbulence in regions where the airflow is normally laminar which in turn diverts inspired air to unobstructed airways. Therefore, a low amount of drug is deposited in obstructed airways. It was concluded that in an obstructed lung, the aerosol will be deposited more centrally by inertial impaction if compared with the uniform distribution achieved in a non-obstructed lung [72]. It was demonstrated that the depth of aerosol deposition was positively correlated with the patient's FEV1 [73]. COPD patients have a significantly lower aerosol penetration than healthy volunteers [74–76]. Aerosol distribution was extremely uneven with a predominate central airway deposition in severely obstructed airways (low FEV1) if compared with unobstructed airways showing a uniform distribution [62].

Moreover, the air-flow restriction can determine the position of aerosol deposition within the lung [64]. Respiratory diseases, such as CF and bronchiectasis, change the architecture of the lung through alterations in bifurcation angles and mucus accumulation, which modify the aerosol deposition and its distribution pattern. Chronic pulmonary infection with *Pseudomonas Aeruginosa* in patients with CF or non-CF bronchiectasis occurs in the airway lumen with a limited invasion of parenchyma. Therefore, the optimal deposition of inhaled antimicrobial therapy would be a uniform distribution on conducting airways. Mucus plugs in the bronchi and bronchioles prevent deposition of small particles in the regions of highest infection which is distal to the airway obstruction and thereby reducing the therapeutic effectiveness [77, 78]. Many researchers reported an inverse correlation between FEV1 and central airway deposition in patients with CF. Moreover, the breathing pattern has a significant effect on aerosol deposition. A wide variation was observed among patients in the deposited aerosol with a coefficient of variation (CV) of 60.2%. When breathing patterns were well-controlled, the variation in deposition decreased to a CV of 18.6% [77]. Also, diffusion of inhaled medications may be altered in smokers, where the tight junctions of the epithelium are damaged, allowing for more transport across the membranes [1].

Additionally, air-way geometry significantly affects the pattern of aerosol deposition. Progressive branching and narrowing of the airways encourage inertial impaction. Also, the high relative humidity of the airway affects aerosol particle deposition due to hygroscopic growth. A hygroscopic aerosol that is delivered at a relatively low temperature and humidity into one of high humidity and temperature would be expected to increase in size when inhaled into the lung. The rate of growth is a function of the initial diameter of the particle, with the potential for the diameter of fine particles <1 μm to increase five fold if compared with two–three fold for particles >2 μm [79].

Also, mucociliary clearance is impaired in many lung diseases such as immotile cilia syndrome, bronchiectasis, CF, and asthma [80]. In immotile cilia syndrome and bronchiectasis, the ciliary function can be either impaired or non-existent. In CF, the ciliary structure and function are normal, but the copious amounts of thick, tenacious mucus present in the airways impair their ability to clear the mucus effectively which in turn impairs aerosol distribution within the lung [81]. In these diseases, clearance of aerosolized medications deposited in the conducting airways is generally decreased and secretions are cleared from the lung by cough [82]. Finally, patients should be monitored before, during, and after the administration of aerosols during mechanical ventilation. Clinicians should also specifically observe patient-ventilator synchrony and airway resistance during aerosol therapy in patients receiving ventilatory support [4].

8.3 Conclusion

Aerosol delivery to patients receiving mechanical ventilation is complex. Many factors are affecting aerosol deposition in the target sites in the lung. The ventilator parameters, circuit heat/humidity and gas density, type and position of the inhalation device, aerosol particle size, drug formulation, presence of lung disease, airway geometry/humidity, and clearance mechanisms are the main factors influencing the extent of aerosol deposition and therefore influencing the therapeutic effectiveness of inhaled medications. To provide an efficient and effective inhalant therapy, all of these factors must be considered, as guided by scientific research recommendations.

Key Major Recommendations

1. Spontaneous modes of breathing during mechanical ventilation are more recommended than controlled modes, when possible, for optimizing aerosol drug delivery. In addition, the use of Vt greater than the circuit volume between nebulizer and patient, low inspiratory flow, a duty cycle of 0.3, and a decreasing ramp or sinusoidal waveforms will together increase aerosol drug delivery to mechanically ventilated patients.
2. If a heated humidifier is used in mechanically ventilated patients, it should be left on during the administration of aerosol drugs except for expensive or critical drugs (short term <10–15 min). If the HME is used, it should be removed during treatment. Low-density gas like heliox should not be used to power a nebulizer but it can be used to entrain the aerosol into the ventilator circuit. In the latter case, the function of the ventilator must be tested and adjusted before its use.

3. JNs should be run intermittently, when possible. If they are run continuously, the flow rate should be set at 6–8 L/min and the ventilator parameters should be adjusted accordingly (Vt and pressure). VMNs is a better alternative for aerosol delivery in mechanically ventilated patients. The JN was most efficient when placed closer to the ventilator. However, other aerosol devices (VMN, USN, and pMDI) were more efficient when placed 6 inches from the Y adapter.
4. Use chamber spacers or bidirectional inline adapters with the pMDIs for aerosol administration to mechanically ventilated patients. pMDIs should be shaken well before administration and the actuation of the pMDI should be synchronized with the beginning of inspiration, with >15 s interval between actuations.
5. Patients should be monitored before, during, and after the administration of aerosols during mechanical ventilation. Clinicians should specifically observe patient-ventilator synchrony and airway resistance during aerosol therapy in patients receiving ventilatory support.

References

1. Pleasants RA, Hess DR. Aerosol delivery devices for obstructive lung diseases. Respir Care. 2018;63(6):708–33.
2. Dhand R. Basic techniques for aerosol delivery during mechanical ventilation. Respir Care. 2004;49(6):611–22.
3. Dhand R, Guntur VP. How best to deliver aerosol medications to mechanically ventilated patients. Clin Chest Med. 2008;29(2):277–96.
4. Ari A, Fink JB. Factors affecting bronchodilator delivery in mechanically ventilated adults. Nurs Crit Care. 2010;15(4):192–203.
5. Harb HS, et al. Update efficacy of aerosol therapy with noninvasive ventilator approach (non-invasive ventilation and nasal high flow). J Drug Deliv Sci Technol. 2020:101922.
6. Dhand R. Special problems in aerosol delivery: artificial airways. Respir Care. 2000;45(6):636–45.
7. MacIntyre NR, et al. Aerosol delivery in intubated, mechanically ventilated patients. Crit Care Med. 1985;13(2):81–4.
8. Fuller H, et al. Pressurized aerosol versus jet aerosol delivery to mechanically ventilated patients. Am Rev Respir Dis. 1990;141(2):440–4.
9. Dhand R, Sohal H. Pulmonary drug delivery system for inhalation therapy in mechanically ventilated patients. Expert Rev Med Devices. 2008;5(1):9–18.
10. Tobin MJ. Principles and practice of mechanical ventilation. Philadelphia: LWW; 2006.
11. Dhand R. Inhalation therapy with metered-dose inhalers and dry powder inhalers in mechanically ventilated patients. Respir Care. 2005;50(10):1331–45.
12. Duarte AG, Fink JB, Dhand R. Inhalation therapy during mechanical ventilation. Respir Care Clin N Am. 2001;7(2):233–60, vi.
13. Fink JB, et al. Aerosol delivery from a metered-dose inhaler during mechanical ventilation. An in vitro model. Am J Respir Crit Care Med. 1996;154(2):382–7.
14. Chatburn RL. Which ventilators and modes can be used to deliver noninvasive ventilation? Respir Care. 2009;54(1):85–101.
15. Hess DR, Dillman C, Kacmarek RM. In vitro evaluation of aerosol bronchodilator delivery during mechanical ventilation: pressure-control vs. volume control ventilation. Intensive Care Med. 2003;29(7):1145–50.

16. Dolovich MA. Influence of inspiratory flow rate, particle size, and airway caliber on aerosolized drug delivery to the lung. Respir Care. 2000;45(6):597–608.
17. Fink JB, et al. Reconciling in vitro and in vivo measurements of aerosol delivery from a metered-dose inhaler during mechanical ventilation and defining efficiency-enhancing factors. Am J Respir Crit Care Med. 1999;159(1):63–8.
18. Miller DD, et al. Aerosol delivery and modern mechanical ventilation: in vitro/in vivo evaluation. Am J Respir Crit Care Med. 2003;168(10):1205–9.
19. McPeck M, O'Riordan T, Smaldone G. Choice of mechanical ventilator: influence on nebulizer performance. Respir Care. 1993;38(8):887–95.
20. ElHansy MH, et al. Inhaled salbutamol dose delivered by jet nebulizer, vibrating mesh nebulizer and metered dose inhaler with spacer during invasive mechanical ventilation. Pulm Pharmacol Ther. 2017;45:159–63.
21. Rabec C, et al. Leak monitoring in noninvasive ventilation. Arch Bronconeumol. 2004;40(11):508–17.
22. Doyle PR. Ventilator adaptable for use with either a dual-limb circuit or a single-limb circuit. 2009, Google Patents.
23. Bach JR, et al. Sleep fragmentation in kyphoscoliotic individuals with alveolar hypoventilation treated by NIPPV. Chest. 1995;107(6):1552–8.
24. Rabec C, et al. Evaluating noninvasive ventilation using a monitoring system coupled to a ventilator: a bench-to-bedside study. Eur Respir J. 2009;34(4):902–13.
25. Ahrens RC, et al. The delivery of therapeutic aerosols through endotracheal tubes. Pediatr Pulmonol. 1986;2(1):19–26.
26. Crogan SJ, Bishop MJ. Delivery efficiency of metered dose aerosols given via endotracheal tubes. Anesthesiology. 1989;70(6):1008–10.
27. O'Riordan TG, et al. Nebulizer function during mechanical ventilation. Am Rev Respir Dis. 1992;145:1117–22.
28. Harvey C, et al. Comparison of jet and ultrasonic nebulizer pulmonary aerosol deposition during mechanical ventilation. Eur Respir J. 1997;10(4):905–9.
29. O'Riordan TG, Palmer LB, Smaldone GC. Aerosol deposition in mechanically ventilated patients. Optimizing nebulizer delivery. Am J Respir Crit Care Med. 1994;149(1):214–9.
30. Lange CF, Finlay WH. Overcoming the adverse effect of humidity in aerosol delivery via pressurized metered-dose inhalers during mechanical ventilation. Am J Respir Crit Care Med. 2000;161(5):1614–8.
31. Duarte AG, Momii K, Bidani A. Bronchodilator therapy with metered-dose inhaler and spacer versus nebulizer in mechanically ventilated patients: comparison of magnitude and duration of response. Respir Care. 2000;45(7):817–23.
32. Mouloudi E, et al. Bronchodilator delivery by metered-dose inhaler in mechanically ventilated COPD patients: influence of end-inspiratory pause. Eur Respir J. 1998;12(1):165–9.
33. Dhand R, et al. Dose-response to bronchodilator delivered by metered-dose inhaler in ventilator-supported patients. Am J Respir Crit Care Med. 1996;154(2):388–93.
34. Wilkes A. Heat and moisture exchangers. Structure and function. Respir Care Clin N Am. 1998;4(2):261–79.
35. Habib DM, Garner SS, Brandeburg S. Effect of helium-oxygen on delivery of albuterol in a pediatric, volume-cycled, ventilated lung model. Pharmacotherapy. 1999;19(2):143–9.
36. Goode ML, et al. Improvement in aerosol delivery with helium–oxygen mixtures during mechanical ventilation. Am J Respir Crit Care Med. 2001;163(1):109–14.
37. Svartengren M, et al. Human lung deposition of particles suspended in air or in helium/oxygen mixture. Exp Lung Res. 1989;15(4):575–85.
38. Anderson M, et al. Deposition in asthmatics of particles inhaled in air or in helium-oxygen. Am Rev Respir Dis. 1993;147:524.
39. Hess DR, et al. The effect of heliox on nebulizer function using a β-agonist bronchodilator. Chest. 1999;115(1):184–9.

40. O'Doherty MJ, et al. Delivery of a nebulized aerosol to a lung model during mechanical ventilation. Am Rev Respir Dis. 1992;146(2):383–8.
41. Harvey C, et al. Effect of a spacer on pulmonary aerosol deposition from a jet nebuliser during mechanical ventilation. Thorax. 1995;50(1):50–3.
42. Fink J, et al. Factors influencing aerosol delivery from nebulizers during mechanical ventilation. Am J Respir Crit Care Med. 2000;161:A385.
43. Hess D, et al. Medication nebulizer performance: effects of diluent volume, nebulizer flow, and nebulizer brand. Chest. 1996;110(2):498–505.
44. Hassan A, et al. In-vitro/in-vivo comparison of inhaled salbutamol dose delivered by jet nebulizer, vibrating mesh nebulizer and metered dose inhaler with spacer during non-invasive ventilation. Exp Lung Res. 2017;43(1):19–28.
45. Hill RL. A comparison of inline MDI actuators for delivery of a beta agonist and a corticosteroid with a mechanically ventilated lung model. Respir Care. 1998;43(9).
46. Mitchell JP, et al. The delivery of chlorofluorocarbon-propelled versus hydrofluoroalkane-propelled beclomethasone dipropionate aerosol to the mechanically ventilated patient: a laboratory study. Respir Care. 2003;48(11):1025–32.
47. Harb HS, et al. Performance of large spacer versus nebulizer T-piece in single-limb noninvasive ventilation. Respir Care. 2018;63(11):1360–9.
48. Manthous CA, et al. Metered-dose inhaler versus nebulized albuterol in mechanically ventilated patients. Am Rev Respir Dis. 1993;148:1567.
49. Bishop MJ, Larson RP, Buschman DL. Metered dose inhaler aerosol characteristics are affected by the endotracheal tube actuator/adapter used. Anesthesiology. 1990;73(6):1263–5.
50. Diot P, Morra L, Smaldone GC. Albuterol delivery in a model of mechanical ventilation. Comparison of metered-dose inhaler and nebulizer efficiency. Am J Respir Crit Care Med. 1995;152(4):1391–4.
51. Fuller HD, et al. Efficiency of bronchodilator aerosol delivery to the lungs from the metered dose inhaler in mechanically ventilated patients: a study comparing four different actuator devices. Chest. 1994;105(1):214–8.
52. Harb HS, et al. Is Combihaler usable for aerosol delivery in single limb non-invasive mechanical ventilation? J Drug Deliv Sci Technol. 2017;40:28–34.
53. Harb HS, et al. Real-life assessment of chronic obstructive pulmonary disease patient performance with different inhalers. Int J Clin Pract. 2021;75:e13905.
54. Harb HS, Rabea H, Abdelrahim M. Determinants of incorrect inhaler technique in chronic obstructive pulmonary disease patients. Int J Clin Pract. 2021;75:e14073.
55. Fink J, et al. Enabling aerosol delivery technology for critical care. Proc Respir Drug Deliv. 2002:12–6.
56. Fink J, Schmidt D, Power J. Comparison of a nebulizer using a novel aerosol generator with a standard ultrasonic nebulizer designed for use during mechanical ventilation. In: American Thoracic Society 97th International Conference. San Francisco, CA. 2001.
57. Dhand R. Aerosol delivery during mechanical ventilation: from basic techniques to new devices. J Aerosol Med Pulm Drug Deliv. 2008;21(1):45–60.
58. Bosco AP, Rhem RG, Dolovich MB. In vitro estimations of in vivo jet nebulizer efficiency using actual and simulated tidal breathing patterns. J Aerosol Med. 2005;18(4):427–38.
59. Saeed H, et al. Effects of fill volume and humidification on aerosol delivery during single-limb noninvasive ventilation. Respir Care. 2018;63(11):1370–8.
60. Saeed H, et al. Fill volume, humidification and heat effects on aerosol delivery and fugitive emissions during noninvasive ventilation. J Drug Deliv Sci Technol. 2017;39:372–8.
61. Rau JL. Design principles of liquid nebulization devices currently in use. Respir Care. 2002;47(11):1257–75. discussion 1275
62. Labiris N, Dolovich M. Pulmonary drug delivery. Part I: physiological factors affecting therapeutic effectiveness of aerosolized medications. Br J Clin Pharmacol. 2003;56(6):588–99.
63. Laube BL, et al. What the pulmonary specialist should know about the new inhalation therapies. Eur Respir J. 2011;37(6):1308–31.

64. Lavorini F, et al. Dilemmas, confusion, and misconceptions related to small airways directed therapy. Chest. 2017;151(6):1345–55.
65. Olsson B, et al. Pulmonary drug metabolism, clearance, and absorption, In: Controlled pulmonary drug delivery. Springer; 2011. p. 21–50.
66. Johnson MA, et al. Delivery of albuterol and ipratropium bromide from two nebulizer systems in chronic stable asthma: efficacy and pulmonary deposition. Chest. 1989;96(1):6–10.
67. Rees P, Clark T, Moren F. The importance of particle size in response to inhaled bronchodilators. Eur J Respir Dis Suppl. 1982;119:73–8.
68. Zanen P, Go LT, Lammers J-WJ. The optimal particle size for β-adrenergic aerosols in mild asthmatics. Int J Pharm. 1994;107(3):211–7.
69. Zanen P, Go LT, Lammers J. Optimal particle size for beta 2 agonist and anticholinergic aerosols in patients with severe airflow obstruction. Thorax. 1996;51(10):977–80.
70. Roberts JK, et al. Metabolism of beclomethasone dipropionate by cytochrome P450 3A enzymes. J Pharmacol Exp Ther. 2013;345(2):308–16.
71. Labiris NR, Dolovich MB. Pulmonary drug delivery. Part II: the role of inhalant delivery devices and drug formulations in therapeutic effectiveness of aerosolized medications. Br J Clin Pharmacol. 2003;56(6):600–12.
72. Dolovich M, Nahmias C, Coates G. Unleashing the PET: 3D imaging of the lung. Respiratory drug delivery VII. Biological, pharmaceutical, clinical and regulatory issues relating to optimized drug delivery by aerosol; 2000. p. 215–30.
73. Pavia D, et al. Effect of lung function and mode of inhalation on penetration of aerosol into the human lung. Thorax. 1977;32(2):194–7.
74. Dolovich M, et al. Aerosol penetrance: a sensitive index of peripheral airways obstruction. J Appl Physiol. 1976;40(3):468–71.
75. Dolovich M, Ryan G, Newhouse M. Aerosol penetration into the lung; influence on airway responses. Chest. 1981;80(6 Suppl):834–6.
76. Harb HS, et al. Prevalence and predictors of suboptimal peak inspiratory flow rate in COPD patients. Eur J Pharm Sci, 2020;147: p. 105298.
77. Ilowite JS, Gorvoy JD, Smaldone GC. Quantitative deposition of aerosolized gentamicin in cystic fibrosis. Am Rev Respir Dis. 1987;136:1445–9.
78. Anderson PJ, et al. Effect of cystic fibrosis on inhaled aerosol boluses. Am Rev Respir Dis. 1989;140:1317–24.
79. Swift D. Aerosols and humidity therapy. Generation and respiratory deposition of therapeutic aerosols. Am Rev Respir Dis. 1980;122(5 Pt 2):71–7.
80. Houtmeyers E, et al. Regulation of mucociliary clearance in health and disease. Eur Respir J. 1999;13(5):1177–88.
81. Rossman CM, et al. Nasal ciliary ultrastructure and function in patients with primary ciliary dyskinesia compared with that in normal subjects and in subjects with various respiratory diseases. Am Rev Respir Dis. 1984;129(1):161–7.
82. Robinson M, Bye PT. Mucociliary clearance in cystic fibrosis. Pediatr Pulmonol. 2002;33(4):293–306.

Chapter 9
Inhaled Medications Employed in Critically Ill Patients

Contents

9.1 Introduction

Aerosolization aims to deliver high drug amounts to the target sites within the lung tissue. Aerosol therapy is commonly used as part of the treatment of many respiratory conditions. Also, there is a significant interest in utilizing the respiratory tract as a portal of systemic therapy of other diseases [1]. The number of drugs considered for that mode of application is rapidly growing, based on its high efficiency and safety [2]. Many factors could contribute to the high bioavailability of the

M. E. A. Abdelrahim et al., *Essentials of Aerosol Therapy in Critically ill Patients*,
https://doi.org/10.1007/978-3-030-85026-5_9

aerosolized drug including thin air-blood barrier and vascular epithelium, large surface area, and minimal first-pass metabolism or enzymatic activity [3]. Moreover, rapid onset of action, minimal systemic side effects, and achieving high local drug concentrations at the target sites of the lung has led to a higher tendency of using aerosolized drugs in intensive care units for critically ill patients [4]. Optimal delivery of therapeutic doses is mainly based on applying a proper nominal dose of a proper formulation with the aid of an optimal administration technique through the aerosol generator. To quote from Byron [5]:

"In the near future, it is likely that optimal formulations will be combined with modified aerosol delivery devices to maximize and achieve reproducible values for dose to lung. These will be used as alternatives to parenteral delivery for small through intermediate dose drugs which are not absorbed via the gastrointestinal tract."

Many studies with experimental pneumonia models had demonstrated that pulmonary concentrations of nebulized amikacin through an ultrasonic nebulizer were significantly higher than those resulting from using the intravenous (IV) route [6, 7], and resulted in higher bactericidal effects and sterility rates if compared with IV route [8]. Even though nebulized drug deposition decreased with a higher degree of pneumonia severity, it still resulted in higher pulmonary concentration than that achieved through the IV route [6]. Similarly, frequent nebulization of ceftazidime achieved higher pulmonary concentrations and greater bactericidal activity if compared to continuous IV infusion, in an experimental model of Pseudomonas pneumonia [9]. From these findings, it could be concluded that the pulmonary route of drug administration had proved superior therapeutic outcomes than other routes of administration with different pulmonary diseases [10].

9.2 Discussion and Analysis of Main Topics

9.2.1 Inhaled Medications Employed During Mechanical Ventilation (MV)

There is a variety of aerosolized medications that could be administered during MV. A lot of them are applied for treating certain pulmonary conditions (e.g.: bronchodilators, mucolytics, antibiotics, and corticosteroids), however, many other medications are intended for systemic absorption through the target sites within the lung (e.g.: anticoagulants, insulin, and anesthetic gases). The underlying scientific principles apply to all of them. The choice of one aerosolized medication over another should be based on efficacy, cost, drug properties, availability, and resistance patterns (in the case of antibiotics). The following are examples of the inhaled medications that could be applied in several conditions [11]:

- Bronchodilators
  - Beta-agonist (albuterol, metaproteronol, fenoterol)
  - Anticholinergic (ipratropium bromide)

  - Combination beta-agonist and anticholinergic (albuterol sulfate + ipratropium bromide)
  - Combination long-acting beta-agonist and inhaled corticosteroid (salmeterol + fluticasone; formoterol + budesonide)

- Prostaglandin (alprostadil, prostacyclin, iloprost, treprostinil).
- Dornase alpha.
- Proteins (Pulmozyme).
- Surfactant (Exosurf).
- Antibiotics/Antibacterial (aminoglycosides).
- Antiviral (Ribavirin).
- Antifungal (amphotericin).
- Mucolytics (acetylcysteine).
- Corticosteroids (beclomethasone; budesonide).
- Anticoagulants (Heparin).
- Miscellaneous (immuno-regulatory agents, insulin, gene therapy, anesthetic gases, and others).

9.2.1.1 Bronchodilators

Bronchodilators are the most commonly applied medications in treating mechanically ventilated patients with asthma or chronic obstructive pulmonary disease (COPD). The goals of bronchodilator therapy include: reversing bronchoconstriction, relieving dyspnea, and decreasing the work of breathing. Aerosolized bronchodilators mainly include β_2-adrenergic agonists [12, 13] or anticholinergic bronchodilators [14]. The main indications for bronchodilator therapy in patients receiving MV include [15]:

1. Severe asthma attacks.
2. COPD exacerbations.
3. High airway resistance.
4. Acute bronchospasm/wheezing.
5. Dynamic hyperinflation/intrinsic positive end-expiratory pressure (PEEP).
6. Chronic ventilator-dependence.
7. Difficulty in weaning.

Several important issues regarding inhalation therapy with bronchodilators have been now clarified. Short-acting preparations help in treating occasional dyspnea and bronchospasm, however, long-acting preparations significantly enhance both pulmonary functions and health status and reduces both dyspnea and exacerbation rate. Short-acting β_2-agonists (SABA) provides greater benefits over short-acting muscarinic antagonists (SAMA) [16]. Also, combinations of SABA/SAMA are superior to monotherapy in increasing forced expiratory volume in 1 second (FEV1) [16]. Moreover, combining bronchodilators of different durations of action and mechanisms is more effective and had lower side effects if compared with increasing the dosage of a single bronchodilator [17]. The combination of fenoterol with ipratropium bromide was proved to be more effective than ipratropium alone in improving respiratory mechanics in COPD mechanically-ventilated patients [18]. Many clinical trials have proven the superiority of long-acting muscarinic antagonists (LAMA) in reducing exacerbation rates if compared with long-acting β_2-agonist (LABA) [19]. Moreover, the combination of LABA/LAMA is superior to either medication alone for reducing symptoms, increasing FEV1 [20], and reducing exacerbations [21].

No serious side effects were reported after bronchodilator administration in mechanically-ventilated patients. Bronchodilator administration during MV could be achieved through a pMDI or a nebulizer [12, 13]. Using a spacer with a pMDI significantly improves the efficacy of aerosol delivery through the ventilation circuit with careful attention to synchronizing the pMDI actuation with the onset of inspiration [22, 23]. Moreover, the application of an external PEEP at a level that counterbalanced the intrinsic PEEP improved the albuterol bronchodilator effect in mechanically-ventilated COPD patients [24]. Albuterol reduces time-constant disparity which results in producing alveolar recruitment during tidal ventilation. The application of external PEEP maintains this alveolar recruitment. As a result, the level of intrinsic PEEP is significantly reduced by the combination of albuterol and external PEEP, which explain their additive effects [24].

9.2.1.2 Prostanoids

The use of prostanoids has evoked great interest in mechanically-ventilated patients due to the high occurrence of pulmonary hypertension as an adverse prognostic factor in patients with acute respiratory distress syndrome (ARDS) [25]. Inhaling prostacyclin provides targeted pulmonary vasodilation. In contrast to the IV route of administration [26, 27], inhaled vasodilators selectively enhance blood flow to well-ventilated but poorly-perfused lung regions during MV in patients with ARDS. Consequentially, that enhances oxygenation and decreases pulmonary artery pressures [28]. Inhaled prostacyclin and prostaglandin E1 are selective pulmonary vaso-dilators at doses lower than 10 ng/kg/min, but systemic vaso-dilation occurs at higher doses. Moreover, Low doses of prostacyclin (<10 ng/kg/min) are well-tolerated, but higher doses cause bronchospasm. In mechanically ventilated patients with ARDS, inhaled prostacyclin and prostaglandin E1 are equally effective as nitric oxide in enhancing oxygenation and hemodynamics [29–31]. Similarly, inhaled prostacyclin significantly improved oxygenation and pulmonary hemodynamics in mechanically-ventilated patients with severe pneumonia with no prior interstitial lung disease [32].

Stable prostacyclin analogs (e.g.: Iloprost) were developed as a result of many attempts to prolong the duration of action of prostacyclin. Iloprost was approved for use to treat patients with chronic pulmonary hypertension. Iloprost has a longer half-life than prostacyclin (20–30 min vs 3 min), and it can produce pulmonary vaso-dilatation for 30–90 min. Hemodynamic effects of inhaled iloprost are similar to those of inhaled prostacyclin and nitric oxide [33–35]. In ambulatory patients, it is delivered by either of two delivery devices: I-neb Adaptive Aerosol Delivery (AAD) system or the Prodose AAD system (Cotherix Inc., South San Francisco, California, USA). The inhaled iloprost dose is 2.5–5 mg administered 6–9 times/day during waking hours, depending mainly on the need and tolerability. Combination of inhaled iloprost with oral sildenafil improved and prolonged the pulmonary vasodilator effect of iloprost with no effect on systemic arterial pressure or oxygenation [36].

Also, inhaled treprostinil is an effective prostacyclin analog used as a pulmonary vasodilator in chronic pulmonary hypertension patients. Its main advantage is its prolonged duration of action. A single inhalation of 15 mg of the drug produces a prolonged vaso-dilator effect exceeding 180 min [37]. Owing to their long duration of effect, inhaled iloprost or treprostinil are efficiently employed for the treatment of acute pulmonary hypertension in mechanically ventilated patients with no need for continuous aerosolization.

9.2.1.3 Surfactant

Endogenous lung surfactant consists of a mixture of proteins and lipids. It lines the alveolar surface, reduces surface tension which allows maintaining of alveolar stability. Changes in the endogenous surfactant result in alveolar edema, atelectasis, abnormal respiratory mechanics, and hypoxemia mostly in neonates with ARDS [38]. Surfactant replacement therapy (SRT) was recently introduced as an attempt to correct the lack of functional surfactant either in neonates or adults with acute lung injury [38]. SRT depends on applying exogenous surfactants which are mixtures of synthetic phosphor-lipids (Exosurf) or modified natural surfactants, obtained from animal lung or alveolar lavage extracts, which consists of phosphor-lipids in combination with a naturally-derived surfactant proteins B and C (e.g., Survanta; Ross/Abbot Laboratories, Columbus, Ohio, USA). More recently, synthetic surfactants were developed with recombinant surfactant protein B (Surfaxin; Discovery Laboratories, Warrington, Pennsylvania, USA) or recombinant protein C (e.g., Venticute; Altana Pharma, Florham Park, New Jersey, USA). Exogenous surfactants do not contain protein A or D and have different functional and morphologic properties if compared to natural surfactants [39].

Techniques of delivery of exogenous surfactant include; liquid-bolus dripping through endotracheal tube followed by a short period of manual ventilation [40], dripping via an intra-tracheal catheter [41], dripping via a bronchoscope [42, 43], or by aerosolization through a nebulizer system [44, 45]. Aerosolized surfactant produces more uniform dispersion in the lung and fewer bolus effects than the liquid-bolus dripping method. Delivery of lower quantities of surfactant to parenchyma is sufficient to reduce the surface tension and enhance pulmonary functions when it is aerosolized if compared to liquid-bolus dripping. Unfortunately, the high viscosity of exogenous surfactants causes a difficulty of aerosolization. Surfactants tend to foam with stable bubbles during the process of nebulization. The majority of surfactant is lost within the aerosol generator and the ventilator circuit, which reduces the efficiency of nebulizer delivery of surfactant to the lower respiratory tract. Furthermore, exhaled aerosol tends to deposit and interfere with the function of monitors and valves of the ventilator. This obstacle could be avoided by the placement of filters in the expiratory limb to trap any aerosol in the circuit before it reaches the ventilator.

Inhaled surfactant is preferentially deposited within less-injured and well-ventilated lung regions in animals with non-homogeneous lung injury [46]. Similarly, in ARDS the pattern of injury is not uniform, so the more affected lung regions may not receive appropriate doses of the inhaled surfactant. Two trials evaluated the efficacy of Exosurf in patients with sepsis-induced ARDS. There was no improvement in oxygenation, length of stay in the intensive care unit (ICU), duration of MV, or survival in both trials [44, 45]. Moreover, the cause of lung injury may affect the response to exogenous surfactant. Patients with direct lung injury caused by pneumonia or aspiration had reduced mortality in contrast to patients with sepsis-induced lung injury [47]. Improvements in the design of delivery systems and exogenous surfactants are needed to make aerosolized surfactant an effective treatment of ARDS.

9.2.1.4 Antibiotics/Antibacterial

Very limited pulmonary penetration of antibiotics after IV administration contributes to treatment failure and a high mortality rate caused by ventilator-associated pneumonia [48]. For that reason, alternative routes of antibiotic administration are being developed to enhance its efficacy. Using aerosolized antibiotics is appealing as a result of allowing the administration of a greater antibiotic dose to the airways than other routes of administration [8, 49], in addition to maintaining a low risk of systemic side effects or toxicity [10]. Another role of aerosolized antibiotics could be to decrease the formation of microbial biofilm on the inner walls of the endotracheal tube, which reduces bacterial seeding of the pulmonary parenchyma [50]. Aerosolization of this biofilm deep into the lung is contributing to the development of ventilator-associated pneumonia [51].

The choice of one inhaled antibiotic against another should be based on specific properties of the antibiotic together with the resistance patterns. Beta-lactams require frequent administration because they are rapidly cleared from airways. Aerosolized aminoglycosides enhance pulmonary functions, reduce the frequency of lung infections, relieve symptoms, and reduce hospitalization rate in spontaneously breathing cystic fibrosis (CF) patients [52]. Likewise, aerosolized tobramycin (TOBI; Chiron Corp., Emeryville, California, USA) is now employed by CF patients [53].

Aminoglycosides require tissue concentrations that are >ten fold higher than the minimum inhibitory concentration (MIC) to be maximally effective. Moreover, serum aminoglycoside concentrations must be monitored to avoid systemic toxicity, because its molecular weight is low and airway inflammation increases its systemic absorption. Aminoglycosides are concentration-dependent therefore their bactericidal activity is best described by Cmax/MIC ratio [54]. Many studies proved that IV administration of aminoglycosides has poor penetration into the epithelial lining fluid [7, 55]. Aerosolized amikacin achieved significant lung concentrations in an Escherichia coli inoculation pneumonia model [7]. Furthermore, there was no accumulation effect or toxicity concerns with repeated administration of aerosolized amikacin [56]. Moreover, serum amikacin concentration was higher in the pneumonia model [7], if compared to that of healthy lungs [56]. A combination of IV and aerosolized aminoglycosides didn't increase curative rates if compared to that of aerosolized antibiotics only. Based on these findings, antibiotic aerosol therapy of ventilator-associated pneumonia (VAP), may be sufficient with no need for IV therapy to minimize systemic toxicity [57].

Similar to aminoglycosides, colistin is a concentration-dependent antibiotic widely applied in an aerosolized form. It has poor lung penetration after IV administration. Many studies showed that a high and rapid bactericidal activity can be achieved with aerosolized colistin. Aerosolized Colistin is not FDA-approved and is not licensed for use in China. The advantage of using aerosolized colistin is to avoid nephrotoxicity with systemic colistin [58]. In an inoculation pneumonia model, low serum concentrations resulted from the aerosolized colistin leading to minimal risk of toxicity [49]. Similar curative rates were found when susceptible P. aeruginosa or A. baumannii were treated with IV colistin alone and multi-drug resistant (MDR) strains were treated with nebulized colistin, in patients with VAP [57]. Combined IV aminoglycoside with aerosolized colistin didn't show superiority over aerosolized colistin alone [58].

Colistin is administered in its anionic form "colistimethate" (one million units of colistimethate contain 80 mg of colistimethate which is equivalent to 33 mg of colistin base). Despite high doses administered in colonized patients with bronchiectasis (up to one million units of colistimethate every 8 h), lung epithelial fluid concentrations are not exceeding 4 mg/L after 8 h (upper threshold of European committee on antimicrobial susceptibility testing (EUCAST) MIC breakpoint for Pseudomonas) or even above 2 mg/L after 8 h in many patients (EUCAST MIC breakpoint for Klebsiella sp. and Acinetobacter baumannii). Therefore, high doses should be considered in pneumonia (five million units every 8 h) [10].

In contrast, the efficacy of aerosolized antibiotics during MV is controversial and not well-defined [59, 60]. An increased mortality rate was observed after administration of aerosolized polymyxin to patients in the ICU, as a result of higher development of polymyxin resistant organisms which disappeared after discontinuation of inhaled antibiotic therapy [59]. However, more recent studies suggest that the aerosolized aminoglycosides could be used in a selected group of patients during MV. The combination of aerosolized colistin with IV antibiotics had beneficial effects with no emergence of resistant organisms, in case of pneumonia caused by multi-resistant gram-negative bacteria [61, 62]. Inhaled antibiotic therapy during MV appears to be promising but still regarded as investigational, pending further work on examining drug distribution within the lung, inhalation versus IV routes, the emergence of antibiotic-resistant organisms, and local toxicity. At present, the use of aerosolized antibiotics is reserved for adjunctive therapy in the treatment of patients with severe pneumonia not responding to the conventional therapy, patients with multi-resistant organisms, or patients with tracheobronchitis after a long-term MV [60].

9.2.1.5 Antiviral

Delivery of aerosolized ribavirin for up to 7 days was associated with a decrease in the duration of MV in mechanically-ventilated neonates and infants with respiratory syncytial virus infection. However, special precautions should be given to avoid crystallization of the drug within the respiratory equipment [63].

9.2.1.6 Mucolytic Agents

Retention of pulmonary secretions increases the risk of pneumonia. However, mechanical suction to clear secretions is extremely painful and may lead to tracheal injury. Acetylcysteine is a mucolytic agent that enhances the clearance of secretions by modifying sputum viscosity. An increase in the inspiratory airway resistance after delivery of mucolytic agents by bolus dripping [64, 65], or aerosol [66] is a problem with using these agents. Recombinant human DNase (Pulmozyme) improves mucus clearance in mechanically-ventilated patients with spinal cord injury and those with recurrent atelectasis refractory to standard therapy [65]. Pulmozyme can't be recommended for the routine management of mechanically-ventilated patients due to its high cost. Moreover, a mucolytic may encourage the prevention of lung collapse or hypoxemia in mechanically-ventilated patients with thick secretions who are refractory to types of treatment.

9.2.1.7 Corticosteroids

Using inhaled corticosteroids (ICS) was recommended in neonates/infants with broncho-pulmonary dysplasia. However, aerosolized budesonide didn't decrease the duration of MV in preterm babies if compared with infants receiving a placebo inhalation [67]. Similarly, inhaled beclomethasone didn't reduce the frequency of broncho-pulmonary dysplasia in premature infants receiving MV if compared with the placebo group [68]. Therefore, ICS may have a limited role in the management of mechanically-ventilated premature infants.

9.2.1.8 Miscellaneous

The aerosol therapy is also being evaluated for a variety of anti-inflammatory agents, immuno-regulatory agents, insulin, gene therapy, anesthetic gases, and others. Soon, many of these agents may be employed for the treatment of patients receiving MV [69]. Firstly, interferon alpha-2b (INFα 2b) is used for the treatment of hepatitis B, hepatitis C and many types of cancer. Injection of INFα 2b is associated with many systemic side effects and irritation at the site of injection. A study compared the pharmacokinetics (PK) and pharmacodynamics (PD) of INFα 2b administered either by injection or inhalation route through Aradigm's AERx system. It found that the relative bioavailability through the inhaled route was 10–12%. Also, the increase in the levels of β2 microglobulin was very high [70]. According to these findings, the biological effects of macromolecular immune-modulators delivered to the lung are much greater than that of conventional measures of bioavailability due to the great extent of absorption of the immune-modulators into the systemic blood circulation [71].

Administration of insulin through the inhalation route has attracted the particular attention of many researchers. However, there is very little data on the PK and PD properties of this new inhaled substance in elderly people. Also, the effect of aging of the lung and co-pathologies are not well-known [2]. Insulin has a relatively narrow therapeutic index. Either over-dosing or under-dosing can lead to serious side effects. Therefore, the control of insulin delivery through inhalation should be as good or even better than delivery through subcutaneous injection. That includes the robustness of the aerosol delivery system, its size, and weight for better portability. Also, the aerosol delivery systems should cater to a variety of people of different ages and different types of the disease [71]. Large numbers of patients and longer studies are required to develop confidence in both the safety and efficacy of inhaled insulin. The most advanced programs, to date, employ aerosol generators utilizing a patient-independent source of energy to create aerosol-cloud [72]. Mainly, there are two developed systems for inhaled insulin delivery: The dry powder system "Exubera" (pioneered by Nektar, formerly Inhale, in partnership with Pfizer and Aventis) and the aqueous insulin inhalation delivery system "AERx iDMS" (developed initially by Aradigm Corporation, and partnered with Novo Nordisk).

Exubera combines a formulation of mannitol-stabilized insulin with a hand-held portable dry powder aerosol generator driven by compressed air and a holding chamber in which the aerosol cloud is formed before patient inhalation [73]. This pulmonary insulin system was investigated in phase 3 of many studies applied in both type 1 and type 2 diabetic patients. It was then concluded that long-term treatment of type 2 diabetic patients with Exubera was well-tolerated and effective in the control of glucose levels, over 2 years, in a joint press release between Pfizer and Aventis. The most common side effect with Exubera was transient and mild cough. There were previous reports of deterioration of lung functions in patients using Exubera, however, confidence intervals for changes in FEV1 and carbon monoxide diffusing capacity (DLCO), after 2 years of treatment, showed no significant differences between the group using inhaled insulin and control groups. Another study of type 1 diabetic patients compared prandial Exubera with a single daily long-acting subcutaneous injection versus 2–3 subcutaneous injections of regular insulin plus long-acting subcutaneous injection [74]. Treatment satisfaction was higher in the inhaled insulin group. Also, there was a similar reduction in the glycated hemoglobin (Hb A1C) level and a smaller number of hypoglycemic events in the inhaled insulin group. Mild to moderate cough was more frequent in the Exubera group if compared with the injection-only group but it decreased during treatment. There was no significant difference in pulmonary function between the Exubera and control groups except for a greater decrease in DLCO in the inhaled insulin group. Understanding the effects of inhaled insulin on the long-term changes of pulmonary function in diabetic patients is complicated due to the effect of this disease on pulmonary functions and microcirculation.

The AERx iDMS insulin inhalation delivery system is an electro-mechanical device that allows titration of the delivered dose. It was developed after extensive clinical testing in type 1 and type 2 diabetic patients. It is ideal for deep lung delivery. It also guides the patient visually to achieve an optimal breathing maneuver [72, 75, 76]. Further, it can download an electronic log of the delivery to help with compliance and overall disease management. Owing to this technology, the intra-subject variability in absorption of insulin appears to be comparable or slightly lower (approximately 20%) in smokers and nonsmokers if compared with subcutaneous insulin injections [77]. However, asthmatic patients using the AERx system get less insulin than non-asthmatics [78]; inhaling even higher doses of aerosolized insulin didn't exacerbate the airway hyper-reactivity state in these patients. Nonsmokers with type 2 diabetes were included in a trial, for 3 months, in which they received inhaled insulin through the AERx device or subcutaneous injections at mealtimes with one long-acting insulin injection at night [79]. There was no significant difference in the overall glycaemic control, pulmonary functions, or chest X-rays between the two study groups. In another trial, type 2 diabetic patients were treated with either inhaled or subcutaneous regular insulin before each meal with intermediate-acting insulin at night in both groups. Total insulin antibodies (non-neutralizing IgGs) greatly rise in the inhaled group while a little rise was observed in the injection-only group [80]. This antibody level was unrelated to insulin dosage requirements or metabolic control. Insulin antibodies were observed also with other routes of administration of insulin but with no apparent side effects, except for a hint in some studies about an increase in the insulin dose requirement [81]. No reports of anaphylaxis or allergic reactions to inhaled insulin were found with either the Exubera or AERx iDMS.

Towards the end of the twentieth century, the rapidly growing biotechnology industry developed several therapeutic recombinant human proteins (e.g.: human growth hormone (hGH) and erythropoietin (EPO)). Also, several new therapeutic peptides were recently approved for human use. Due to the molecular properties of these agents, they can't be administered conveniently by oral route. They must be injected. Massive research efforts were made to find a non-invasive route of administration of these valuable compounds. By the beginning of the 1990s, the pulmonary route of delivery was developed for peptides/proteins and many delivery devices and formulations were investigated [82]. Then the recombinant human deoxyribonuclease (rhDNase) was approved for the treatment of CF by inhalation [83]. Pulmonary delivery of homologous copies of human proteins was not reported to have any safety concerns [71].

Induction of general anesthesia by inhalation of highly soluble gases (ether, nitrous oxide, and chloroform) was also possible in the era of modern medicine. It could be applied in transformed surgery for people of all ages. Contemporary anesthetic gases reduced the risks of surgery for frail older patients [84]. Also, the administration of inhaled opiates through a small droplet bolus aerosol-generating system with breath-control (AERx, Aradigm Corp.) leads to deep pulmonary deposition followed by a rapid absorption into the systemic circulation [85]. The blood levels of these drugs are very similar to those obtained by IV injections. It is therefore suggested that this noninvasive mode of delivery is more suitable for the treatment of severe breakthrough pain. A high level of satisfaction was reported in cancer patients who received fentanyl through this route [86]. The mean time for pain relief was about 12 min. This rapid onset of action may be an advantage when treating male erectile dysfunction. A dry powder inhaler was developed by Vectura to deliver apomorphine hydrochloride and showed median onset of action of about 8 min.

9.2.2 *Common Applications of Aerosol Therapy in Critical Care*

With great developments in aerosol delivery devices and drug formulations, more is clear now about the optimal conditions required for effective aerosol therapy. Despite these improvements, there are many concerns that there is no best evidence applied for administration, particularly for inhaled antibiotics [87, 88]. Table 9.1 summarizes the common applications of aerosol therapy in critical care. Inhaled bronchodilators and ICS have been effectively utilized in critical care. Aerosolized antibiotics are rapidly gaining more data to support their use in critical care.

9.2.3 *Effect of Dosing*

With the use of the inhaled route for drug delivery, significant extra-pulmonary loss usually occurs. The actual delivered drug dose may be <60% of the total emitted dose (TED) in the trachea and even less in the alveolar space [49]. This should be considered when calculating doses. The inhaled drug dose is likely to be significantly higher than expected due to concerns about drug losses. Experimental studies showed effective drug nebulization during MV with good PK properties and high local concentrations if compared to IV route e,g: teicoplanin and ceftazidime [89–91]. Doses should be different in patients with tracheobronchitis, colonization, or pneumonia. Increasing the dose (e.g. five million units in case of colistin) requires a longer time for nebulization (~1 h) which is not well-tolerated in patients with ARDS [10]. On the other hand, administration of high doses of β_2-agonists is associated with serious arrhythmias and hypokalemia. Episodes of ventricular ectopy and supraventricular

Table 9.1 Common applications of aerosol therapy in critical care [10]

	Drug class			
Feature	Bronchodilators	Anti-inflammatory	Anti-microbial agents	Vasoactive agents
Indications	Bronchospasm (e.g. COPD exacerbation, acute asthma)	Airway inflammation (e.g. COPD exacerbation, acute asthma, acute interstitial lung disease)	MDR trachea-bronchitis MDR Pneumonia Aspergillus prevention (lung transplant)	Pulmonary Hypertension Right ventricular Failure
Site of action	Airways	Airways/alveoli	Airways/alveoli	Alveoli
Preferred device	pMDI plus spacer	pMDI plus spacer	VMN	VMN
Drugs	Beta2-agonists (e.g. salbutamol, salmeterol) Anticholinergics (e.g. ipratropium, tiotropium)	Fluticasone Budesonide	Antibiotics (e.g. colistin, Tobramycin, amikacin, amphotericin B, ceftazidime)	Iloprost Epoprostenol

Heliox helium and oxygen, *COPD* chronic obstructive pulmonary disease, *MDR* multi-drug resistant, *pMDI* pressurized metered-dose inhaler, *VMN* vibrating mesh nebulizer

tachycardia have occurred after administration of 3–6 times the normal dose of albuterol by a nebulizer [92], but no arrhythmia was observed after administration of 4–10 puffs of albuterol with a pMDI [12]. When using pMDIs in very high doses or when pMDI is directly delivered beyond the endotracheal tube through an attached catheter to the canister nozzle, its propellants may cause local ulceration and serious cardiac arrhythmias [93, 94]. Most mechanically-ventilated patients don't show incremental effects with increasing drug doses of bronchodilators [12]. However, other classes of aerosolized drugs may show a linear dose-response relationship. Further PK–PD studies are needed to guide inhaled drug dosing regimen.

9.2.4 Effect of Administration Technique

The optimal techniques for the administration of inhaled drugs to mechanically-ventilated patients are presented in Table 9.2. They were established based on many studies focusing on factors affecting aerosol delivery through common aerosol generators [11, 15, 69]. When these techniques are applied, adequate aerosol deposition in the lung would be achieved [95–97], and a significant clinical response could be observed. The employed technique should be adjusted between the optimum operating device characteristics and the patient's condition. For example, in patients with airflow limitation, a higher duty cycle increases aerosol delivery [95, 98], but it may worsen dynamic hyperinflation [99]. The main aspects of the pMDI technique are to

Table 9.2 Optimal technique for aerosol delivery through commonly used aerosol generators in mechanically-ventilated patients [11]

pMDI	Air-jet Nebulizer
1. Review order, identify patient, and assess the need for the drug 2. Assess airway, remove excess secretions if present 3. Shake pMDI and warm to hand temperature (prime if not used within 24 h) 4. Place pMDI in the adapter in the ventilator circuit 5. Remove HME (Don't disconnect humidifier) 6. Coordinate pMDI actuation with the beginning of inspiration 7. Administer total dose; wait at least 15 s between actuations 8. Monitor for adverse effects 9. Reconnect HME 10. Document clinical outcome	1. Review order, identify patient, and assess the need for the drug 2. Assess airway, remove excess secretions if present 3. Place the drug in the nebulizer, do not exceed manufacturer recommendations 4. Place nebulizer in the inspiratory line 18 in from the patient or proximal to the ventilator 5. Use minimal flow-by or continuous flow during operation 6. Remove HME from the circuit (do not disconnect humidifier) 7. Set the gas flow to nebulizer at 2–10 L/min, based on manufacturer label a. Use a ventilator to power the nebulizer if it meets the nebulizer flow requirements and cycles on inspiration, or b. Use continuous flow from an external source (*50 psi) 8. Adjust ventilator volume or pressure limit and alarms to compensate for added flow 9. Run until the nebulizer begins to sputter 10. Remove nebulizer from the circuit, rinse with sterile water and run dry, store in a safe place 11. Reconnect humidifier or HME, return ventilator settings and alarms to previous values 12. Monitor the patient for adverse effects 13. Assess outcomes and document findings

pMDI metered-dose inhaler, *HME* heat and moisture exchanger

place an adequate adapter 15 cm from the endotracheal tube and to synchronize actuation with the inspiratory flow. For nebulizers, it is important to use the device as recommended by the manufacturer and to place it at a distance from the patient.

9.2.5 Limitations of Aerosol Therapy in Critical Care

Firstly, the adverse events, associated with the use of aerosol therapies, are the main limitation of their use. Indeed, there is the potential of systemic toxicity (e.g. nephrotoxicity by aminoglycosides), local toxicity (e.g.: airway irritation, bronchospasm, and cough) [100], pulmonary injury, worsening hypoxemia as well as secondary arrhythmias [101]. Moreover, obstruction of expiratory filters and ventilator malfunction was reported and contraindicate using drugs with lactose sugar or lipid components in the formulation (e.g.: zanamivir and lipid-based amphotericin formulations). Careful monitoring of the airway pressure and oxygen saturation is needed to anticipate severe adverse effects [102]. However, modification of ventilator parameters for appropriate jet-nebulizer use is not well-tolerated by some patients, leading to higher work of breathing and ventilator dys-synchrony which require additional sedation. Poor tolerance may preclude using aerosolized antibiotics in patients with high PEEP requirements or $PaO_2/FiO_2 < 200$ mmHg.

Initial concerns of drug resistance resulting from intratracheal or nebulized use of antibiotics (polymyxin B) were investigated and don't appear to be supported. Aerosolized antibiotics are applied through newer devices no more likely than IV therapy to confer bacterial resistance [103]. This was probably linked to previous generation nebulizers and the administration technique. Tolerance of aerosolization is different when drugs were nebulized for different durations of time. As a result, this may limit the use of aerosolization in patients with ARDS, severe hypoxemia, and severe pneumonia (in contrast to ventilator-associated tracheobronchitis), who often have poor tolerance.

When higher doses of colistin are nebulized, it may take 1 h of nebulization and many patients need relaxation or added sedatives (with potential increased risk of hypotension or myopathy). This requirement would be associated with a longer MV time and length of stay. Therefore, further studies should use pre-defined outcome parameters (instead of surrogates), careful recording of adverse effects, and control by hypoxemia [102].

Environmental contamination caused by the aerosolization of drugs in an open circuit represents a significant risk to the caregivers. To overcome this problem, expiratory filters with valves in the aerosol delivery devices should be used. This occupational risk exposure must be assessed and interventions to minimize these risks should be performed [10]. It is recommended to change the filter after every use, especially when giving aerosolized antibiotics.

Optimization of the above-mentioned factors may enhance effective drug delivery. However, it is critical to realize that aerosolization of drugs doesn't automatically lead to beneficial effects and sometimes may be harmful [104]. Furthermore, it was showed that the decrease in praxis, cognition, and executive function have a detrimental effect on inhaler technique because accurate and reliable inhalation would not be achieved. That was highly prevalent in elderly people. Therefore, it is more expected that elderly patients may not be able to use aerosolized drugs targeted for alveolar absorption. On the other hand, it is more likely that cognitively intact older people with acceptable neurological, musculoskeletal, and pulmonary performance would be able to use inhaled therapies like younger individuals [2].

9.3 Conclusion

The pulmonary route of drug administration had proved superior therapeutic outcomes than other routes of administration. The choice of one aerosolized medication over another should be based on efficacy, cost, drug properties, availability, and resistance patterns (in the case of antibiotics). A variety of aerosolized medications could be administered during mechanical ventilation (MV) including; bronchodilators, prostaglandins, mucolytic, proteins, surfactant, antibiotics, antibacterial, antiviral, antifungal, corticosteroids, anticoagulants, and miscellaneous. Optimal delivery of therapeutic doses is mainly based on applying a proper nominal dose of a proper formulation with the aid of an optimal administration technique through the aerosol generator.

Key Major Recommendations

1. Combining bronchodilators of different durations of action and mechanisms is more effective and had lower side effects if compared with increasing the dosage of a single bronchodilator.
2. Application of an external PEEP at a level that counterbalanced the intrinsic PEEP improved albuterol bronchodilator effect in mechanically-ventilated COPD patients.
3. Owing to their long duration of effect, inhaled iloprost or treprostinil are efficiently employed for the treatment of acute pulmonary hypertension in mechanically ventilated patients with no need for continuous aerosolization.
4. Placement of filters in the expiratory limb is recommended to trap any aerosolized surfactant in the circuit before it reaches the ventilator.
5. The use of aerosolized antibiotics is reserved for adjunctive therapy in the treatment of patients with severe pneumonia not responding to the conventional therapy, patients with multi-resistant organisms, or patients with tracheobronchitis after a long-term MV.
6. Special precautions should be given to avoid the crystallization of inhaled ribavirin within the respiratory equipment.
7. Long-term treatment of type 2 diabetic patients with Exubera was well-tolerated and effective in the control of glucose levels.
8. Inhalation of opiates is a preferable non-invasive route for the treatment of severe breakthrough pain in cancer patients.
9. Optimal delivery of therapeutic doses is mainly based on applying a proper nominal dose of a proper formulation with the aid of an optimal administration technique through the aerosol generator.
10. Careful monitoring of the airway pressure and oxygen saturation is needed during aerosol therapy of mechanically-ventilated patients to anticipate severe adverse effects.
11. Expiratory filters with valves in the aerosol delivery devices should be used to minimize environmental contamination caused by the aerosolization of drugs in an open circuit, and filter is recommended to be changed after every use, especially when giving aerosolized antibiotics.

References

1. Skyler JS, et al. Efficacy of inhaled human insulin in type 1 diabetes mellitus: a randomised proof-of-concept study. Lancet. 2001;357(9253):331–5.
2. Allen S. Are inhaled systemic therapies a viable option for the treatment of the elderly patient? Drugs Aging. 2008;25(2):89–94.

3. Byron PR, Patton JS. Drug delivery via the respiratory tract. J Aerosol Med. 1994;7(1):49–75.
4. Lipworth BJ. Pharmacokinetics of inhaled drugs. Br J Clin Pharmacol. 1996;42(6):697–705.
5. Byron PR. Determinants of drug and polypeptide bioavailability from aerosols delivered to the lung. Adv Drug Deliv Rev. 1990;5(1–2):107–32.
6. Elman M, et al. Influence of lung aeration on pulmonary concentrations of nebulized and intravenous amikacin in ventilated piglets with severe bronchopneumonia. J Am Soc Anesthesiol. 2002;97(1):199–206.
7. Goldstein I, et al. Lung deposition and efficiency of nebulized amikacin during Escherichia coli pneumonia in ventilated piglets. Am J Respir Crit Care Med. 2002;166(10):1375–81.
8. Goldstein I, et al. Mechanical ventilation-induced air-space enlargement during experimental pneumonia in piglets. Am J Respir Crit Care Med. 2001;163(4):958–64.
9. Ferrari F, et al. Nebulized ceftazidime in experimental pneumonia caused by partially resistant Pseudomonas aeruginosa. Intensive Care Med. 2009;35(10):1792–800.
10. Dhanani J, et al. Fundamentals of aerosol therapy in critical care. Crit Care. 2016;20(1):1–16.
11. Dhand R, Guntur VP. How best to deliver aerosol medications to mechanically ventilated patients. Clin Chest Med. 2008;29(2):277–96.
12. Dhand R, et al. Dose-response to bronchodilator delivered by metered-dose inhaler in ventilator-supported patients. Am J Respir Crit Care Med. 1996;154(2):388–93.
13. Duarte AG, Momii K, Bidani A. Bronchodilator therapy with metered-dose inhaler and spacer versus nebulizer in mechanically ventilated patients: comparison of magnitude and duration of response. Respir Care. 2000;45(7):817–23.
14. Yang SC, Yang SP, Lee TS. Nebulized ipratropium bromide in ventilator-assisted patients with chronic bronchitis. Chest. 1994;105(5):1511–5.
15. Ari A, Fink JB, Dhand R. Inhalation therapy in patients receiving mechanical ventilation: an update. J Aerosol Med Pulm Drug Deliv. 2012;25(6):319–32.
16. Appleton S, et al. Ipratropium bromide versus short acting beta-2 agonists for stable chronic obstructive pulmonary disease. The Cochrane Library. 2006.
17. Cazzola M, Molimard M. The scientific rationale for combining long-acting β 2-agonists and muscarinic antagonists in COPD. Pulm Pharmacol Therap. 2010;23(4):257–67.
18. Fernandez A, et al. Comparison of one versus two bronchodilators in ventilated COPD patients. Intensive Care Med. 1994;20(3):199–202.
19. Vogelmeier C, et al. Tiotropium versus salmeterol for the prevention of exacerbations of COPD. N Engl J Med. 2011;364(12):1093–103.
20. Tashkin DP, et al. Formoterol and tiotropium compared with tiotropium alone for treatment of COPD. J Chron Obstruct Pulm Dis. 2009;6(1):17–25.
21. GOLD. Global strategy for prevention, diagnosis and management of copd. 2020 [cited 2020 October 2020]. https://goldcopd.org/wp-content/uploads/2020/03/GOLD-2020-POCKET-GUIDE-ver1.0_FINAL-WMV.pdf.
22. Dhand R. Inhalation therapy with metered-dose inhalers and dry powder inhalers in mechanically ventilated patients. Respir Care. 2005;50(10):1331–45.
23. Dhand R, Tobin MJ. Inhaled bronchodilator therapy in mechanically ventilated patients. Am J Respir Crit Care Med. 1997;156(1):3–10.
24. Tzoufi M, et al. The effects of nebulized salbutamol, external positive end-expiratory pressure, and their combination on respiratory mechanics, hemodynamics, and gas exchange in mechanically ventilated chronic obstructive pulmonary disease patients. Anesth Analg. 2005;101(3):843–50.
25. Villar J, et al. Pulmonary hypertension in acute respiratory failure. Crit Care Med. 1989;17(6):523–6.
26. Bihari D, et al. The effects of vasodilation with prostacyclin on oxygen delivery and uptake in critically ill patients. N Engl J Med. 1987;317(7):397–403.
27. Radermacher P, et al. Prostacyclin for the treatment of pulmonary hypertension in the adult respiratory distress syndrome: effects on pulmonary capillary pressure and ventilation—perfusion distributions. J Am Soc Anesthesiol. 1990;72(2):238–44.

28. Meyer J, et al. Inhaled prostaglandin E1 for treatment of acute lung injury in severe multiple organ failure. Anesth Analg. 1998;86(4):753–8.
29. Putensen C, et al. Cardiopulmonary effects of aerosolized prostaglandin E1 and nitric oxide inhalation in patients with acute respiratory distress syndrome. Am J Respir Crit Care Med. 1998;157(6):1743–7.
30. Walmrath D, et al. Direct comparison of inhaled nitric oxide and aerosolized prostacyclin in acute respiratory distress syndrome. Am J Respir Crit Care Med. 1996;153(3):991–6.
31. Zwissler B, et al. Inhaled prostacyclin (PGI2) versus inhaled nitric oxide in adult respiratory distress syndrome. Am J Respir Crit Care Med. 1996;154(6):1671–7.
32. Walmrath D, et al. Effects of aerosolized prostacyclin in severe pneumonia. Impact of fibrosis. Am J Respir Crit Care Med. 1995;151(3):724–30.
33. Hoeper MM, et al. Long-term treatment of primary pulmonary hypertension with aerosolized iloprost, a prostacyclin analogue. N Engl J Med. 2000;342(25):1866–70.
34. Olschewski H, et al. Inhaled iloprost for severe pulmonary hypertension. N Engl J Med. 2002;347(5):322–9.
35. Leuchte HH, et al. Hemodynamic response to sildenafil, nitric oxide, and iloprost in primary pulmonary hypertension. Chest. 2004;125(2):580–6.
36. Ghofrani HA, et al. Combination therapy with oral sildenafil and inhaled iloprost for severe pulmonary hypertension. Ann Intern Med. 2002;136(7):515–22.
37. Voswinckel R, et al. Inhaled treprostinil for treatment of chronic pulmonary arterial hypertension. Ann Intern Med. 2006;144(2):149–50.
38. Lewis JF, Jobe AH. Surfactant and the adult respiratory distress syndrome. Am Rev Respir Dis. 1993;147:218.
39. Davidson WJ, et al. Exogenous pulmonary surfactant for the treatment of adult patients with acute respiratory distress syndrome: results of a meta-analysis. Crit Care. 2006;10(2):1–9.
40. Spragg RG, et al. Acute effects of a single dose of porcine surfactant on patients with the adult respiratory distress syndrome. Chest. 1994;105(1):195–202.
41. Spragg RG, et al. Treatment of acute respiratory distress syndrome with recombinant surfactant protein C surfactant. Am J Respir Crit Care Med. 2003;167(11):1562–6.
42. Walmrath D, et al. Bronchoscopic surfactant administration in patients with severe adult respiratory distress syndrome and sepsis. Am J Respir Crit Care Med. 1996;154(1):57–62.
43. Wiswell TE, et al. Bronchopulmonary segmental lavage with surfaxin (KL4-surfactant) for acute respiratory distress syndrome. Am J Respir Crit Care Med. 1999;160(4):1188–95.
44. Anzueto A, et al. Aerosolized surfactant in adults with sepsis-induced acute respiratory distress syndrome. N Engl J Med. 1996;334(22):1417–22.
45. Weg JG, et al. Safety and potential efficacy of an aerosolized surfactant in human sepsis-induced adult respiratory distress syndrome. JAMA. 1994;272(18):1433–8.
46. Lewis JF, et al. Physiologic responses and distribution of aerosolized surfactant (Survanta®) in a nonuniform pattern of lung injury. Am Rev Respir Dis. 1993;147(6_pt_1):1364–70.
47. Spragg RG, et al. Effect of recombinant surfactant protein C–based surfactant on the acute respiratory distress syndrome. N Engl J Med. 2004;351(9):884–92.
48. Chastre J, Fagon J-Y. Ventilator-associated pneumonia. Am J Respir Crit Care Med. 2002;165(7):867–903.
49. Lu Q, et al. Nebulized and intravenous colistin in experimental pneumonia caused by Pseudomonas aeruginosa. Intensive Care Med. 2010;36(7):1147–55.
50. Adair C, et al. Eradication of endotracheal tube biofilm by nebulised gentamicin. Intensive Care Med. 2002;28(4):426–31.
51. Adair C, et al. Implications of endotracheal tube biofilm for ventilator-associated pneumonia. Intensive Care Med. 1999;25(10):1072–6.
52. Campbell PW, Saiman L. Use of aerosolized antibiotics in patients with cystic fibrosis. Chest. 1999;116(3):775–88.
53. Ramsey BW, et al. Intermittent administration of inhaled tobramycin in patients with cystic fibrosis. N Engl J Med. 1999;340(1):23–30.

54. Solé-Lleonart C, et al. Intratracheal administration of antimicrobial agents in mechanically ventilated adults: an international survey on delivery practices and safety. Respir Care. 2016;61(8):1008–14.
55. Panidis D, et al. Penetration of gentamicin into the alveolar lining fluid of critically ill patients with ventilator-associated pneumonia. Chest. 2005;128(2):545–52.
56. Ferrari F, et al. Lack of lung tissue and systemic accumulation after consecutive daily aerosols of amikacin in ventilated piglets with healthy lungs. J Am Soc Anesthesiol. 2003;98(4):1016–9.
57. Lu Q, et al. Efficacy of high-dose nebulized colistin in ventilator-associated pneumonia caused by multidrug-resistant Pseudomonas aeruginosa and Acinetobacter baumannii. J Am Soc Anesthesiol. 2012;117(6):1335–47.
58. Abdellatif S, et al. Efficacy and toxicity of aerosolised colistin in ventilator-associated pneumonia: a prospective, randomised trial. Ann Intensive Care. 2016;6(1):1–11.
59. Feeley T, et al. Aerosol polymyxin and pneumonia in seriously ill patients. N Engl J Med. 1975;293(10):471–5.
60. Palmer LB, et al. Aerosolized antibiotics in mechanically ventilated patients: delivery and response. Crit Care Med. 1998;26(1):31–9.
61. Hamer DH. Treatment of nosocomial pneumonia and tracheobronchitis caused by multidrug-resistant Pseudomonas aeruginosa with aerosolized colistin. Am J Respir Crit Care Med. 2000;162(1):328–30.
62. Michalopoulos A, et al. Aerosolized colistin for the treatment of nosocomial pneumonia due to multidrug-resistant gram-negative bacteria in patients without cystic fibrosis. Crit Care. 2005;9(1):1–7.
63. Smith DW, et al. A controlled trial of aerosolized ribavirin in infants receiving mechanical ventilation for severe respiratory syncytial virus infection. N Engl J Med. 1991;325(1):24–9.
64. Fernandez R, et al. The effect of short-term instillation of a mucolytic agent (mesna) on airway resistance in mechanically ventilated patients. Chest. 1995;107(4):1101–6.
65. Merkus P, et al. DNase treatment for atelectasis in infants with severe respiratory syncytial virus bronchiolitis. Eur Respir J. 2001;18(4):734–7.
66. Zandstra D, Stoutenbeek C, Miranda D. Effect of mucolytic and bronchodilator aerosol therapy on airway resistance in mechanically ventilated patients. Intensive Care Med. 1985;11(6):316–8.
67. Merz U, et al. Inhaled budesonide in ventilator-dependent preterm infants: a randomized, double-blind pilot study. Neonatology. 1999;75(1):46–53.
68. Cole CH, et al. Early inhaled glucocorticoid therapy to prevent bronchopulmonary dysplasia. N Engl J Med. 1999;340(13):1005–10.
69. Dhand R. Inhalation therapy in invasive and noninvasive mechanical ventilation. Curr Opin Crit Care. 2007;13(1):27–38.
70. Balwani G, et al. Evaluation of the AERx system for the pulmonary delivery of recombinant human interferon alfa-2b to healthy subjects. In: 29th annual meeting of the Controlled Release Society, Seoul, Korea; 2002.
71. Gonda I. Systemic delivery of drugs to humans via inhalation. J Aerosol Med. 2006;19(1):47–53.
72. Owens DR, Bolli GB, Zinman B. Alternative routes of insulin delivery. International textbook of diabetes mellitus; 2003.
73. Clark AR. Dry powder inhalation systems from inhale therapeutic systems. Drugs Pharm Sci. 2003;126:903–12.
74. Hollander PA, et al. Efficacy and safety of inhaled insulin (Exubera) compared with subcutaneous insulin therapy in patients with type 2 diabetes: results of a 6-month, randomized, comparative trial. Diabetes Care. 2004;27(10):2356–62.
75. Schuster J, Farr SJ. The AERx pulmonary drug delivery system. Drugs Pharm Sci. 2003;126:825–34.

76. Gonda I, et al. Inhalation delivery systems with compliance and disease management capabilities. J Control Release. 1998;53(1–3):269–74.
77. Mellén A, et al. Pharmacokinetics and intra-subject variability of inhaled insulin in healthy smokers and non-smokers. Diabetes. 2001;50.
78. Henry RR, et al. Inhaled insulin using the AERx insulin diabetes management system in healthy and asthmatic subjects. Diabetes Care. 2003;26(3):764–9.
79. Hermansen K, et al. Intensive treatment with pulmonary insulin using the AERx® insulin diabetes management system-a proof of concept trial in type 2 diabetic patients. Diabetes. 2002;51.
80. Adamson U, et al. Inhaled human insulin via the AERx ((R)) insulin Diabetes Management System in combination with NPH insulin offers the same metabolic control as intensive sc therapy. A proof of concept trial in type 2 diabetic patients. In: Diabetologia. New York: Springer; 2002.
81. Stoever JA, Palmer JP. Inhaled insulin and insulin antibodies: a new twist to an old debate. Diabetes Technol Ther. 2002;4(2):157–61.
82. Gonda I. The ascent of pulmonary drug delivery. J Pharm Sci. 2000;89(7):940–5.
83. Gonda I. Deoxyribonuclease inhalation. Lung Biol Health Dis. 1997;107:355–66.
84. Sanders M. Inhalation therapy: an historical review. Prim Care Respir J. 2007;16(2):71–81.
85. Farr SJ, et al. AERx-development of a novel liquid aerosol delivery system concept to clinic. Respir Drug Deliv. 1996;1:175–85.
86. Boyle F, et al. Inhaled fentanyl via the AERx system for the treatment of breakthrough cancer pain. In: Poster presented at: 19th Annual Scientific Meeting, American Pain Society. 2000.
87. Solé-Lleonart C, et al. Global survey on nebulization of antimicrobial agents in mechanically ventilated patients: a call for international guidelines. Clin Microbiol Infect. 2016;22(4):359–64.
88. Ehrmann S, et al. Aerosol therapy during mechanical ventilation: an international survey. Intensive Care Med. 2013;39(6):1048–56.
89. Guillon A, et al. Aerosol route to administer teicoplanin in mechanical ventilation: in vitro study, lung deposition and pharmacokinetic analyses in pigs. J Aerosol Med Pulm Drug Deliv. 2015;28(4):290–8.
90. Ferrari F, et al. Comparison of lung tissue concentrations of nebulized ceftazidime in ventilated piglets: ultrasonic versus vibrating plate nebulizers. Intensive Care Med. 2008;34(9):1718–23.
91. Tonnellier M, et al. Intravenous versus nebulized ceftazidime in ventilated piglets with and without experimental bronchopneumonia: comparative effects of helium and nitrogen. J Am Soc Anesthesiol. 2005;102(5):995–1000.
92. Manthous CA, et al. Metered-dose inhaler versus nebulized albuterol in mechanically ventilated patients. Am Rev Respir Dis. 1993;148:1567.
93. Spahr-Schopfer I, et al. Proximate delivery of a large experimental dose from salbutamol MDI induces epithelial airway lesions in intubated rabbits. Am J Respir Crit Care Med. 1994;150(3):790–4.
94. Silverglade A. Cardiac toxicity of aerosol propellants. JAMA. 1972;222(7):827–9.
95. Fink JB, et al. Aerosol delivery from a metered-dose inhaler during mechanical ventilation. An in vitro model. Am J Respir Crit Care Med. 1996;154(2):382–7.
96. Fink JB, et al. Reconciling in vitro and in vivo measurements of aerosol delivery from a metered-dose inhaler during mechanical ventilation and defining efficiency-enhancing factors. Am J Respir Crit Care Med. 1999;159(1):63–8.
97. Miller DD, et al. Aerosol delivery and modern mechanical ventilation: in vitro/in vivo evaluation. Am J Respir Crit Care Med. 2003;168(10):1205–9.
98. O'Riordan TG, Palmer LB, Smaldone GC. Aerosol deposition in mechanically ventilated patients. Optimizing nebulizer delivery. Am J Respir Crit Care Med. 1994;149(1):214–9.
99. Guerin C, et al. Inhaled bronchodilator administration during mechanical ventilation: how to optimize it, and for which clinical benefit? J Aerosol Med Pulm Drug Deliv. 2008;21(1):85–96.

100. Katzman M, et al. High incidence of bronchospasm with regular administration of aerosolized pentamidine. Chest. 1992;101(1):79–81.
101. Van Heerden P, et al. Pulmonary toxicity of inhaled aerosolized prostacyclin therapy—an observational study. Anaesth Intensive Care. 2000;28(2):161–6.
102. Lu Q, et al. Nebulized ceftazidime and amikacin in ventilator-associated pneumonia caused by Pseudomonas aeruginosa. Am J Respir Crit Care Med. 2011;184(1):106–15.
103. Palmer LB, Smaldone GC. Reduction of bacterial resistance with inhaled antibiotics in the intensive care unit. Am J Respir Crit Care Med. 2014;189(10):1225–33.
104. Zitter JN, et al. Inhaled Dornase alfa (Pulmozyme) as a noninvasive treatment of atelectasis in mechanically ventilated patients. J Crit Care. 2013;28(2):218.e1–7.

Chapter 10
Aerosol Therapies During High Flow Oxygen Therapy

Contents

10.1 Introduction

Recently, combining inhaled drug delivery with high flow nasal cannula (HFNC) is greatly used in hospital settings to allow the administration of scheduled doses of inhaled drugs without the discontinuation of gas flow in critically ill patients. These systems enable the delivery of the drug in a significant amount producing the desired therapeutic effect without stopping the gas. Many benefits arise from combining oxygen therapy with inhaled drug delivery as allowing the release of only smaller particles while large particles (>4 μm) are deposited within the device and also improving the patient tolerability to the whole procedure [1–4]. The loss of aerosol within these systems was found to be significantly high which was proven by various studies and might be returned to the humidification and heating of medical gas used. Narrow therapeutic indexed and expensive drugs are greatly affected by such limitations [3, 5–7]. Enhanced condensational growth technique can reduce the aerosol loss within HFNC system from 50% to only 20% by providing submicrometer-sized aerosol droplets rather than micrometer-sized droplets but the

M. E. A. Abdelrahim et al., *Essentials of Aerosol Therapy in Critically ill Patients*,
https://doi.org/10.1007/978-3-030-85026-5_10

clinical evidence of such technique is still debated [2, 8, 9]. Factors that determine the amount of aerosol delivery within a high flow system are the flow rate of gas, gas density, type of aerosol generator, and its position and interface type.

10.2 Factors Affecting Aerosol Delivery Within High Flow Oxygen System

10.2.1 Flow Rate of Gas

High flow systems can deliver gas flow rates up to 60 L/min but with increasing the gas flow rate, the amount of delivered dose is significantly decreased. The lower aerosol delivery is thought to be due to the increased turbulence within the HFNC circuit which results in particle deposition by the inertial impaction, especially within the nasal cannula [1–3, 10]. Aerosol loss noticed when HFNC is used in pediatrics is much lower than that noticed in adults as the maximum gas flow delivered in most pediatric situations is equal to 8 L/min [5, 11]. A previous study had tested the effect of different gas flow rates (5, 10, 20, and 40 L/min) on the delivered inhaled dose using an adult-sized cannula within the Vapotherm system and had demonstrated that the inspired dose of the drug was inversely proportional to gas flow while a negligible amount of drug was approximately estimated at the cannula outlet at a gas flow rate of 40 L/min [7]. Also, Reminiac et al. had tested the optimal conditions for implementing aerosol nebulization within the HFNC system (OptiflowTM system). They emphasized the inverse relationship between gas flow and the inspired dose but they found that respiratory distress conditions (open-mouth breathing) had resulted in a higher respirable mass than quiet breathing patterns (closed mouth breathing) at higher gas flow rates tested (30, 45, and 60 L/min) [6]. In contrast, one study reported the increase of aerosol delivery with increasing gas flow rate in simulated distressed breathing patterns [12]. The loss of inhaled dose within this system can be returned to the deposition in the small-diameter nasal cannula or humidifier or large-diameter tubing. Previous work performed on animal models simulating full-term newborn and 9-month toddler had observed that increasing gas flow rate was associated with an increase in nasal cannula deposition as 2.6% of nasal cannula deposition was estimated at a gas flow rate of 2 L/min versus 28.8% at 8 L/min. Conversely, aerosol deposition in the humidifier was increased with low gas flow rates (37.3% at 2 L/min versus 13.9 at 8 L/min) [5]. Additionally, the use of oxygen gas was found to improve the aerosol delivery within the HFNC system if compared with that without any oxygen delivery using the same system [1]. Future studies are needed to identify the regional deposition of nebulized drugs in lungs delivered by a mean HFNC system to ensure the efficiency of such technique [13]. Madney et al. had compared the delivery of a vibrating mesh nebulizer and jet nebulizer within a high flow system but at a selected low oxygen flow of 5 L/min and 100% oxygen concentration in acutely exacerbated chronic obstructive pulmonary disease (COPD) patients through the use of urinary pharmacokinetic quantification method [2]. They demonstrated encouraging results of this technique which were comparable to aerosol nebulization within non-invasive ventilation (NIV) circuit in COPD [14–21].

10.2.2 *The Type of Aerosol Generator and Its Position Within the HFNC Circuit*

Aerosol generators such as nebulizers and pressurized metered-dose inhalers (pMDIs) can be used within the HFNC system to deliver the inhaled drugs to patients where they are placed in upstream position just before the humidifier or in downstream position immediately after the humidifier or just before the patient interface as illustrated in Fig. 10.1 [1–3, 5, 6, 13, 22]. Of note, this type of open system design is offered by Fisher-Paykel Healthcare Corporation.

Previous studies showed the superiority of the upstream position over the other two positions as large particles are trapped within the humidifier which can reduce nasal and oropharyngeal aerosol deposition allowing only particles with smaller sizes to effectively reach the patient [1, 6]. In contrast, the Vapotherm high flow system only offers one position for placing an aerosol generator which is just before

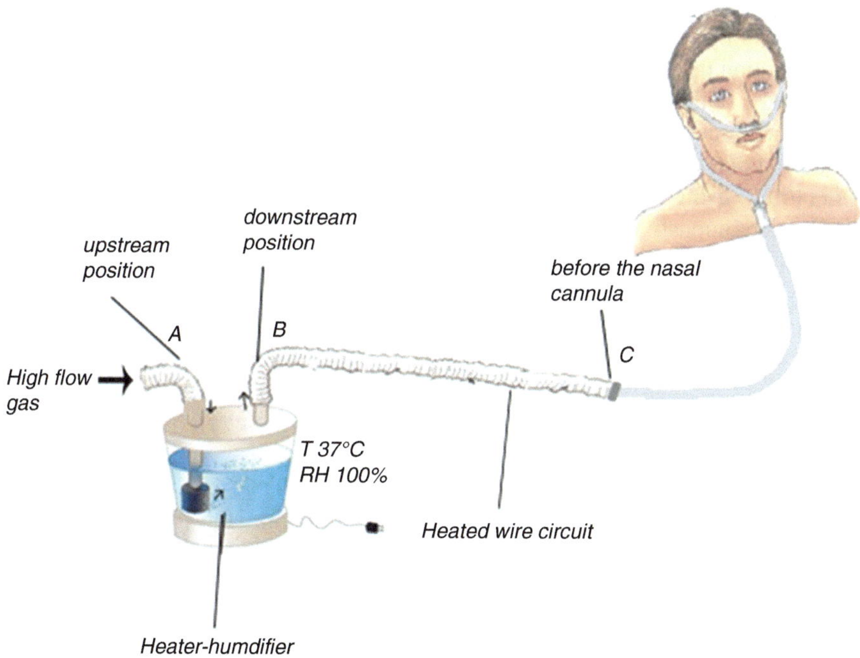

Fig. 10.1 A diagram illustrating three positions available for placing the aerosol generator

the nasal cannula since it is a closed system which may account for its lower aerosol delivery when compared with that of Fisher-Paykel [1, 3, 7, 22]. Lower aerosol delivery can be returned to forcing the high flow gas through a small diameter cannula which increases gas flow turbulence leading to high drug deposition in the nebulizer adapter and lower drug fraction to reach the patient [7].

Vibrating mesh nebulizers are considered the best aerosol generators to be used within the high flow system where jet nebulizers exhibit some limitations as high residual volume and aerosol loss which can be solved partly by the dilution of inhaled drugs with saline or water with a noticeable increase in the time of nebulization. Previous studies reported the lower efficiency of jet nebulizers to deliver inhaled salbutamol dose when compared with vibration mesh nebulizer in COPD patients [2, 3]. Furthermore, the drug solution in jet nebulizer can be nebulized either by the delivered high gas flow or through the use of a compressor where the airflow is added to the total flow delivered by the system [24–26]. Unfortunately, testing pMDIs with holding chambers within the HFNC system showed unsatisfactory results which returned to the effect of gas density on the evaporation of propellant [3].

10.2.3 Density of Gas

The density of the gas has a negative impact on the aerosol delivery within high flow systems similar to NIV circuits. Heliox (80% helium:20% oxygen) is the highest concentration that can be safely administered in the clinical setting. The heliox can provide the optimal impact on aerosol delivery within the HFNC system since its effects are concentration-dependent which lowers the flow turbulence and the loss of aerosol due to impaction. When the use of heliox was compared with pure oxygen (100%) using HFNC system, heliox had resulted in the higher aerosol deposition of continuously nebulized drugs than pure oxygen in both adult and pediatric patients [10, 12]. Also, pMDIs exhibit lower aerosol delivery efficiency when the density of the gas delivered is increased. The maximum effect of denser gases on pMDI aerosol delivery is noticed at selected low gas flows since it decreases both the shearing force applied on gas layers and the evaporation rate of propellant [3].

10.2.4 Interface

The nasal cannula is the standard interface used within a high flow system while the size of the nasal cannula can affect the aerosol delivery. Cannulas with pediatric, infant, and adult sizes are available while adult cannula delivers higher aerosol doses than infant and pediatric ones [27]. Interfaces like facemask and mouthpiece can guarantee better aerosol delivery than nasal cannula but with great concern regarding tolerability and patient comfort since mouthpiece, use needs patient cooperation and is difficult to be maintained during sleep. On the other hand, a facemask increases the risk for facial and ocular aerosol deposition and claustrophobic feelings besides interference with daily activity. These interfaces can exclusively be used within high flow systems for mouthbreathers or only during the time of nebulization, especially for expensive or narrow therapeutic index drugs [1, 28].

References

1. Madney YM, et al. The influence of changing interfaces on aerosol delivery within high flow oxygen setting in adults: an in-vitro study. J Drug Deliv Sci Technol. 2020;55:101365.
2. Madney YM, et al. Aerosol delivery through an adult high-flow nasal cannula circuit using low-flow oxygen. Respir Care. 2019;64(4):453–61.
3. Madney YM, et al. Nebulizers and spacers for aerosol delivery through adult nasal cannula at low oxygen flow rate: an in-vitro study. J Drug Deliv Sci Technol. 2017;39:260–5.
4. Hess DR. Aerosol therapy during noninvasive ventilation or high-flow nasal cannula. Respir Care. 2015;60(6):880–91; discussion 891–3.
5. Reminiac F, et al. Nasal high flow nebulization in infants and toddlers: an in vitro and in vivo scintigraphic study. Pediatr Pulmonol. 2017;52(3):337–44.
6. Reminiac F, et al. Aerosol therapy in adults receiving high flow nasal cannula oxygen therapy. J Aerosol Med Pulm Drug Deliv. 2016;29(2):134–41.
7. Perry SA, et al. Influences of cannula size and flow rate on aerosol drug delivery through the vapotherm humidified high-flow nasal cannula system. Pediatr Crit Care Med. 2013;14(5):e250–6.
8. Golshahi L, et al. Intermittent aerosol delivery to the lungs during high-flow nasal cannula therapy. Respir Care. 2014;59(10):1476–86.
9. Golshahi L, et al. The use of condensational growth methods for efficient drug delivery to the lungs during noninvasive ventilation high flow therapy. Pharm Res. 2013;30(11):2917–30.
10. Ari A, et al. In vitro comparison of heliox and oxygen in aerosol delivery using pediatric high flow nasal cannula. Pediatr Pulmonol. 2011;46(8):795–801.
11. Saslow JG, et al. Work of breathing using high-flow nasal cannula in preterm infants. J Perinatol. 2006;26(8):476–80.
12. Dailey PA, et al. Aerosol delivery through adult high flow nasal cannula with heliox and oxygen. Respir Care. 2017;62(9):1186–92.
13. Alcoforado L, et al. Impact of gas flow and humidity on trans-nasal aerosol deposition via nasal cannula in adults: a randomized cross-over study. Pharmaceutics. 2019;11(7):320.
14. Harb HS, et al. Performance of large spacer versus nebulizer T-piece in single-limb noninvasive ventilation. Respir Care. 2018;63(11):1360–9.
15. Abdelrahim ME. Aerosol delivery to a critically ill patient: a big issue easily solved by developing guidelines. Pulm Ther. 2018;4(2):125–33.
16. Hassan A, et al. In-vitro/in-vivo comparison of inhaled salbutamol dose delivered by jet nebulizer, vibrating mesh nebulizer and metered dose inhaler with spacer during non-invasive ventilation. Exp Lung Res. 2017;43(1):19–28.
17. ElHansy ME, et al. Inhaled salbutamol dose delivered by jet nebulizer, vibrating mesh nebulizer and metered dose inhaler with spacer during invasive mechanical ventilation. Pulm Pharmacol Ther. 2017;45:159–63.
18. Rabea H, et al. Modelling of in-vitro and in-vivo performance of aerosol emitted from different vibrating mesh nebulisers in non-invasive ventilation circuit. Eur J Pharm Sci. 2016;97:182–91.
19. Hussein RR, et al. In vitro/in vivo correlation and modeling of emitted dose and lung deposition of inhaled salbutamol from metered dose inhalers with different types of spacers in noninvasively ventilated patients. Pharm Dev Technol. 2017;22(7):871–80.

20. Abdelrahim ME, Plant PK, Chrystyn H. The relative lung and systemic bioavailability of terbutaline following nebulisation in non-invasively ventilated patients. Int J Pharm. 2011;420(2):313–8.
21. Abdelrahim ME, Assi KH, Chrystyn H. Relative bioavailability of terbutaline to the lung following inhalation, using urinary excretion. Br J Clin Pharmacol. 2011;71(4):608–10.
22. Bhashyam AR, et al. Aerosol delivery through nasal cannulas: an in vitro study. J Aerosol Med Pulm Drug Deliv. 2008;21(2):181–8.
24. Lewis RA, Fleming JS. Fractional deposition from a jet nebulizer: how it differs from a metered dose inhaler. Br J Dis Chest. 1985;79:361–7.
25. Waldrep J, Dhand R. Advanced nebulizer designs employing vibrating mesh/aperture plate technologies for aerosol generation. Curr Drug Deliv. 2008;5(2):114–9.
26. Saeed H, et al. Fill volume, humidification and heat effects on aerosol delivery and fugitive emissions during noninvasive ventilation. J Drug Deliv Sci Technol. 2017;39:372–8.
27. Harb HS, et al. Update efficacy of aerosol therapy with noninvasive ventilator approach (non-invasive ventilation and nasal high flow). J Drug Deliv Sci Technol. 2020;59:101922.
28. Madney YM, et al. Aerosol delivery aspects within a high flow therapy system in chronic obstructive pulmonary disease patients. ERJ Open Res; 2020.

Chapter 11
Methods of Detecting Aerosol Delivery to the Lung

Contents

11.1 Introduction

Assessment of inhaled drug formulation and the device that generates the aerosol is essential to determine the efficacy of aerosol delivery. These could involve in-vitro, ex-vivo, and in-vivo studies which detect and measure the amount of emitted drug

M. E. A. Abdelrahim et al., *Essentials of Aerosol Therapy in Critically ill Patients*,
https://doi.org/10.1007/978-3-030-85026-5_11

and also the amount of the drug that deposited in the patient lung. Also, the portion of the drug that had been absorbed systemically after swallowing the drug could be determined [1–3].

In-vitro studies for assessment of inhaled medications characterization mainly focus on two main factors that influence aerosol delivery, these factors are the range of aerosol particle size distribution and the total released dose.

The distribution of the size of the released aerosol particles or droplets could be described in different ways. Ways of description depend on one of the following parameters, the volume, number, and mass of aerosol particles. The frequencies of occurrence of each parameter are recorded and the final expression includes the value that half of the particles follow at least. Scientific expressions of each parameter are the volume median diameter (VMD), Count median diameter (CMD), and mass median diameter (MMD) [4, 5]. In case all particles of the released aerosol have the same density, the CMD and VMD will have the same value or will be identical [6]. The CMD is not usable or useful in measuring the amount of inhaled drug that is delivered or emitted from the aerosol-producing devices as the droplet that has a large size contains more drugs than that has a small size or small diameter. The aerodynamic diameter (the spherical aerosol droplets diameter) is the optimum way to describe the aerodynamic characteristics of aerosol generated. The emitted doses of an inhaled medication have polydispersity and it is best to be described by mass median aerodynamic diameter (MMAD) using inertial impaction because it could describe the behavior of the aerosol particles in certain airflow. Geometric standard deviation (GSD) is also used with MMAD to describe the range of polydispersity. Increasing polydispersity is reflected by the large GSD value [4].

11.2 Particle Size Distribution

The distribution of the aerosol particle size could be determined by two methods the first is the inertial impaction and the second method is the laser diffraction. Laser diffraction measures the aerosol particle volume while inertial impaction measures the amount of drug entrained within the released droplets [7].

11.3 Measuring Aerosol Particle Distribution with Inertial Impaction

An impactor device is a device that consists of many stages each stage has smaller pores compared to the one before. Air passes through the device by connecting it to a pump, the airflow is determined using a flow meter. Each stage traps aerosol particles with particles size more than their permeability ability as shown in Fig. 11.1.

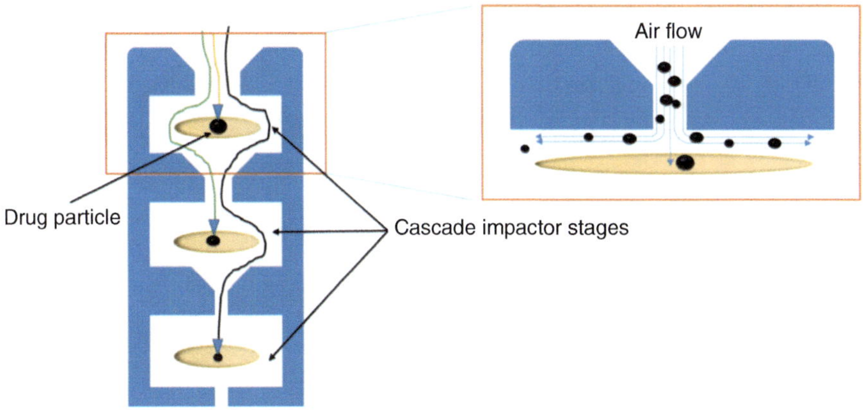

Fig. 11.1 Schematic design explaining the principle of operation for cascade impactors

The last stage of the impactor is a filter that collects all small particles that passed through all the above stages and were not affected with impaction. The more the number of cascade stages the higher the accuracy and validity of the aerodynamic characterization and the distribution of particle size will be clear. Regarding the size analysis of aerosol particles, cascade impactors are the most commonly used devices [8]. There are many types of cascade impactors [9–11].

11.4 Twin Stage Impinger

This type of impactors as shown in Fig. 11.2a could be operated at certain flow rates, 30 and 90 L/min. It is not expensive and also a simple device that could be used for quality control analysis of aerosol-products. However, the impinger is simple but also it cannot provide sufficient and accurate resolution of aerodynamic characterization for aerosol particles in the range between half and five micrograms and this is due to the low number of stages [13].

11.5 Marple-Miller Cascade Impactor

Marple-Miller Cascade Impactor (MMI) was originally designed to meet the needs of the pharmaceutical application particularly the evaluation of medical inhalers, but it could be used in other fields as well. The operating method, with flow rates of 30, 60, and 90 liters per minute, was designed to speed and facilitate the preparation of samples for the quantitative and chemical analyzes needed for multi-component sprays [14]. The low losses of aerosol particles in the interstage space of the impactor was a prime consideration to simplify data analysis and allow the accurate sum

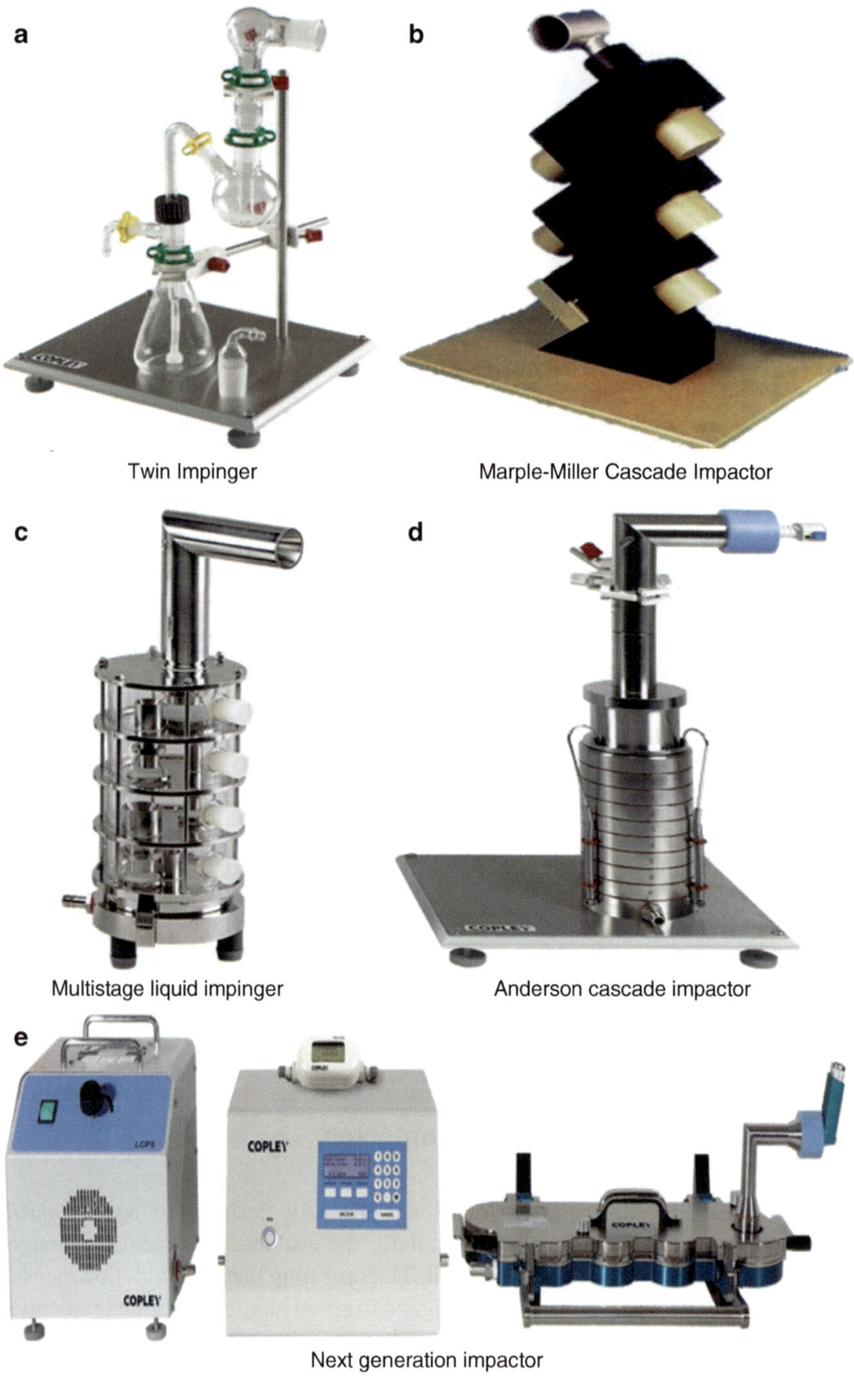

Fig. 11.2 Several types of cascade impactors (**a**) Twin impinger (**b**) Marple-Miller Cascade Impactor (**c**) Multistage liquid impinger (**d**) Anderson cascade impactor (**e**) Next-generation impactor [12]

of the drug portions collected on each stage to measure the total emitted dose. The port of entry to the cascade is intended to imitate the human throat holdup characteristics for a pressurized metered-dose inhaler (pMDI), (Fig. 11.2b) [14] and it is of the required geometry to serve as a pre-separator and a means of allowing the suspended spray particles as long as it remains in the throat of the patient. The distribution of mass and size of aerosol particles contained on the recovery surfaces of the different stages will thus closely correlate to the mass and dimensions of the material moving through the human throat. This device is a five-stage impactor, the MMI is therefore unconventional in its stream, making it simpler for removable external collection cups rather than impaction plates to be used. The outside removable collection cups enable for simple and fast removal of MMI drug deposits from the impactor without the cumbersome dismantling of the entire impactor, as with traditional cascading impactors. There are two available models of MMI, the first is the high flow rate impactor (model 160) that operates at a flow rate of 60 or 90 liters per minutes, while the second version (model 150) is a low flow rate impactor that acts at 30 liters per minute.

11.6 Multistage Liquid Impinger

Multistage liquid impinger (MSLI) is more accurate than twin stage impinger as it has a higher number of stages but still an insufficient number of stages to provide detailed information about generated aerosol particles. MSLI consists of five stages, the last one contains only a filter as shown in Fig. 11.2c.

11.7 Anderson Cascade Impactor

Anderson cascade impactor (ACI) is a multistage impactor that consists of eight plates as shown in Fig. 11.2d. All ACI plates have pores that are accurately drilled with different cut-off diameters. Decreasing cut-off diameters of the plates starting from higher pores diameter in the upper stage moving to the final filter that collects the smallest particle sizes. The ACI produce a more detailed report about the inhaled aerosol particle generated by different aerosol generators due to the larger number of stages with different cut off pores compared to MSLI and twin stage impinger [15, 16].

ACI could be used with different inhalation or flow rates by doing some rearrangement in the cascade stages [17]. Normal plates or stages distribution of ACI should be used with a flow rate of less than 30 L/min but higher flow rates like 60 and 90 L/min need stage replacement. For an inhalation rate equal to 60 L/min two stages should be removed (stage 0 and stage 7) and another two stages should be added at the top (stage −1 and stage −0). For an inhalation rate equal to 90 L/min, three stages should be removed (stage 0, 6, and 7) and should be replaced by (stage −0, −1, and −2).

Another method of using ACI with high flow rates greater than 30 L/min is by adjusting the cut-off diameters of stages of the ACI according to the following equation $ECD_{F2} = ECD_{28.3}\ (28.3/F2)^{0.5}$. Where ECD_{F2} is the Effective Cut off Diameter at the higher flow, $ECD_{28.3}$ is the ECD at the stander flow (28.3 L/min) and F2 is the higher flow rate in L/min [18]. The previous setting differs from the settings used with the dry powder inhaler (DPI). In the case of aerodynamic characterization of aerosol particles generated by DPIs, a pre-separator should be added to the ACI to prevent aerosol particles larger than 10 μg from bouncing to stages of the impactor [19].

11.8 Next-Generation Impactors

The next generation impactor (NGI) (Fig. 11.2e) was developed for testing aerosol-producing devices. This type of impactors could act with any inhalation flow rate that lies between 30 and 100 L/min. The design of NGI allows for rapid analysis of the samples and easy collection of deposited particles inside the different collection cups. The results of ACI with modifications could be comparable to that of the NGI [19].

11.9 Light Diffraction Methods

To characterize aerosols in the atmosphere as well as in specific applications, optical particle counters (OPCs) in which particle size discrimination is based on variations in scattered light intensity within a well-defined angle are commonly used. However, sampling issues seriously restrict their applicability to the study of aerosols from different pharmaceutical inhalers, as many laser emitting instruments require the concentrating of individual particles in the light path as they are measured, which limits the flow rate that can be achieved in the OPC [20]. OPC systems also are prone to a range of environmental factors, such as optical contamination in the window while there is a sampling cell, which alters either the light intensity of the illuminating beam or the scattered light detected [20].

11.10 Laser Diffraction

The laser diffraction method depends on emitting aerosol from aerosol-producing devices and passing it through the laser beam produced by the laser emitting device. Aerosol particles cause a great scattering of the laser beam, scattered laser rays then pass through a specific lens to be detected and analyzed by a detector. The size of the emitted aerosol droplet is inversely proportional to the angle of light diffraction. Laser diffraction is suitable for the determination of geometric characterization of the aerosol, not the aerodynamic characterization. It calculates the volume of

Table 11.1 Advantages and disadvantages of laser diffraction techniques

Advantages	Disadvantages
For a given optical configuration, it has a wide measurement range	The mass of active pharmaceutical ingredients is not explicitly traceable
It depends on the volume (mass)–weighted measurements rather than the number-weighted size distribution	Aerosol particles are presumed to be spherical
The time required for sample analysis is shorter than that required by cascade impactor which requires further investigation after aerosol distribution inside the impactor	"Vignetting" can occur in several configurations, especially when used in open bench mode, in which light scattered at large angles misses the array of detectors, and thus results in bias due to the lack of the finest particles in the distribution
Lazer diffraction techniques are noninvasive in open bench mode	Multiple scattering from highly concentrated aerosols can lead to bias associated with the true size distribution being over-broadened
The reproducibility between subsequent measurements of the same aerosol-producing device is excellent	In measuring aerosols where volatile substances (water or ethanol) are present, droplet evaporation during measurement may result in a bias to finer aerosol sizes
Analysis of aerosol samples did not require the preparation of other calibrating samples in contrast to cascade impactors	As a result of changes in the refractive index of the support gas for the measured aerosol, beam steering can occur

released aerosol [21, 22]. The use of a laser diffractor for the assessment of particle size of medical inhalers has certain advantages but also, there are more limitations (Table 11.1) [23].

11.11 Pulmonary Function Tests

The function of the lung could be evaluated by several tests that assess the ability of the lung to inhale and exhale the air and determine the extent of lung obstruction. These tests are used in classifying obstructive lung disease into different classes of severity. Monitoring the efficacy of respirable drugs also could be determined by pulmonary function tests [24].

11.12 Spirometry

Spirometry is a quick and simple technique in which the spirometer device (Fig. 11.3) is used to measure the patients' rate and amount of exhaled gas. The patient should exhale through the spirometer mouthpiece after a full inhalation to determine the volume of air exhaled at a certain time. This procedure should be done while the patient is in a sitting position [26].

Forced expiratory volume in one second is described as the air volume expressed in liters that the patient exhales forcibly in one second following full air inhalation [27].

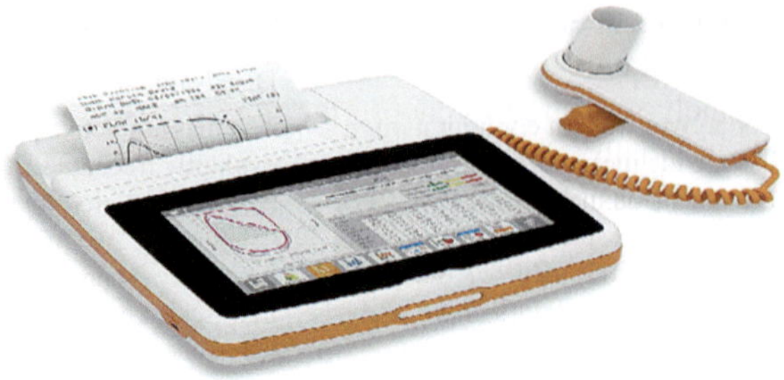

Fig. 11.3 Portable Desktop Spirometer [25]

Forced vital capacity is the liters of air that could be exhaled forcibly by the patient after a full inhalation.

Dividing the forced vital capacity (FEV_1) by forced vital capacity (FVC) will result in a ratio that represents the status of lung obstruction and restriction and also for the diagnosis of interstitial lung diseases. The normal value of this ratio is above 80% [28, 29].

A spirometer could be used for assessment of lung obstruction degree or could be performed after receiving bronchodilators for differentiation between asthma and chronic obstructive pulmonary disease (COPD) or between obstructive and restrictive lung diseases [30, 31].

Uses of spirometry are not limited to COPD and asthma but could be used for measuring pulmonary function before surgery, in case of exposure to chemicals that could cause damage to the lung [32].

Normal values of spirometry are not the same for all patients as these values depend on some parameters that are related to the patient like age, gender, and height. The abnormal values of spirometry reflect the obstruction of airways that are predicted when the FEV_1/FVC ratio is less than 70% of the predicted value (normal value for a certain gender, age, and height) together with a low FEV_1 value. For restrictive diseases, the ratio of FEV_1/FVC would be higher than 70% while the FVC will be reduced more than the normal predicted value like interstitial lung diseases, lung fibrosis, and any disease that causes lung scars [33].

Spirometry results depend on the effort exerted by the patient and also it could be a false result that is not representative of the actual lung function. False spirometry could be noted in case of inability to use the device correctly or in some conditions like abdomen and chest pain in which the patient will exert suboptimal effort. Spirometry should be repeated three times and the average or the higher result should be considered [24].

Tuberculosis patients are eligible to perform the pulmonary function test with a spirometer, but certain precautions should be maintained to prevent cross-contamination. Regarding those patients, the test should be done in the room of the patient at the end of the day to prevent the contamination possibility in the laboratory room and to allow more time for device cleaning and disinfection [24].

General instruction to patients performing spirometry should be ensured like stopping smoking 1 h at least before the test, also not to wear tight clothes or eat a heavy meal 2 h before the test [34].

11.13 Models Used for Aerosol Delivery Quantification

There are several models available for analysis of aerosol and aerosol-generating devices, modes are in-vitro, in-vivo, or ex-vivo based studies. Ach model has some advantages that could not be achieved with other models (Table 11.2) but also all models act together for better aerosol analysis.

Table 11.2 Characteristics of different models for the analysis of aerosol delivery

Model	Characteristics
In-vitro total emitted	Used for quantification of the total emitted aerosol from certain devices as a step for the evaluation of the device efficacy. It is useful for comparing the efficacy of different aerosol generators without recruiting human subjects, besides, it is the model of choice for determining the dead (residual) volume of different nebulizers The results produced by this model are representative of the in-vivo results, but the magnitude of significance in results is different between the two models. Besides, the amount of aerosol detected by this model is greatly higher than that would be detected by the in-vivo models which are considered a limitation for this model
In-vitro aerodynamic characterization	This model is a bench study that uniquely determines the aerodynamic characteristics of emitted aerosol from certain devices. This model gives more specific details regarding the effectiveness of different aerosol generators regarding the production of sufficient amounts of aerosol particles with inhalable diameters. Also, this model could predict the oropharyngeal deposition of different aerosol formulations The main drawback for this model is the time required for analysis of the aerosol samples especially it requires the quantitative analysis of the collected samples with a different instrument
In-vivo pharmacokinetics model	This is a clinical model which involves the recruitment of human subjects. The results of this model are reflecting the actual efficacy of the aerosol generators. However, the high certainty level of this model's findings, but also, many limitations surround the model such as the need for a specific analytical method for extraction of drugs from the biological samples. Another limitation is the sensitivity of sample drawing time, delayed withdrawal of the biological sample might lead to over-estimated amounts of the drugs This model is sensitive to the nebulization time, hence to the volume of the nebulized solution so a large volume of nebulized solution cannot be tested by this model Similar to the previous model it requires additional instruments for quantitative analysis of drug amount
Ex-vivo model	This is the intermediate model between the in-vitro total emitted and in-vivo model, which is able of detecting the total inhaled amounts of the aerosolized medications without delivering aerosol to the subject's lung. The results of this model are more accurate regarding the type of recruited subjects because it depends on the actual inhalation and exhalation rates. Also, this model requires further quantitative analysis for measuring the measured amounts

11.14 In-Vitro Models

These models mimic the conditions and characteristics of inhaled medications delivery for patients that require aerosol therapy and suffering from a respiratory disease such as asthma or COPD. In addition to determining the quantity of aerosol delivered by certain aerosol devices, they aim to characterize aerosols produced by different devices with the aerodynamic characterization of aerosolized particles with an evaluation of how those particles transit and deposit through different pathways under different conditions.

The effect of different nebulizers [jet nebulizer (JN) and vibrating mesh nebulizer (VMNs)] designs on the aerosol delivery from each design during non-invasive ventilation (NIV) was tested using a breathing simulator to mimic the breathing pattern of the subject [35]. This in-vitro model demonstrated that different designs of JNs (3 designs) have a significant effect on the delivery of aerosolized medications, while all tested VMN designs (3 designs) were similar in aerosol delivery efficacy [35]. The comparison between different nebulizer designs was judged by measuring the total emitted dose and residual volume inside nebulizers' chambers.

11.15 In-Vitro Determination of Emitted Dose

The total amount of drug released from the inhaler could be determined by collecting the released amount on a filter then analyzing the amount of the drug by measuring devices like High-performance liquid chromatography (HPLC) or other spectrophotometric methods. Also measuring the weight of the inhaler before and after emitting the drug could be used for quantification of the emitted dose. Inhaled and exhaled amounts of the emitted medications also could be detected by connecting the filters to the lung simulator device. The amount of the drug remaining in the nebulizer chamber also could be measured for the determination of the dead volume or the amount that could not be inhaled [1, 36].

The procedure of these models depends on the existence of three crucial elements; aerosol-generating device, breathing simulator, and ventilator in case of assessment of aerosol delivery to mechanically ventilated patients [37]. The spontaneous breathing model is more simple than the ventilation model because the latter is affected by ventilator settings and the circuit elements. Different ventilation modes exist and are chosen differently to suit the patient situation where two types of inhalers can be used for the distribution of aerosol inside NIV circuits; pressure measured dose inhalers (pMDIs) and nebulizers [38]. Within this model, the presence of a breathing simulator system is meant to reflect the behavior of the patient's lung when the aerosolized medication is inhaled, where various inhalation/exhalation ratios could be demonstrated by this breathing machine to accommodate the simulated subject's population. The purpose of these models is to measure the delivered drug amount that has been emitted from the aerosol-generating device by collecting the inhaled amount released to the inhalation filter, which should be set directly before the lung simulator to gather the inhaled aerosol (Fig. 11.4). By putting a filter above the expiration port mounted on a pump that operates to get rid of exhaled air and collect the suspended aerosol at an average gas flow rate of 25 L/min when in the dual limb circuit of mechanical ventilation. Besides, the exhaled aerosol could be estimated in a single limb ventilator circuit; its location is at the end of the ventilator exhalation limb (Fig. 11.4b).

An in-vitro model by Abdelrahim et al. was intended to assess the efficacy of different nebulizers on delivering aerosol particles, also to evaluate the effect of different nebulizer positions during single limb NIV [40]. Nebulizers were mounted in two separate positions; the first position was before the expiration port while the other was after it, in a single limb NIV circuit with a tidal volume of 500 ml, inspiratory: expiratory gas pressures of 20:5 cmH_2O, 15 breaths per minute [40]. This in-vitro model has been used in numerous other aerosol-related studies e.g. to evaluate aerosol delivery from pMDI, JN, VMN, [36] effect of drug fill volume placed in JN and VMN, and the effect of humidity of the ventilator circuit while delivering aerosol [41].

11.16 In-Vitro Model for Characterization of Aerosol Particle Size Via Inertial Impaction

Particle size distribution and mass median aerodynamic diameter (MMAD) is among the particle size characteristics calculated by this model. It is suspected that aerosol particles less than 5 μm enter deep pulmonary zones, but those of 5 μm or more are ideally deposited in the oropharyngeal region, not deposited deeply in the lungs. To evaluate the aerosol particle characteristics and the aerosol particle size distribution, these in-vitro models depend on the existence of a separate system called a cascade impactor such as ACI and NGI. These instruments will precisely determine the size of the emitted particles and identify the distribution of aerosolized particles from different formulations within the lung. In addition to the cascade impactor, the in-vitro particle size characterization model merely includes an electrostatic filter in a holder, a breathing simulator to simulate patient condition, two T-pieces attached. In the case of the ACI, the cascade impactor should first be put in

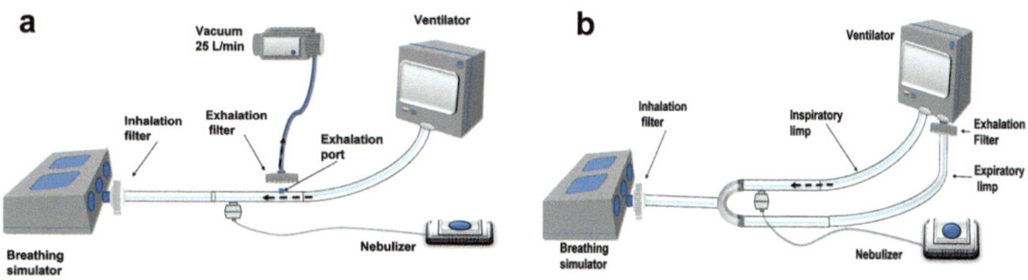

Fig. 11.4 Invitro models during a single (**a**) and dual limb (**b**) mechanical ventilation [39]

the refrigerator before use for 1 h, whereas the NGI takes 1.5 h [42, 43]. Figure 11.5a shows the exact arrangement of these parts for aerosol delivery in a single limb NIV circuit, where Fig. 11.5b shows that of a dual limb. As noted, at an average flow rate of 15 L/min, the cascade impactor is connected to a vacuum pump to draw air, which in turn enhances the patient's inspiratory flow rate (quiet breathing pattern) and allows analysis of the entry of an inhaled drug sample into the cascade impactor system at the same time. Characterization of aerosol particles is conducted only for the inhaled drug sample reached the cascade impactor, not for all the aerosol released from the generating device, which is considered to be the main limitation of the setup mentioned above. Using the Anderson cascade impactor to calculate fine particle fraction and MMAD, Hassan et al. calculated the aerodynamic characteristics of aerosol droplets emitted from four separate nebulizers during NIV [36]. The previous model consisted of a breathing simulator, a ventilator, an Anderson cascade impactor, and an NIV breathing circuit consisting of a corrugated tubing 180 cm in length (22 mm in diameter) and a fixed leak expiration port. The maximum fine particle doses were provided by the VMNs [36].

Within the NIV circuit, one modification could be made to allow the characterization of all aerosol delivered by using the mixing inlet (Fig. 11.5c), where a Y-tube is used to connect an additional air source delivered at a gas flow rate of 15 liters per minute, a breathing simulator, and a mixing inlet to the cascade impactor [44]. This modification was only checked with a dual-limb NIV circuit with the prospect of a single-limb application. The existence of this mixing inlet enables the delivery of additional air at the same flow rate as that removed by the vacuum pump linked to the cascade impactor, resulting in a zero-flow rate removed from the ventilation circuit. Using this configuration, the inhalation profile is restated within the

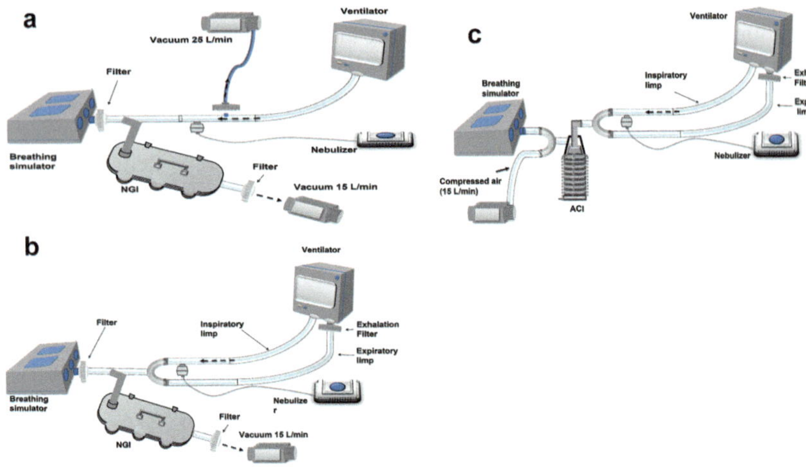

Fig. 11.5 Schematic of breathing simulator and bi-level ventilator circuit for aerodynamic particle size characterization of the respirable dose, (**a**) single limb, (**b**) dual limb and (**c**) for determination of the whole aerosol emitted [39]

ventilator circuit, when the inspiratory phase of the breathing simulator machine was withdrawn from the additional air; and because of the steady flow of air being withdrawn through the cascade impactor. Hence, the inhaled medication could be removed from the circuit which is then introduced to the cascade impactor. It added more airflow to the supplementary air when the expiratory process began. Owing to the continuous flow of air being removed through the cascade impactor, the inhalation profile is replayed again inside the ventilation circuit. So, until the next inspiratory point, the aerosolized drug is kept inside the circuit, resampling what happens when the patient is administered aerosol therapy [44]. In a study by Elhansy et al., this model has been used to evaluate the emitted dose of aerosolized medications. An in-vitro analysis was performed for comparison of VMN and JN with the spacer [44]. Similar to what was observed in the previous analysis, the highest fine particle doses were seen in VMNs.

To model the human lung, the cascade impactor consists of several circular stages organized in a descending way according to the diameter of the pores in each stage where the stage containing the largest pores is positioned at the top near the system of the mouth inlet followed by that of the smaller diameter and so on until the last stage is reached [17]. As aerosol particles pass through the different stages of the cascade impactor, aerosolized particles with adequate inertia will impact within a particular stage while the rest of aerosolized particles go through the pores of the stage toward the following stages until the settling of all emitted aerosol particles. By washing all cascade stages with a particular solvent carefully selected to match the solubility of the studied medication, the amount of inhaled drug that deposited on each stage could be eluted and then determined by using analytical methods such as the HPLC or ultra-violet (UV) spectrophotometer. Then, in each step, the mass values of the measured drug are inserted into some software provided by the manufacturer of the cascade impactor to convert them into the aerodynamic characteristics of the aerosol administered; MMAD, geometric standard deviation (GSD), fine particle dose (FPD), and fine particle fraction (FPF). The MMAD is a central tendency metric that corresponds to the cutoff size where half the aerosol particles are smaller than that diameter and the other half is larger than it. GSD is used to define the distribution spectrum of inhaled aerosol particles where a higher GSD number shows the strongly destructed or dispersed aerosol. FPD refers to a proportion of the inhaled amount with a particle size of fewer than 5 μm, where the percentage of FPD is simply FDF. As previously mentioned, large aerosol particles of 5 μm or more will affect and deposit in the oropharyngeal region and, if orally ingested, may participate in the systemic drug effects in addition to raising its adverse effects. However, particles smaller than 2 μm in diameter are mostly deposited by sedimentation in the alveolar zone, so many respiratory diseases still prefer inhaled aerosols with smaller MMADs (<2 μm).

Saeed et al. performed an ex-vivo analysis on two types of nebulizers during mechanical ventilation, Obstructive pulmonary diseases subjects were recruited into the study and allocated into four groups receiving inhaled, nebulized medication under different, inhalation filters were placed to capture the total amount emitted before the patient facemask [3]. Study findings showed a high significance of adding more fill volume for both nebulizers on the aerosolized medication delivery, but there was no substantial difference concerning humidification [3].

11.16.1 In-Vivo Models

In-vivo studies of aerosol deposition were performed in one of two concepts, first is the determination of aerosol distribution on the lung, the other concept is the quantitative analysis of inhaled medications [45]. Aerosol distribution in human lungs could be determined by imaging devices like three-dimensional single-photon emission computed tomography (SPECT), two-dimensional planar scintigraphy which is the most commonly used with children due to its safety regarding radiation exposure, and the positron emission tomography (PET). These techniques give data that represent the inhalation pattern of the patient and also determine the characteristics of aerosol-producing devices [46–48]. Inhaled drugs in these studies were labeled with radioisotopes to be detected with gamma scintigraphy.

Technetium (Tc^{99m}) is the radioisotope that was commonly used during these studies. Tc^{99m} has a short half-life of about 6 h systemically and less than 20 min in the lung, providing a rapid clearance from the biological system [49, 50].

These imaging studies were used mainly with nebulizers as Tc^{99m} could be added to the nebulized solution in a nebulization chamber easily compared with DPIs and pMDIs [51].

Aerodynamic characterization of inhaled medications before and after labeling with radioactive isotopes is an important step to ensure that the radioisotope did not interfere with the inhaled drug distribution. This will ensure that the images obtained by scintigraphy will be truly indicative for the drug deposition and distribution. Also, these imaging methods should follow specific guidelines [6, 52, 53].

The second method that could be used for aerosol particle deposition is the pharmacokinetics method. Samples in this method could be plasma or urine drawn from the patient to be extracted by solid-phase extraction (SPE) then be analyzed by spectrophotometry. The main drawback with the pharmacokinetic method is the high volume of distribution of the inhaled medications that results in a low concentration of the inhaled medications. The principle of this method depends on taking the samples in the absorption lag time or the time in which the drug could not be absorbed systemically to ensure that all the amount detected is representative of the lung bioavailability. The amount of drug absorbed systemically could be determined by collecting urine for 24 h after inhalation of the aerosolized drug. While lung bioavailability of the drug could be determined by collecting a urine sample after half an hour from starting the nebulization [3, 54–56].

An important component of these experiments is the human subjects, either a volunteer or a patient, where the subject inhales the aerosolized medication dose and then biological samples are drawn for quantitative analysis studies, primarily to

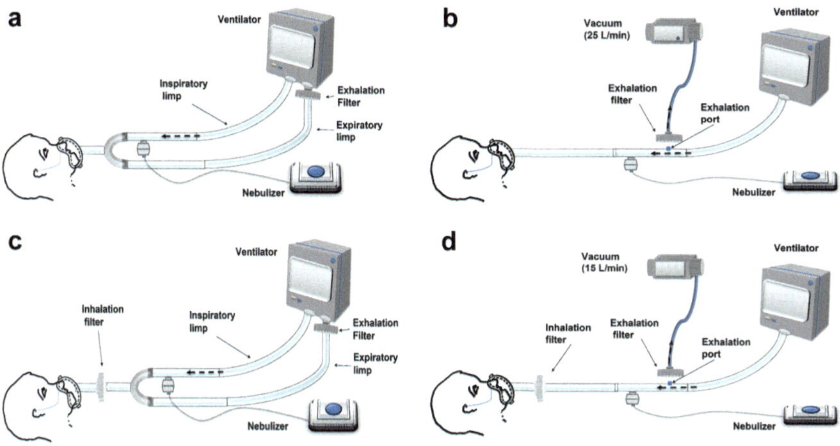

Fig. 11.6 In-vivo (**a**, **b**) and Ex-vivo (**c**, **d**) models during single and double limp ventilation [39]

measure the inhaled mass and assess the potential drug activity (Fig. 11.6). Besides, some in-vivo models also allow the assessment of aerosol distribution within different zones of the patient lung. Before the start of the analysis, it is important to temporarily stop the administration of inhaled medication being tested to allow a washout time to ensure accurate outcomes of the administered drug dose, where the exact stopping period depends on the pharmacokinetics of the studied medication. Noteworthy, a drug substitute should be administered during the washout period to fulfill the health needs of the recruited subjects.

11.16.2 Pharmacokinetics Model

Pharmacokinetic studies are generally designed to measure drug bioavailability, metabolism, and clearance. The application of clinical kinetic analysis for the evaluation of aerosol therapy is specifically orient toward quantification of the lung and systemic bioavailability of the aerosolized medications.

The concept of pharmacokinetic studies depends on performing laboratory analysis of the drawn biological samples from the recruited subjects either plasma [57] or urine samples from the subject after inhaling the aerosolized drug by certain aerosol generators for the period of its absorption lag time to measure the inhaled dose. Nevertheless, because of the relatively large volume of distribution of the tested medications and the smaller the blood samples, the analysis of these samples drawn during the absorption lag time of the inhaled medication usually accounts for lower or undetectable drug concentration. Based on drawing urine samples, the pharmacokinetic study can be carried out in two separate ways where the first relies on the co-administration of oral charcoal beside the inhaled medication to adsorb every swallowed fraction of the drug, and then the samples of urine drawn will contain only the fraction of the inhaled drug delivered to the lung. Even worse, not only does the administered charcoal obstruct and prevent the absorption of the studied medication, but also other patient-administered medications that are frequently seen in critically ill patients and mechanically ventilated. Furthermore, the second urine model route focuses mostly on the lag time for drug absorption, where the patient typically provides two urine samples at different times, first to present the pulmonary bioavailability and the other sample to reflect the systemic absorption [3]. Concerning salbutamol bronchodilator which used mainly for testing the efficacy of different aerosol generators, this time is calculated to be approximately 30 min as the first urine sample is taken 30 min after the start of inhalation to suggest the delivery of pulmonary salbutamol and the second sample is obtained up to 24 h collection after inhalation in containers to indicate delivery of systemic salbutamol. The effectiveness of this in-vivo determination pathway hinges on the duration of drug nebulization, which is not more than 8 min to ensure that all the drug amount delivered to the lung can appear in 30 min after urine sample inhalation, after this time a fraction of the amount of salbutamol detected in urine would be results from systemic absorption of the tested drug [58]. Eight minutes of drug nebulization could deliver variable amounts of inhaled medications depending on the type of nebulizer used. Ultrasonic and VMN have a short nebulization time compared with the traditional and most commonly used JN. This nebulization time of 8 min is considered acceptable for nebulizing approximately 2 mL of the inhaled medication with traditional JN, the time of nebulization would be longer with greater fill volumes, which also is uncomfortable for the patient. The volume of the urine samples collected is recorded and the drug found in these samples should be extracted and determined using the methods of analysis available. Solid-phase extraction (SPE) is among the most suitable methods for extracting the drug from a urine sample and introducing it to quantitative analysis. With urinary pharmacokinetic models, HPLC is the most widely utilized method where urine samples are required to be subjected to prior SPE processing until injection into the HPLC system. SPE technique tries to get rid of undesirable endogenous substances that are included with the collected urine samples such as proteins and waste products and only maintains the studied drug on specifically selected cartilage where the presence of these unwanted substances will cause damage to the column of the HPLC or eventually mask the desired drug peak. Noteworthy, when dealing with 24 h urine samples before SPE is carried an additional step is needed; ester-type or other potential forms to be determined in the free drug through a pre-hydrolysis step to break down any drug conjugate [59].

An in vivo pharmacokinetic model research was performed by Harb et al. to illustrate the effect of different aerosol device connections (T-adapter and Spacer) on delivery of aerosolized drug during mechanical ventilation of obstructive lung diseases patients [60]. VMN nebulized 1 mL of salbutamol solution with three separate settings T-piece, large spacer, and large spacer plus pMDI; two urine samples were obtained and analyzed for the subject using any of the different settings. The results indicated that both T-piece and the spacer were equally successful for VMN aerosol delivery in COPD patients during mechanical ventilation. Besides, the addition of two bronchodilator puffs before inhaled drug nebulization enhanced the delivery of the inhaled medication to the lung [60]. A further pharmacokinetic study was performed in the spontaneous mode of mechanical ventilation with an initial inspiration of exhalation pressure of 20/5 cmH_2O, 15 breaths/min, and 1:3 inspiratory to expiratory pressure, using the bi-level ventilator connected to the dry single-limb circuit [61]. Devices that produce aerosol have been put next to the COPD subject's face masks. Two forms of nebulizers JN and VMN were loaded with 1 mL of respirable salbutamol solution. After extracting the inhaled drug from the two different urine samples by SPE, amounts of the drug in both samples were determined. Study findings showed that the delivery of VMN was higher than the conventional JN [61].

The effect of humidity on delivered aerosol dose was studied in a previous study using this model, in dual limb ventilation circuit and observed no significant difference between heated humidity and dry conditions on aerosol delivery [62]. Besides, this model has been also used in comparing the performance of large valved holding chambers versus traditional nebulizer T-adapter using single-limb ventilator, [60] different VMNs in NIV circuit, [63] pMDI with different connections in NIV, [64] Low-flow oxygen aerosol delivery via adult High flow nasal cannula (HFNC), [65] delivery of inhaled medications during invasive mechanical ventilation, [66] and they have been linked to in-vitro and ex-vivo methods of comparison in most studies.

The use of inspiratory synchronization of the VMN was studied by Michotte et al., as a way to increase the availability of pulmonary aerosols delivery and deposition compared to the conventional continuous nebulization of VMN which is associated with high drug loss during the expiration phase [67]. The research was based on a pharmacokinetic model that involved the recruitment of human subjects and was based on the entire urine sample collection.

11.16.3 Ex-Vivo Models

The ex-vivo model could be viewed as an intermediate step between in-vitro and in-vivo studies in which an additional viewpoint is added to the calculation of the total dose emitted over the in-vitro model, which is the presence of a realistic breathing pattern in the patient and takes the individual differences into account. While all runs are similar for the in-vitro model using a mechanical breath simulator to mimic the patient, the ex-vivo model has a mean difference from the in-vitro model, the presence of participating subjects that represents more delegate outcomes. In some cases, the results of the in-vitro models could be different from that of ex-vivo or in-vivo models. A previous in-vitro study investigating the effect of the presence of a humidifier and changing the inhaled drug fill volume during mechanical ventilation on the total emitted amount from the tested nebulizer reported findings that differed from that of the ex-vivo study for evaluation of the same factors [3, 41]. Such a study also allows the investigator to create associations between in-vitro and in-vivo studies and predict the amount of medication that would be delivered to the patient in real practice, hence, there is particular importance of this model for studies involves several dosing systems [68]. Similar to in-vitro studies, ex-vivo models use collecting filters between the aerosol-generating device and airway of a patient, which determine the inhaled amount of the aerosolized drug (Fig. 11.6) [3, 69].

11.16.4 Imaging Models

The importance of imaging models is related to their ability to detect the regional deposition of aerosol particles within the subject's lung which is mainly influenced by aerodynamic characteristics of the emitted aerosol particles. Via various imaging techniques such as single-photon emission computed tomography (SPECT), gamma scan, positron-emission tomography (PET), and aerosol bolus methods, these models provide accurate data on both the overall and regional deposition of pulmonary targeting inhaled medication [45, 70]. The key concept of the two-dimensional (2D) gamma scintigraphy is the co-administration of the inhaled drug understudy combined with a radioactive isotope such as Techtanium-99m, where the added isotope is easily identified by the imaging technique used and the regional deposition of the inhaled medication can therefore be visualized and evaluated [47, 53]. In addition to the accurate measurement of pulmonary drug deposition by subdivision of lungs into many zones based on the size of the airways, several studies used a 2D gamma camera due to its ability to image the regional aerosol deposition [71, 72]. Such images do not, however, explicitly account for the delivery of the inhaled medications in the pulmonary system [73]. Consequently, due to their ability to assess the exact mass of aerosol accumulated inside any pulmonary area and not the relative deposition compared to other regions, 3D imaging techniques such as SPECT and PET are greatly appreciated [74]. Their theory is based on the use of a radioactive atom delivered with the studied drug like other imaging methods, except this time the gamma camera travels around the lung of the patient to gather photographs from all lung angles [75–77]. The distribution of aerosolized drug particles at the 3D level of the lungs can be shown in these images and can also be used as a method to distinguish between peripheral and central inhaled drug deposition [75].

In healthy adults with spontaneous breathing and NIV, a previous study, compared radiolabeled aerosol deposition using JN, reporting no significant difference in lung deposition for inhaled medications but higher tidal volumes with mechanical ventilation [78].

A crossover clinical trial involving 10 healthy volunteers randomly assigned to receive an aerosolized medication during NIV with JN and VMN was reported by Galindo-Filho and colleagues [2]. In the determination of mass balance, VMN demonstrated higher drug deposition of inhaled radio-aerosol compared to conventional JNs and higher percentages of radio-aerosol deposited in the lungs while receiving positive inspiratory and expiratory pressures of 12 and 5 cmH_2O. Both subjects used naso-oro face masks when receiving positive inspiratory and expiratory pressures of 12 and 5 cmH_2O. For JNs, the dead drug volume was higher relative to VMNs [2]. In a similar model, Compared to JN, the peripheral radio-aerosol deposition was substantially greater with VMN. It should be noted that although the inhaled dosage was comparable, COPD subjects had higher lung deposition than healthy adults [79]. Using the imaging model, recruited patients with moderate and severe COPD, the group reported inhaled and lung doses were higher with VMN compared with JN, also the dead volume of the nebulized medication was lower in VMN than JN [79]. The peripheral radio-aerosol deposition was significantly higher with VMN compared with JN. It should be noted that while inhaled dose was similar, the lung deposition was higher in COPD subjects than in healthy adults.

11.16.5 Data Modeling

For further study and optimization, meaningful data acquired from both in-vitro and in-vivo studies can be collected and compared through data modeling techniques. These technologies primarily use advanced mathematical and statistical models that allow very complex data and multivariate parameters to be dealt with. Artificial neural networks (ANNs), often implemented in the field of pharmaceuticals and pharmaceutical development where their usage ensures the ease and pace of analysis of outcomes, are one of the strong examples of data mining technologies. Modeling of data relies on the input of collected data into the modeling program that projects and forecasts how to expand the experimental findings to a wider range of parameters and optimize the outcomes. In-vitro data obtained from studies of various drug formulations and medical devices were applied to ANNs and demonstrated their success in modeling these data and predicting in-vivo actions [36, 64, 80–82]. In addition to the well-known in-vitro and in-vivo studies, this modeling technology has been very useful in comparing aerosol delivery by different inhalers in mechanically ventilated subjects [61, 64].

The valuable application of modeling to combining data from two or three previous studies was reflected in several modeling studies (in-vitro, ex-vivo, and in-vivo). The influence of nebulizer fill volume on aerosol delivery and lung deposition was demonstrated in a study by Saeed et al. [68]

The model of artificial neural networks showed that, relative to the JN, VMN increased both pulmonary bioavailability and systemic absorption of aerosolized medications. Compared to the JN, VMN was less impacted by nebulizer fill-volume adjustment, which should be diluted to improve aerosol delivery from JN. The valuable result of the modeling was that the model proposed a solution of the inhaled drug should be loaded in a VMN with a fill volume of 2 mL to achieve the optimal lung deposition and systemic absorption that was not significantly detected by traditional in-vitro or in-vivo research statistics [68]. Three filling volumes of nebulizers using saline as a diluent combined with a fixed salbutamol volume were used, in the in-vitro, ex-vivo, and in-vivo trials, so the optimum value should be one of the three volumes used, while the appropriate optimum salbutamol volume was inserted into the modeling software during the modeling analysis to generate a filling volume different from that used during the. In contrast with conventional statistical models, the modeling produced better performance. Therefore, with limited sample sizes, the key benefit of data modeling is to get more precise predictions.

A recent study used artificial modeling to compare three types of VMNs that were found to be equivalent by the traditional statistical method; however, one of the VMNs was found to be a bit better than the other two by modeling the in-vitro, ex-vivo, and in-vivo data along with a suggestion that they could be used in an exchangeable manner [63]. The same conclusion was observed when modeling pMDI in-vitro, ex-vivo, and in-vivo data with various spacers inside the non-invasive ventilation circuit [64].

The modeling was therefore efficient in predicting the optimum values of certain variables, essentially expanding the relationship between the data points gathered from the original studies without further experiments being carried out [68].

References

1. Abdelrahim ME, Plant P, Chrystyn H. In-vitro characterisation of the nebulised dose during non-invasive ventilation. J Pharm Pharmacol. 2010;62(8):966–72.
2. Galindo-Filho VC, et al. Radioaerosol pulmonary deposition using mesh and jet nebulizers during noninvasive ventilation in healthy subjects. Respir Care. 2015;60(9):1238–46.
3. Saeed H, et al. Effects of fill volume and humidification on aerosol delivery during single-limb noninvasive ventilation. Respir Care. 2018;63(11):1370–8.
4. Lipworth B. Targets for inhaled treatment. Respir Med. 2000;94:S13–6.
5. Kulkarni P, Baron PA, Willeke K. Aerosol measurement: principles, techniques, and applications. Hoboken: Wiley; 2011.
6. Fonceca AM, et al. Drug administration by inhalation in children. In: Kendig's disorders of the respiratory tract in children, 9th ed. Elsevier; 2019. p. 257–271.e3.
7. Martin A, et al. Laser diffraction characterization of droplet size distributions produced by vibrating mesh nebulization in air and a helium–oxygen mixture. J Aerosol Sci. 2010;41(12):1159–66.
8. Kesavan J, Kesavan M, Rule AM. Sampling efficiencies of two modified viable cascade impactors. Aerosol Sci Technol. 2017;51(11):1296–302.
9. Kang JS, et al. Characterization of a microscale cascade impactor. Aerosol Sci Technol. 2012;46(9):966–72.
10. Chen M, Romay FJ, Marple VA. Design and evaluation of a low flow personal cascade impactor. Aerosol Sci Technol. 2018;52(2):192–7.
11. Jain S, Petrucci GA. A new method to measure aerosol particle bounce using a cascade electrical low pressure impactor. Aerosol Sci Technol. 2015;49(6):390–9.
12. Mitchell JP and Roberts DL. Current approaches to APSD measurements of OIPs based on inertial impaction. In: Good cascade impactor practices, AIM and EDA for orally inhaled products. Springer; 2013. p. 15–55.
13. Vecellio None L, et al. Validation of laser diffraction method as a substitute for cascade impaction in the European Project for a Nebulizer Standard. J Aerosol Med. 2001;14(1):107–14.

14. Marple VA, et al. A low-loss cascade impactor with stage collection cups: calibration and pharmaceutical inhaler applications. Aerosol Sci Technol. 1995;22(1):124–34.
15. Scherließ R. Particle size measurements in aerosols. In: Analytical techniques in the pharmaceutical sciences. Springer; 2016. p. 701–15.
16. Gaspar D, et al. General introduction-Particle engineering by nanoparticle microencapsulation for pulmonary delivery. Microencapsulated lipid nanoparticles for pulmonary delivery of biopharmaceutical agents; 2017. p. 1.
17. Abdelrahim M, Assi KH, Chrystyn H. Dose emission and aerodynamic characterization of the terbutaline sulphate dose emitted from a Turbuhaler at low inhalation flow. Pharm Dev Technol. 2013;18(4):944–9.
18. Van Oort M. In vitro testing of dry powder inhalers. Aerosol Sci Technol. 1995;22(4):364–73.
19. Yoshida H, et al. Comparison of aerodynamic particle size distribution between a next generation impactor and a cascade impactor at a range of flow rates. AAPS PharmSciTech. 2017;18(3):646–53.
20. Mitchell J, Nagel MJKP. Particle size analysis of aerosols from medicinal inhalers. KONA Powder Particle J. 2004;22:32–65.
21. Newman S, Pellow P, Clarke S. Droplet size distributions of nebulised aerosols for inhalation therapy. Clin Phys Physiol Meas. 1986;7(2):139.
22. Pilcer G, Vanderbist F, Amighi K. Correlations between cascade impactor analysis and laser diffraction techniques for the determination of the particle size of aerosolised powder formulations. Int J Pharm. 2008;358(1–2):75–81.
23. Mitchell JP, et al. Laser diffractometry as a technique for the rapid assessment of aerosol particle size from inhalers. J Aerosol Med. 2006;19(4):409–33.
24. Pellegrino R, et al. Interpretative strategies for lung function tests. Eur Respir J. 2005;26(5):948–68.
25. Cawley MJ, et al. Spirometry: tool for pharmacy practitioners to expand direct patient care services. J Am Pharm Assoc. 2013;53(3):307–15.
26. Goldman L, Schafer AI. Goldman's cecil medicine e-book. Elsevier Health Sciences; 2011.
27. Patil VB, et al. A brief introduction on asthma. Pharma Sci Monitor. 2014;5(2).
28. Swanney MP, et al. Using the lower limit of normal for the FEV1/FVC ratio reduces the misclassification of airway obstruction. Thorax. 2008;63(12):1046–51.
29. DeCato TW, et al. Correlation between Fev1/FVC ratio, total lung capacity, and single-breath diffusing capacity. In: A76. What's in the tool box to assess lung function. American Thoracic Society; 2017. p. A2516.
30. Moore V. Spirometry: step by step. Breathe. 2012;8(3):232–40.
31. Hegewald M, et al. Time of maximal spirometric change after bronchodilator inhalation. Eur Respir J. 2017;50:PA3007.
32. Nishimura Y, et al. Long-term pulmonary complications of chemical weapons exposure in former poison gas factory workers. Inhal Toxicol. 2016;28(8):343–8.
33. Vestbo J, et al. Global strategy for the diagnosis, management, and prevention of chronic obstructive pulmonary disease: GOLD executive summary. Am J Respir Crit Care Med. 2013;187(4):347–65.
34. Welch L. A guide to spirometry best practice for community nurses. J Commun Nurs. 2016;30(1):58–65.
35. Saeed H, et al. Effect of nebulizer designs on aerosol delivery during non-invasive mechanical ventilation: a modeling study of in vitro data. Pulm Ther. 2017;3(1):233–41.
36. Hassan A, et al. In-vitro characterization of the aerosolized dose during non-invasive automatic continuous positive airway pressure ventilation. Pulm Ther. 2016;2(1):115–26.
37. Boukhettala N, et al. In vitro performance of spacers for aerosol delivery during adult mechanical ventilation. J Aerosol Med Pulm Drug Deliv. 2015;28(2):130–6.
38. Bello G, De Pascale G, Antonelli MJ. Noninvasive ventilation: practical advice. Curr Opin Crit Care. 2013;19(1):1–8.

39. Saeed H, et al. Aerosol delivery via noninvasive ventilation: role of models and bioanalysis. Ann Transl Med. 2021;9(7):589.
40. Abdelrahim ME, et al. In-vitro characterisation of the nebulised dose during non-invasive ventilation. J Pharm Pharmacol. 2010;62(8):966–72.
41. Saeed H, et al. Fill volume, humidification and heat effects on aerosol delivery and fugitive emissions during noninvasive ventilation. J Drug Deliv Sci Technol. 2017; 39:372–8.
42. Abdelrahim ME, Chrystyn H. Aerodynamic characteristics of nebulized terbutaline sulphate using the next generation impactor (NGI) and CEN method. J Aerosol Med Pulm Drug Deliv. 2009;22(1):19–28.
43. Abdelrahim ME. Aerodynamic characteristics of nebulized terbutaline sulphate using the Andersen Cascade impactor compared to the next generation impactor. Pharm Dev Technol. 2011;16(2):137–45.
44. ElHansy MHE, et al. In vitro aerodynamic characteristics of aerosol delivered from different inhalation methods in mechanical ventilation. Pharm Dev Technol. 2017;22(6): 844–9.
45. Tay ZW, et al. In vivo tracking and quantification of inhaled aerosol using magnetic particle imaging towards inhaled therapeutic monitoring. Theranostics. 2018;8(13): 3676.
46. Sá RC, et al. Regional ventilation is the main determinant of alveolar deposition of coarse particles in the supine healthy human lung during tidal breathing. J Aerosol Med Pulm Drug Deliv. 2017;30(5):322–31.
47. Ditcham W, et al. Lung deposition of 99mTc-radiolabeled albuterol delivered through a pressurized metered dose inhaler and spacer with facemask or mouthpiece in children with asthma. J Aerosol Med Pulm Drug Deliv. 2014;27(S1):S63–75.
48. Roller C, et al. Spacer inhalation technique and deposition of extrafine aerosol in asthmatic children. Eur Respir J. 2007;29(2):299–306.
49. Hickey AJ. Practical aspects of imaging techniques employed to study aerosol deposition and clearance. In: Pharmaceutical inhalation aerosol technology. 2nd ed. Boca Raton: CRC Press; 2016. p. 180–221.
50. Sanchez-Crespo A. Lung scintigraphy in the assessment of aerosol deposition and clearance. In: Seminars in nuclear medicine. Elsevier; 2018.
51. Réminiac F, et al. Nasal high flow nebulization in infants and toddlers: an in vitro and in vivo scintigraphic study. Pediatr Pulmonol. 2017;52(3):337–44.
52. Newman S, et al. Standardization of techniques for using planar (2D) imaging for aerosol deposition assessment of orally inhaled products. J Aerosol Med Pulm Drug Deliv. 2012;25(S1):S10–28.
53. Devadason SG, et al. Validation of radiolabeling of drug formulations for aerosol deposition assessment of orally inhaled products. J Aerosol Med Pulm Drug Deliv. 2012;25(S1):S6–9.
54. Hindle M, Chrystyn H. Determination of the relative bioavailability of salbutamol to the lung following inhalation [see comments]. Br J Clin Pharmacol. 1992;34(4):311–5.
55. Borgström L, Nilsson M. A method for determination of the absolute pulmonary bioavailability of inhaled drugs: terbutaline. Pharm Res. 1990;7(10):1068–70.
56. Abdelrahim M, Plant P, Chrystyn H. The relative lung and systemic bioavailability of terbutaline following nebulisation in non-invasively ventilated patients. Int J Pharm. 2011;420(2):313–8.
57. Sangwan S, et al. Aerosolized protein delivery in asthma: gamma camera analysis of regional deposition and perfusion. J Aerosol Med. 2001;14(2):185–95.
58. Silkstone V, Corlett S, Chrystyn HJ. Determination of the relative bioavailability of salbutamol to the lungs and systemic circulation following nebulization. Br J Clin Pharmacol. 2002;54(2):115–9.
59. Silkstone V, et al. An investigation of in vitro/in vivo correlations for salbutamol nebulized by eight systems. J Aerosol Med. 2002;15(3):251–9.
60. Harb HS, et al. Performance of large spacer versus nebulizer T-piece in single-limb noninvasive ventilation. Respir Care. 2018;63(11):1360–9.

61. Hassan A, et al. In-vitro/in-vivo comparison of inhaled salbutamol dose delivered by jet nebulizer, vibrating mesh nebulizer and metered dose inhaler with spacer during non-invasive ventilation. Exp Lung Res. 2017;43(1):19–28.
62. Moustafa IO, et al. Lung deposition and systemic bioavailability of different aerosol devices with and without humidification in mechanically ventilated patients. Heart Lung. 2017;46(6):464–7.
63. Rabea H, et al. Modelling of in-vitro and in-vivo performance of aerosol emitted from different vibrating mesh nebulisers in non-invasive ventilation circuit. Eur J Pharm Sci. 2017;97:182–91.
64. Hussein RR, et al. In vitro/in vivo correlation and modeling of emitted dose and lung deposition of inhaled salbutamol from metered dose inhalers with different types of spacers in non-invasively ventilated patients. Pharm Dev Technol. 2017;22(7):871–80.
65. Madney YM, et al. Aerosol delivery through an adult high-flow nasal cannula circuit using low-flow oxygen. Respir Care. 2019;64(4):453–61.
66. ElHansy MH, et al. Inhaled salbutamol dose delivered by jet nebulizer, vibrating mesh nebulizer and metered dose inhaler with spacer during invasive mechanical ventilation. Pulm Pharmacol Ther. 2017;45:159–63.
67. Michotte J-B, et al. Pulmonary drug delivery following continuous vibrating mesh nebulization and inspiratory synchronized vibrating mesh nebulization during noninvasive ventilation in healthy volunteers. J Aerosol Med Pulm Drug Deliv. 2018;31(1):33–41.
68. Saeed H, et al. Modeling and optimization of nebulizers' performance in non-invasive ventilation using different fill volumes: comparative study between vibrating mesh and jet nebulizers. 2018;50:62–71.
69. Lin HL, et al. Aerosol delivery during spontaneous breathing with different types of nebulizers-in vitro/ex vivo models evaluation. 2018;48:225–31.
70. Yeo LY, et al. Ultrasonic nebulization platforms for pulmonary drug delivery. Expert Opin Drug Deliv. 2010;7(6):663–79.
71. Newman SP, Chan H-K. In vitro/in vivo comparisons in pulmonary drug delivery. J Aerosol Med Pulm Drug Deliv. 2008;21(1):77–84.
72. Newman SP, Wilding IR, Hirst PH. Human lung deposition data: the bridge between in vitro and clinical evaluations for inhaled drug products? Int J Pharm. 2000;208(1–2):49–60.
73. Bur M, et al. Inhalative nanomedicine—opportunities and challenges. Inhal Toxicol. 2009;21(suppl 1):137–43.
74. Kim CS. Methods of calculating lung delivery and deposition of aerosol particles. Respir Care. 2000;45(6):695–711.
75. Cryan S-A, Sivadas N, Garcia-Contreras L. In vivo animal models for drug delivery across the lung mucosal barrier. Adv Drug Deliv Rev. 2007;59(11):1133–51.
76. Jaafar-Maalej C, et al. Assessment methods of inhaled aerosols: technical aspects and applications. Expert Opin Drug Deliv. 2009;6(9):941–59.
77. Kwok PCL, et al. Studies of Radioaerosol deposition in the respiratory tract. In: Seminars in nuclear medicine. Elsevier; 2019.
78. França EE, et al. Nebulization associated with bi-level noninvasive ventilation: analysis of pulmonary radioaerosol deposition. Respir Med. 2006;100(4):721–8.
79. Galindo-Filho VC, et al. A mesh nebulizer is more effective than jet nebulizer to nebulize bronchodilators during non-invasive ventilation of subjects with COPD: a randomized controlled trial with radiolabeled aerosols. Respir Med. 2019;153:60–7.
80. Ali AMA, Abdelrahim MEA. Modeling and optimization of terbutaline emitted from a dry powder inhaler and influence on systemic bioavailability using data mining technology. J Pharm Innov. 2014;9(1):38–47.
81. Jacobson GA, et al. SULT 1A3 single-nucleotide polymorphism and the single dose pharmacokinetics of inhaled salbutamol enantiomers: are some athletes at risk of higher urine levels? Drug Test Anal. 2015;7(2):109–13.
82. Sun Y, et al. Application of artificial neural networks in the design of controlled release drug delivery systems. Adv Drug Deliv Rev. 2003;55(9):1201–15.

Chapter 12
Monitoring Plans and Weaning Protocols for Critically Ill Patients

Contents

12.1 Introduction

While critically ill patients are treated, ventilator requirements get changed. Therefore, ventilator settings must be reviewed through close monitoring of clinical parameters and ventilator parameters of the patients to meet their new criteria and prevent ventilator-induced lung injury (VILI). While on NIV, more

M. E. A. Abdelrahim et al., *Essentials of Aerosol Therapy in Critically ill Patients*,
https://doi.org/10.1007/978-3-030-85026-5_12

parameters must be monitored to early predict non-invasive ventilation (NIV) failure for the decision of intubation or assess weanability as soon as possible. Moreover, some technical issues must be applied first to optimize ventilation settings before considering NIV failure [1]. Spontaneous breathing must start at a certain point during mechanical ventilation. Taking into consideration that spontaneous breathing has a high risk of lung injury known as "patient self-inflicted lung injury (P-SILI)", in addition to the injury of diaphragm known as "myotrauma" [2, 3]. Such injuries lead to difficult weaning, prolonged ventilation, and high mortality [4, 5]. Most of these injuries can be detected by monitoring the respiratory effort. This emphasizes the potential for such monitoring to guide clinicians to ensure safe spontaneous breathing during mechanical ventilation [6]. Safe spontaneous breathing represents a complex challenge to clinicians because treatment goals include minimizing both volume and transpulmonary pressure (PL) to avoid P-SILI, and at the same time, maintaining an appropriate respiratory effort to avoid diaphragm atrophy. Therefore, respiratory monitoring is essential during both NIV and invasive mechanical ventilation (IMV) [7, 8]. Different types and phases of acute respiratory failure require different priorities: in early ARDS close monitoring is needed to avoid the high inspiratory effort to minimize VILI and P-SILI. Adjustments of ventilation parameters should be made as early as possible to obtain a low level of inspiratory effort and to avoid myotrauma. Once patient clinical parameters/lung functions get normalized, a weaning plan could be started safely [9].

12.2 Discussion and Analysis of Main Topics

12.2.1 Monitoring Patient During Invasive Mechanical Ventilation (IMV)

First of all, the treatment of a critically ill patient must be guided by his clinical condition. It is important to be able to early detect when the patient's respiratory status is compromised. The familiar "look, listen and feel" approach could be applied to evaluate the efficacy of breathing, chest movement, work of breathing (WOB), accessory muscle use, and efficiency of ventilation [10], in addition to the mental status, general appearance (particularly skin color), presenting symptoms, heart rate (HR), characteristics of dyspnea and coexisting clinical features (fever, palpitations, swollen and painful calf, and ankle swelling). Moreover, many regular investigations are essential for patient monitoring including; pulse-oximetry, blood-gas analysis, and peak-flow measurements [11]. Besides monitoring the patient's clinical parameters, many approaches are needed to assess the efficiency and safety of the ventilation. These include monitoring of; ventilator parameters, spontaneous breathing, and endotracheal tube (ETT) / tracheostomy tube (TST).

12.2.1.1 Monitoring of Ventilator Parameters During IMV

During IMV careful monitoring of the following measurements is recommended hourly and after any modifications in the ventilator settings [11]:

- Respiratory rate (RR): Normal respiratory rate in adults is about 12 breaths/min; tachypnoea (RR > 12 breaths/min) indicates respiratory distress. Bradypnoea (RR < 10 breaths/min) may be caused by central nervous system (CNS) depression, fatigue, hypothermia, or drugs, e.g. opiates.
- Fractional inspired concentration of oxygen (FiO_2).
- Tidal volume (Vt): It should be equal to or slightly greater than preset Vt. Vt of 6–8 mL/kg is recommended. In case that inspired Vt does not match with expired Vt in volume-cycled ventilation, check that the cuff on the ETT is well-inflated, check for possible leaks within the circuit and check the ventilator inner valves. While if Vt is high, there is a possible added gas into the circuit such as when nebulizing medicated aerosols or the patient is breathing spontaneously.
- Positive end-expiratory pressure (PEEP): It should be 5–20 cmH_2O. PEEP is over and above inspiratory pressure, i.e. if PEEP is 5 cmH_2O and pressure is 20 cmH_2O, PIP will be 25 cmH_2O.
- Minute volume: It must always be equal to preset Vt multiplied by the preset rate (Minute volume = Vt × rate).
- Peak inspiratory pressure (PIP): It should always be at the lowest possible value to ensure adequate ventilation, reduce the risks of barotrauma and minimize cardiovascular side effects of IMV.
- Inspiratory:expiratory ratio (I:E ratio): Normal I:E ratio is 1:2. Alteration of the I:E ratio affects the alveolar gas exchange.
- End-tidal carbon dioxide (ETCO2) levels: Measuring ETCO 2 indicates the adequacy of ventilation.
- Humidifier temperature: It should be 37 °C.
- Regularly ensure that all low and high alarm limits are set appropriately.

Table 12.1 summarizes the numerical values of ventilator parameters used to predict successful IMV weaning.

Table 12.1 Ventilator parameters used to predict successful IMV weaning [12]

Parameter	Target value
Minute ventilation	<10 L/min
Vital capacity/weight	>10 mL/kg
Respiratory frequency	<35 bpm
Tidal volume/weight	>5 mL/kg
Maximum inspiratory pressure	< −25 cmH_2O
Pa_{O2}/PA_{O2}	>0.35
Respiratory rate/tidal volume	<100/L
Pa_{O2}/FI_{O2}	>20 mmHg (26.3 KPa)

Pa_{O2} Partial pressure of arterial oxygen, PA_{O2} Partial pressure of alveolar oxygen, FI_{O2} fractional inspired concentration of oxygen

12.2.1.2 Monitoring Spontaneous Breathing During IMV

There are several available techniques for monitoring respiratory drive and inspiratory effort during IMV to guide for safe spontaneous breathing patients [7]:

Monitoring through Esophageal Pressure (*P*es)

In patients with acute respiratory distress syndrome (ARDS) undergoing passive mechanical ventilation, *P*es monitoring is advised to monitor the safety of spontaneous breathing [13]. *P*es monitoring is the gold standard to assess a patient's WOB and respiratory effort. Its use is uncommon as a result of neglecting the utility of the information derived from *P*es monitoring by many researchers.

Transpulmonary Pressure (PL)

Firstly, *P*L can be calculated by the use of *P*es instead of pleural pressure (*P*pl) (*P*L = positive airway pressure (*P*aw) − *P*pl), by replacing *P*pl with *P*es [14]. *P*L can easily reach an extremely high value during assisted mechanical ventilation. To limit the risk of lung injury, a "precautionary" peak inspiratory value of 20 cmH_2O is an acceptable target in an injured lung [15]. The measured value of *P*L will underestimate lung stress in the presence of the pendelluft phenomenon and regional ventilation heterogeneity. While the quasi-static plateau *P*L (obtained during an end-inspiratory occlusion) reflects lung stress during passive ventilation, the dynamic swing in *P*L (Δ*P*L) would be more reflective of injury risk during spontaneous breathing [16]. Δ*P*L represents the upper limit of mechanical stress experienced in dorsal regions of the lung under dynamic conditions [17]. The dynamic (tidal increase) in lung stress is a more important driver of lung injury than the global (peak) lung stress [18, 19].

Inspiratory Muscle Pressure (Pmus)

The proper definition of *P*mus is "the global force generated by the inspiratory muscles including the diaphragm which is the most important respiratory muscle, and the accessory inspiratory muscles (sternomastoid, rib cage, and scalene muscles)". *P*es and the additional pressure needed to overcome the chest wall elastic recoil (*P*cw) allow measurement of the inspiratory effort. *P*mus is computed from the difference between *P*es and *P*cw (*P*mus = *P*cw − *P*es).

Recent data recommended that *P*mus optimal values are similar to those of healthy subjects breathing at rest to prevent diaphragm atrophy during assisted mechanical ventilation (5–10 cmH_2O) [20, 21]. However, in actual clinical practice, one can neglect the correction of *P*cw because chest wall elasticity is usually relatively low (even when *P*pl is high). Therefore, a target Δ*P*es of about 3–8 cmH_2O can be considered comparable to a normal *P*mus of about 5–10 cmH_2O. The integral of *P*mus over the inspiration duration (pressure-time product [PTP]) is the gold standard measurement of patient respiratory effort. PTP is more correlated to inspiratory muscle energy expenditure. PTP values of 50–100 $cmH_2O/s/min$ indicate acceptable oxygen consumption and adequate respiratory effort [22]. In actual clinical practice, the frequency and magnitude of the ΔPes swing are adequately sufficient for respiratory effort monitoring.

Transdiaphragmatic Pressure (Pdi)

The pressure generated by the diaphragm is known as *P*di. It could be quantified by applying a double-balloon catheter that monitors inspiratory swings in *P*es and gastric pressure (*P*ga). During inspiration, the diaphragm's contractile effort expands the thoracic cavity (negative swing in *P*es) and moves the abdominal organs downwards, increasing abdominal pressure (positive swing in *P*ga). Even when thoracoabdominal motion is similar to the diaphragm upward movement during inspiration (i.e., *P*ga decreases), the contractile effort of the diaphragm is proven by the fact that *P*ga declines less than *P*es (*P*di increases). This parameter is not applied in actual clinical practice [6].

Monitoring Through Occlusion Maneuvers

Occlusion maneuvers during both inspiration and expiration represent noninvasive reliable maneuvers to monitor spontaneous breathing during assisted mechanical ventilation.

Inspiratory Occlusion Maneuver

Plateau pressure (*P*plat) can be measured through end-inspiratory occlusion maneuvers in passive mechanical ventilation. The driving pressure (ΔP) could be calculated as the difference between PEEP and *P*pl. Of note, ΔP reflects both the dynamic lung-stress and lung-injury risk, in addition to high correlation to mortality in patients with ARDS [19]. It was suggested that reliable measurements of *P*plat could be obtained through end-inspiratory occlusion maneuver even in assisted mechanical ventilation [23]. In which, the contracting inspiratory muscles are relaxed at the end of inspiration, leading to high ΔPaw, which could be easily detected on the ventilator waveform. If the patient is over-assisted with low respiratory effort, *P*aw decreases during the occlusion. High ΔP and *P*plat measured in this condition indicate hyperdistention with possible lung injury. It was recently reported that ΔP measured by brief inspiratory occlusion maneuvers during assisted mechanical ventilation can predict the rate of mortality, which supports both relevance and validity of these measures [23]. There are some limitations of this measurement technique. The first is that it may underestimate regional lung-injury risk as a result of the pendelluft mechanism of P-SILI because the measurement is obtained under quasi-static conditions [17]. The second limitation is the fact that the stability and pattern of the *P*aw tracing during the occlusion needs a careful evaluation to determine if the measurement is affected by the abdominal muscles or not. Abdominal muscles may lead to a rapid increase of *P*aw at the onset of neural expiration.

Expiratory Occlusion Maneuver

Expiratory occlusion maneuvers could be applied to measure intrinsic PEEP (iPEEP) during passive mechanical ventilation or to measure maximal inspiratory pressure during spontaneous breathing during maximal voluntary ventilation. The inspiratory effort could be assessed through the airway pressure swing during a brief end-expiratory occlusion maneuver. The airway pressure swing is highly correlated to pleural pressure swing, under occluded conditions. Therefore, the presence and magnitude of pleural pressure swings resulting from patient respiratory effort could be assessed through the airway pressure swing during the occlusion (ΔPocc), with special consideration of the differences in pleural pressure swing in occluded versus dynamic conditions. Accordingly, ΔPocc can be employed to assess *P*mus, ΔPes, and ΔPL during the respiratory cycle as long as the patient's respiratory drive is unchanged by a brief unexpected end-expiratory occlusion during the tidal breath [24, 25]. The end-expiratory occlusion maneuver is proven to be a non-invasive practical routine method that helps in the evaluation of respiratory effort and *P*L during assisted mechanical ventilation [26, 27].

Airway Occlusion Pressure (P0.1)

The airway pressure in the first 100 ms of inspiration against an expiratory occlusion is known as *P*0.1. Certainly, it measures the patient's respiratory drive [28]. An occlusion cannot modify respiratory output until inspiration is prolonged beyond 200 ms [29]. Respiratory pressure generation is independent of diaphragm function or pulmonary mechanics during the first 100 ms [29, 30]. An acceptable value of *P*0.1 of 1.5–3.5 cmH_2O was concluded for guiding clinicians about ventilation adjustment during assisted mechanical ventilation [31–35]. *P*0.1 values lower than 1.5 cmH_2O indicate that respiratory effort may be inadequate [36], however, values more than 3.5 cmH_2O indicate that respiratory drive is high [31].

Measurement of *P*0.1 has many advantages: being easy, practical method and available through most of the modern ventilators. The method for adjusting the pressure support based on the *P*0.1 measurement has been recorded [37]. Taking into consideration that repeated measurements of *P*0.1 are needed with the calculation of mean value to overcome intra-patient variability. Moreover, iPEEP delays the fall in *P*aw in hyper-inflated patients, which results in underestimation of *P*0.1. In this condition, start the 100 ms for the *P*0.1 measurement when the expiratory flow is equal to zero to overcome this issue [38].

Monitoring Through Electrical Activity of the Diaphragm (EAdi)

Continuous monitoring of EAdi is allowed through using a special catheter fitted to electromyography (EMG) electrodes [39]. EAdi is comparable to *P*di measurement and is more practical than surface EMG [40]. When ventilation is driven by EAdi such as neurally adjusted ventilatory-assist (NAVA), patient-ventilator interaction is enhanced [41, 42]. Also, EAdi guides clinicians to detect any asynchrony [41, 43]. EAdi measurement can be used to early recognize weaning failure [44]. EAdi alterations start before signs of fatigue. It gradually increases with the spontaneous breathing failure, while diaphragm-activity remains stable in patients who pass spontaneous breathing trials [44].

Being an electrical signal, EAdi indicates CNS activation of the diaphragm (respiratory motor-output) and not the diaphragm force generation (effort). In healthy subjects, EAdi greatly varies between 5 and 30 μV, during resting breathing [45]. Owing to this great variation, it is impossible to refer to a target EAdi value during mechanical ventilation. Instead, EAdi can be applied to measure *P*mus under many conditions of ventilator assistance by coupling electrical activity with pressure generation constant. Then EAdi allows a breath by breath assessment of *P*mus during the normal breathing cycle [46].

"Neuro-mechanical coupling = *P*mus/EAdi obtained during expiratory occlusion".

Monitoring Through Diaphragm Ultrasound

Diaphragm ultrasound is easy, non-invasive, and reproducible technique. There is a variation in the diaphragm thickness (thickening fraction, TFdi) during the respiratory cycle. TFdi is closely correlated to EAdi and respiratory pressure generation. Consequentially, it can be applied to measure diaphragm weakness. TFdi values <30% during a maximal inspiratory effort highly indicate diaphragm weakness [47]. Regular measurement of end-expiratory diaphragm thickness may recognize the respiratory muscles' structural changes. During IMV, a gradual increase in diaphragm thickness with time had a direct correlation with excessive effort and may indicate under-assistance myotrauma [3]. TFdi of 15–30% during tidal ventilation was associated with the shortest duration of ventilation and stable diaphragm thickness [21]. Diaphragm ultrasound could be used for intermittent patient assessment; it is not suitable for continuous monitoring.

Table 12.2 summarizes different available methods to monitor both the respiratory drive and inspiratory effort during assisted mechanical ventilation with possible target values for safe spontaneous breathing. The applications and interpretations of these measurements must be guided by the clinical condition of the patient. Clinicians should be aware of patient respiratory effort and need to estimate the benefits and risks of manipulation of patient respiratory effort during acute respiratory failure. It is still unknown if it is possible to achieve an acceptable respiratory effort during the acute phase of illness, suggesting more clinical investigation.

Table 12.2 Potential target values for safe spontaneous breathing during mechanical ventilation [6]

Technique	Parameter	Target values for safe spontaneous breathing
Pes	Peak end-inspiratory transpulmonary pressure (*P*L)	≤20 cmH_2O
	Swing in transpulmonary pressure (Δ*PL*)	≤15 cmH_2O
	Peak inspiratory muscle pressure (*P*mus)	5–10 cmH_2O
	Esophageal pressure swing (Δ*Pes*)	3–8 cmH_2O
	Transdiaphragmatic pressure swing (Δ*P*di)	5–10 cmH_2O
	Pressure time product (PTP)	50–100 cmH_2O/s/min
Occlusion maneuvers	Inspiratory occlusion for plateau airway pressure (*P*plat)	≤30 cmH_2O
	Inspiratory occlusion for driving pressure (Δ*P*aw = *P*plat − PEEP)	≤15 cmH_2O
	Expiratory occlusion for estimated Pmus	5–10 cmH_2O
	Airway occlusion pressure (*P*0.1)	1.5–3.5 cmH_2O
EMG	Diaphragm electrical activity (EAdi)	Uncertain

PEEP positive end-expiratory pressure, *EMG* Electromyography, *Pes* Esophageal pressure

12.2.1.3 Monitoring of ETT

On the management of a critically ill patient through an ETT, there are main principles that must be considered [11]:

- Maintain patency of the tube through close monitoring of ventilation with immediately available suction.
- Secure the ETT to the patient's head and face with an adhesive or cotton tape.
- Modify the tube position at the lips daily to minimize pressure ulcerations.
- Record the length at which the tube is cut and tied at the lips then check regularly for migration from these markers.
- Apply regular ETT suction with or without hyper-inflation, to minimize sputum retention.
- Secure/support the ventilator tubing to reduce excess weight on the ETT.
- Adhere to continuous pulse-oximetry to detect hypoxemia.
- Adhere to the continuous electrocardiogram (ECG) with respiratory waveform.
- Regular auscultation for breath sounds to confirm equal inflation and exclude the possibility of slipping off the ETT into one main bronchus with unilateral ventilation.
- Check emergency equipment at least once a shift for accidental extubation, such as intubation equipment, suction and manual rebreathe circuits.
- Use ETTs with high-volume, low-pressure cuffs to reduce the risk of tracheal stenosis/ischemia.
- Regularly check cuff pressures by the use of cuff manometers.
- Check for the possible complications of ETT. The acronym DOPE helps detect problems: "Displacement of the tube, Obstruction of the tube, Pneumothorax,

and Equipment". Other complications of ETT include; esophageal or right main bronchus intubation, vocal folds damage, soft palate and lips damage, herniation of the cuff, tracheal stenosis, and tracheal ulceration.
- Maintain regular oral hygiene with a soft toothbrush and toothpaste to prevent the proliferation of bacteria.

12.2.1.4 Monitoring of TST

The need for a temporary TST is frequent in critically ill settings. A patient who required a temporary TST is often a patient with a severe and extensive illness leading to severe debilitation. These patients are usually suffering a significantly impaired muscle strength and physical energy. They remain susceptible to serious infections. Therefore, they require continuous monitoring even in the post-intensive care period. Monitoring principles are [11, 48]:

- Ensure continuous observation of the patient.
- Continually monitor the patency and position of TST: observe the patient for signs of respiratory distress.
- Adhere to regular physiological monitoring including RR, HR, blood pressure (BP), oxygen saturation (SaO_2), temperature, and level of consciousness.
- Record the amount, consistency, and color of secretions on the tracheal suction.
- Do suction as required, for the shortest possible duration.
- Observe the amount, consistency, and color of sputum within the inner tube when cleaned with sterile 0.9% NaCl.
- Clean according to the requirements (at least three times a day).
- Regularly monitor the microbiological results of sputum samples.
- Monitor both water level and the temperature of the humidifier, confirming that water traps are empty and positioned below the height of the patient's head.
- Monitor nutritional status; keep a food diary if not receiving enteral nutrition.
- Observe the tracheal stoma for signs of irritation, infection, or granulation. If there is a risk of stoma breakdown, get in contact with a wound specialist.
- Early detection and prevention of serious complications. The use of TST with a removable inner-tube for cleansing can significantly decrease the risk of a blocked tube and compromised airway [49].

12.2.2 Weaning from IMV

If the patient parameters get stabilized and meet the criteria for extubation, a weaning plan must start as soon as possible. When patients are ready to wean, the best method to evaluate their ability to breathe on their own is by undertaking a spontaneous breathing trial (SBT) which accelerates the weaning process. SBT is the traditional approach for patient weaning from IMV. This could be applied by disconnecting the patient from the ventilator and connecting to another device such as a T-piece. Also, SBTs may include the application of continuous positive airway pressure (CPAP), which keeps the functional residual capacity, and a low level of pressure support ventilation (PSV) to overcome resistance to breathing via an ETT (tube compensation). Moreover, SBT could be conducted by increasing the duration with/without disconnecting the patient from the ventilator to aid the weaning process (Fig. 12.1) [12].

If the patient completed an SBT, he is encouraged to proceed to extubation. However, those who fail an SBT need a slower weaning process with SBTs of gradual increase of duration. The best ventilatory choices for weaning patients that fail their initial SBT include the following: (1) T-piece trials; (2) synchronized intermittent mandatory ventilation (SIMV); or (3) PSV. Finally, NIV allows prevention of

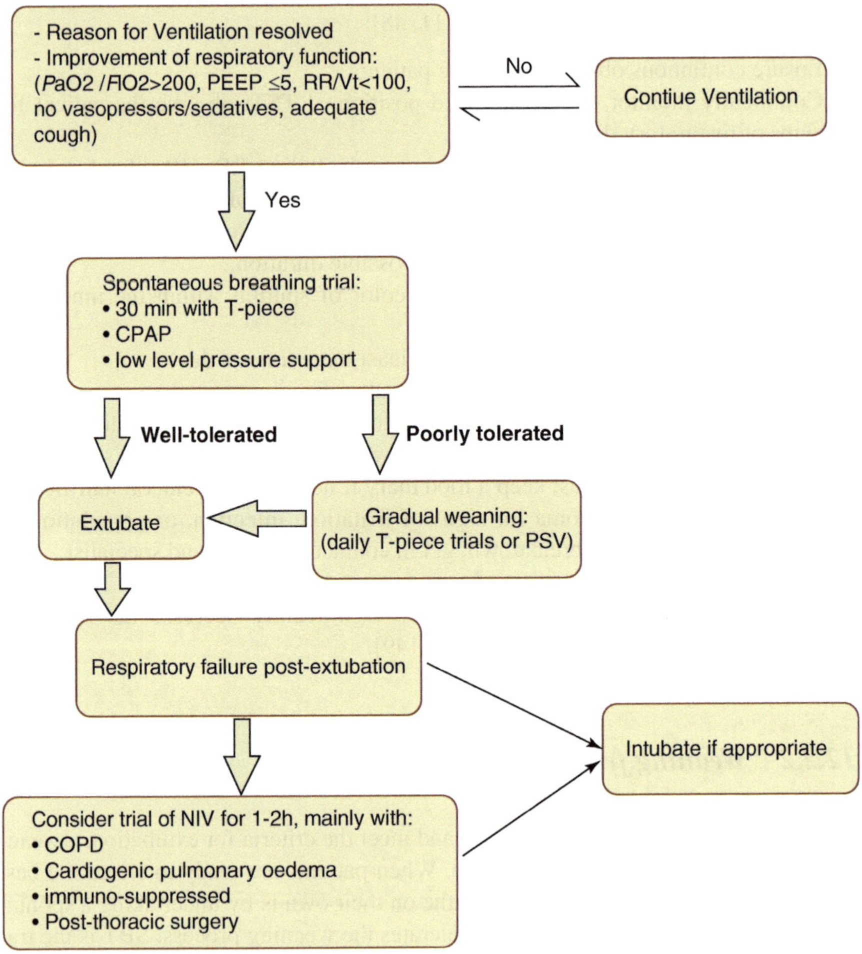

Fig. 12.1 Algorithm for weaning of IMV

re-intubation in patients who have failed extubation, mainly applied with chronic obstructive pulmonary disease (COPD), immunosuppressed patients with bilateral infiltrates, and in those with cardiogenic pulmonary edema [50].

12.2.3 Monitoring of Patient During NIV

Inappropriate NIV settings may lead to NIV failure and high morbidity. NIV patients need close monitoring to early detect signs of NIV failure. Therefore, close monitoring of patient clinical parameters and lung functions during NIV is essential to provide effective and safe ventilation and to minimize any potential injury with adequate weaning at a suitable time. Mechanical characteristics of the ventilated lung can only be interpreted if elastic properties, the volume of the lung, and the degree of obstruction have been accurately quantified by the measurement of lung functions. Evaluation of clinical parameters and lung functions provides a diagnostic and therapeutic tool to guide the selection of adequate ventilator settings in case of patient-ventilator dyssynchrony (PVD) or to assess patient weanability. PVD usually results from great mask leak, inappropriate inspiratory time (Ti) or expiratory time (Te), inadequate inspiratory positive airway pressure (IPAP), extremely sensitive triggers, or high iPEEP levels [51].

12.2.3.1 Monitoring of Clinical Parameters During NIV

A monitoring plan of several clinical parameters is applied for NIV patients to recognize if there is a need for intubation or not especially within the first 4 h of ventilation [7]:

- pH and ABG measurement before and following starting NIV.
- RR and HR.
- Continuous SaO_2 monitoring with intermittent measurement of partial pressure of carbon dioxide (pCO_2) during NIV.
- ECG monitoring is advised especially with dysrhythmia, cardiomyopathy, or HR >120 bpm.
- Transcutaneous pCO_2 ($TcpCO_2$) monitoring is a common investigation in-home ventilation units and is increasingly employed in hospitals.

The schedule of the recommended monitoring plan during the first 12 h of NIV is summarized in Table 12.3.

12.2.3.2 Monitoring of Special Laboratory Indices during NIV

Laboratory indices may be more sensitive than clinical parameters for monitoring of NIV patients, they include [53]:

Table 12.3 Schedule for monitoring plan of patient clinical parameters during the first 12 h of NIV (reproduced from [52])

Clinical parameter	Schedule
– RR – HR – ABG	– Baseline observations
– Pulse oximetry – ECG[a]	– Continuous measurement during the first 12 h
– RR – HR – Level of consciousness – Ventilator synchrony – Mask fit (skin condition and degree of leak) – Compliance – Patient comfort – Chest wall movement – Accessory muscle use	Frequent clinical monitoring (acutely ill patients): – Every 15 min in the first hour – Every 30 min in the 1–4 h period – Hourly in the 4–12 h period
Repeat ABG	– After 1 h of NIV therapy and 1 h after every subsequent change in settings – Further ABG at 4 h or earlier in patients who are not improving clinically

ABG arterial blood gas measurements, *RR* respiratory rate, *HR* heart rate, *ECG* electrocardiogram, *NIV* non-invasive ventilation
[a]With existing cardiomyopathy

- Partial pressure of arterial oxygen/fractional inspired concentration of oxygen ratio (Pa_{O2}/FI_{O2}): unimproved or worsened ratio during the first 1 h of NIV highly predicts NIV failure.
- Oxygenation index (OI): it provides an excellent estimate of lung function involvement. OI is better than the Pa_{O2}/FI_{O2} ratio for the prediction of NIV failure.

12.2.3.3 Monitoring of Lung Functions and Ventilator Parameters During NIV

Special restrictions are important to be considered by the therapist when treating critically ill patients. The most important one is the safety and the patient's ability to cooperate during spirometry. Therefore limited lung functions and several ventilator parameters could be employed for NIV monitoring as follow [8]:

- Basic measurements include maximal inspiratory pressure (MIP), maximal voluntary ventilation (MVV), vital capacity (VC), Vt, and exhaled volume/breath (VE), which are commonly made to assess weanability.
- WOB, PTP, P0.1, and oxygen cost of breathing (O_2COB) may be of potential value for the difficult to wean patient (lack evidence).
- Measurement of air leaks, compliance, resistance, discomfort, mean airway pressure (MAP), and unintended positive end-expiratory pressure (autoPEEP) provides useful therapeutic and diagnostic information.

- Waveform monitoring reveals important patient-ventilator interactions such as lung overdistension, autoPEEP, presence of secretions, and patient effort. Waveform monitoring highlights important issues involved in the management of NIV patients to the close attention of the therapists.

12.2.4 Optimizing Ventilator Settings During NIV

The most common reasons for NIV failure include insufficient pressure support (PS) and PVD [54]. Before considering the failure of NIV, it is important to check that common technical issues have been identified and ventilator settings are optimized. While critically ill patients are treated, ventilator requirements get changed. Therefore, ventilator settings must be reviewed regularly. This allows optimizing ventilatory support through several interventions including; increasing PS, increasing inspiratory-flow trigger, adding PEEP, and using low RR for the helmet. Certainly, NIV settings must be optimized before increasing FiO_2 because the gas exchange will be enhanced with increased alveolar ventilation. If that is ineffective, or results in respiratory distress, FiO_2 must be temporarily increased with a senior review of all settings. Also, NAVA preserves spontaneous breathing and blood gases and minimizes PVD by reducing the cycling and triggering delays, especially at the high level of assistance [1]. Additionally, regular patient monitoring ensures a continuous check of the contributing factors for PVD such as water in the circuit, air leaks, and noise to make prompt corrections. The leak could be minimized by changing the mask type or making mask adjustments. Positional upper airway obstruction leads to ineffective NIV due to variable mask leak. Care is needed to ensure that head flexion is avoided, particularly in sleep (Table 12.4).

Table 12.4 Technical issues to optimize NIV delivery [7]

Problem	Causes	Solutions
Ventilator not triggering despite the visible patient effort	– Great mask leak – Inspiratory trigger sensitivity is very low	– Minimize mask leak – Adjust trigger – For NMD, switch to PCV
Ventilator cycling independently of patient effort	– Inspiratory trigger sensitivity is very high – Great mask leak	– Adjust trigger – Minimize mask leak
Chest/abdominal paradox	– Upper-airway obstruction	– Avoid neck flexion – Increase EPAP
Inadequate chest expansion despite apparent triggering	– Inadequate Vt	– Increase IPAP. – In NMD or CWD, apply longer Ti
Premature expiratory effort by patient	– Excessive IPAP or Ti	– Adjust as necessary

NMD neuro-muscular disease, *PCV* pressure-controlled ventilation, *EPAP* expiratory positive airway pressure, *Vt* tidal volume, *IPAP* inspiratory positive airway pressure, *CWD* chest wall disease, *Ti* inspiratory time

Finally, Patients who get benefits from NIV support during the first 4 h of treatment should receive NIV support for as long as possible (minimum of 6 h) during the first 24 h, and treatment is indicated until the acute cause is resolved (commonly 2–3 days). However, applying NIV support must not delay escalation to IMV if there is a deterioration of the case or persistent acidosis ($pH < 7.15$) despite attempts to optimize NIV support. The decision of patient intubation should be made within the first 4 h of starting NIV or sooner. Changes in ABG, RR, and HR are usually significant within this time. Moreover, IMV must be considered in patients suffering late NIV failure (failure after 48 h of NIV) rather than further NIV support [1].

12.2.5 Weaning from NIV

A weaning plan for NIV should start after normalization of pH and pCO_2 or a general improvement in the patient's clinical parameters as presented by $SpO_2 > 90\%$ on $FiO_2 \leq 50\%$, arterial $pH \geq 7.35$, $RR \leq 25$/min, systolic $BP \geq 90$ mmHg, $HR \leq 120$/min and absence of signs of respiratory distress (diaphoresis, agitation, and anxiety) following the first 24 h of treatment or longer [9].

The first possible NIV weaning strategy includes a stepwise reduction of the duration of NIV use. This strategy involves a gradual increase of the NIV free intervals over few days (usually 2–3 days) followed by complete removal of NIV (Fig. 12.2) [55]. British Thoracic Society/ Royal College of physicians (BTS/RCP) recommend a protocol which takes 4 days for weaning in which [9]:

- Day (1): patients receive NIV for as much as possible.
- Day (2): patients receive NIV for 16 h (including 6–8 h overnight).
- Day (3): patients receive NIV 12 h (including 6–8 h overnight).
- Day (4): NIV could be discontinued unless is clinically indicated.

The second NIV weaning strategy includes a stepwise reduction in the PS through a gradual reduction of IPAP and EPAP (2–4 cmH_2O) every 4–6 h. The NIV could be discontinued once the patient can tolerate IPAP of 6–8 cmH_2O and EPAP

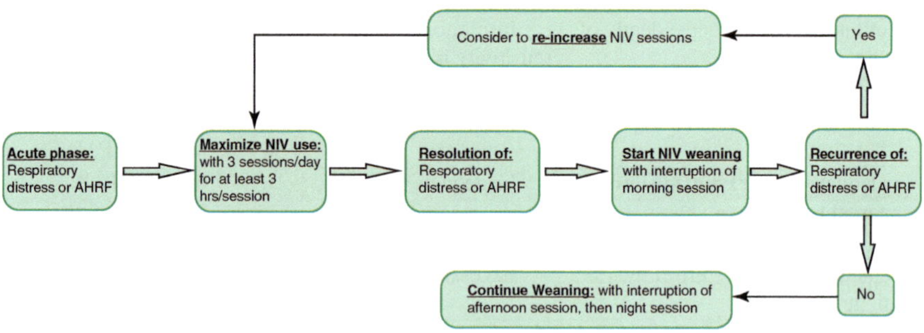

Fig. 12.2 Stepwise reduction of the duration of NIV use

of 4–6 cmH_2O [9]. The last NIV weaning strategy includes an immediate withdrawal of NIV once the patient meets the above-mentioned weaning criteria. It is not favored by clinicians owing to the highest failure rate leading to the reinstitution of NIV [9].

12.3 Conclusion

In conclusion, critically ill patients should be closely monitored until adequately stabilized. During IMV, the familiar "look, listen and feel" approach should be applied to assess the patient's clinical condition. Moreover, many regular investigations are essential including; pulse-oximetry, blood-gas analysis, peak-flow measurements, and regular check of ventilator parameters, spontaneous breathing, and ETT/TST. If the patient parameters meet the criteria for extubation, a weaning plan must start as soon as possible. SBT is the best method to evaluate patients' ability to breathe on their own. During NIV, clinicians must pay attention not only to gas exchange and vital signs but also to patient-ventilator interaction, air leaks, resistance, compliance, discomfort, lung functions, and ventilator parameters. Optimizing ventilatory support with patient requirements, accurate clinical/instrumental monitoring of PVD and proper choice of the patient interface is essential to minimize NIV failure risk. Once patient clinical parameters/lung functions get normalized, a NIV weaning plan could be started safely. NIV weaning strategies include a stepwise reduction of NIV duration, a stepwise reduction in PS, and immediate withdrawal of NIV.

Key Major Recommendations

1. In early ARDS, close monitoring is needed to avoid the high inspiratory effort to minimize VILI and P-SILI.
2. Adjustments of ventilation parameters should be made as early as possible to obtain a low level of inspiratory effort and to avoid myotrauma.
3. All patients started on IMV should be monitored closely for the efficacy of breathing, chest movement, WOB, accessory muscle use, the efficiency of ventilation, mental status, general appearance (particularly skin color), presenting symptoms, HR, dyspnea, and coexisting clinical features. Moreover, many regular investigations are essential including; pulse-oximetry, blood-gas analysis, peak-flow measurements and regular check of ventilator parameters (RR, FiO_2, Vt, PEEP, Minute ventilation, PIP, I:E ratio, ETCO2, humidifier temperature), spontaneous breathing (*P*es, occlusion maneuvers, EAdi and diaphragm ultrasound) and ETT / TST.
4. Daily screening of respiratory function ($PaO_2 / FIO_2 > 200$, PEEP ≤ 5, respiratory rate/ tidal volume < 100 with no vasopressors or sedatives) is an appropriate guide for starting an SBT as a start of IMV weaning.
5. All patients started on NIV should be monitored closely for SaO_2, pCO_2, pH, ABG, RR, HR, ECG monitoring (for possible cardiomyopathy), waveform

monitoring until adequately stabilized beside measurements of air leaks, resistance, compliance, discomfort, MAP, and autoPEEP.

6. Before considering NIV to have failed, NIV settings should be optimized by optimizing ventilatory support (increasing PS, adding PEEP, increasing inspiratory flow trigger, and using low respiratory rates for the helmet) and checking factors for PVD (air leaks, water in circuit, noise) and taken care of promptly (preferring NAVA). If that is ineffective then FiO_2 should be increased.
7. Basic measurements such as MIP, MVV, VC, Vt, and VE are commonly made to assess NIV weanability.

References

1. Spahija J, et al. Patient-ventilator interaction during pressure support ventilation and neurally adjusted ventilatory assist. Crit Care Med. 2010;38(2):518–26.
2. Yoshida T, et al. Spontaneous breathing during lung-protective ventilation in an experimental acute lung injury model: high transpulmonary pressure associated with strong spontaneous breathing effort may worsen lung injury. Crit Care Med. 2012;40(5):1578–85.
3. Goligher EC, et al. Evolution of diaphragm thickness during mechanical ventilation. Impact of inspiratory effort. Am J Respir Crit Care Med. 2015;192(9):1080–8.
4. Goligher EC, et al. Diaphragmatic myotrauma: a mediator of prolonged ventilation and poor patient outcomes in acute respiratory failure. Lancet Respir Med. 2019;7(1):90–8.
5. Dres M, et al. Coexistence and impact of limb muscle and diaphragm weakness at time of liberation from mechanical ventilation in medical intensive care unit patients. Am J Respir Crit Care Med. 2017;195(1):57–66.
6. Bertoni M, SS, Goligher EC. Monitoring patient respiratory effort during mechanical ventilation: lung and diaphragm-protective ventilation. In: Vincent JL, editor. Annual update in intensive care and emergency medicine. Springer; 2020.
7. Davidson AC, et al. BTS/ICS guideline for the ventilatory management of acute hypercapnic respiratory failure in adults. Thorax. 2016;71(Suppl 2):ii1–ii35.
8. Adams A. Pulmonary function in the mechanically ventilated patient. Respir Care Clin N Am. 1997;3(2):309–31.
9. Hadda V, Kumari R. Protocols for weaning from NIV: appraisal of evidence. Insights Chest Dis. 2016;1:14.
10. Steen C. Prevention of deterioration in acutely ill patients in hospital. Nurs Stand. 2010;24(49):49–57.
11. Jevon P, Ewens B, Pooni JS. Monitoring the critically ill patient. Wiley Online Library; 2012.
12. Lermitte J, Garfield MJ. Weaning from mechanical ventilation. Contin Educ Anaesth Crit Care Pain. 2005;5(4):113–7.
13. Fish E, et al. The esophageal pressure-guided ventilation 2 (EPVent2) trial protocol: a multicentre, randomised clinical trial of mechanical ventilation guided by transpulmonary pressure. BMJ Open. 2014;4(10):e006356.
14. Grieco DL, Chen L, Brochard L. Transpulmonary pressure: importance and limits. Ann Transl Med. 2017;5(14):285.
15. Kassis EB, Loring SH, Talmor D. Mortality and pulmonary mechanics in relation to respiratory system and transpulmonary driving pressures in ARDS. Intensive Care Med. 2016;42(8):1206–13.
16. Yoshida T, et al. Esophageal manometry and regional transpulmonary pressure in lung injury. Am J Respir Crit Care Med. 2018;197(8):1018–26.

17. Yoshida T, Amato MB, Kavanagh BP. Understanding spontaneous vs. ventilator breaths: impact and monitoring. Intensive Care Med. 2018;44(12):2235–8.
18. Protti A, et al. Lung stress and strain during mechanical ventilation: any difference between statics and dynamics? Crit Care Med. 2013;41(4):1046–55.
19. Amato MB, et al. Driving pressure and survival in the acute respiratory distress syndrome. N Engl J Med. 2015;372(8):747–55.
20. Carteaux G, et al. Bedside adjustment of proportional assist ventilation to target a predefined range of respiratory effort. Crit Care Med. 2013;41(9):2125–32.
21. Goligher EC, et al. Mechanical ventilation–induced diaphragm atrophy strongly impacts clinical outcomes. Am J Respir Crit Care Med. 2018;197(2):204–13.
22. Mauri T, et al. Esophageal and transpulmonary pressure in the clinical setting: meaning, usefulness and perspectives. Intensive Care Med. 2016;42(9):1360–73.
23. Bellani G, et al. Plateau and driving pressure in the presence of spontaneous breathing. Intensive Care Med. 2019;45(1):97–8.
24. Goldman M, et al. Mechanics of the human diaphragm during voluntary contraction: dynamics. J Appl Physiol. 1978;44(6):840–8.
25. Grassino A, et al. Mechanics of the human diaphragm during voluntary contraction: statics. J Appl Physiol. 1978;44(6):829–39.
26. Spadaro S, et al. A methodological approach for determination of maximal inspiratory pressure in patients undergoing invasive mechanical ventilation. Minerva Anestesiol. 2015;81(1):33–8.
27. Bertoni M, et al. A novel non-invasive method to detect excessively high respiratory effort and dynamic transpulmonary driving pressure during mechanical ventilation. Crit Care. 2019;23(1):1–10.
28. Telias I, Damiani F, Brochard L. The airway occlusion pressure (P 0.1) to monitor respiratory drive during mechanical ventilation: increasing awareness of a not-so-new problem. Intensive Care Med. 2018;44(9):1532–5.
29. Whitelaw WA, Derenne J-P, Milic-Emili J. Occlusion pressure as a measure of respiratory center output cm conscious man. Respir Physiol. 1975;23(2):181–99.
30. Holle R, Schoene RB, Pavlin E. Effect of respiratory muscle weakness on P0. 1 induced by partial curarization. J Appl Physiol. 1984;57(4):1150–7.
31. Rittayamai N, et al. Effect of inspiratory synchronization during pressure-controlled ventilation on lung distension and inspiratory effort. Ann Intensive Care. 2017;7(1):1–10.
32. Vargas F, et al. Respiratory failure in chronic obstructive pulmonary disease after extubation: value of expiratory flow limitation and airway occlusion pressure after 0.1 second (P0. 1). J Crit Care. 2008;23(4):577–84.
33. Kera T, Aihara A, Inomata T. Reliability of airway occlusion pressure as an index of respiratory motor output. Respir Care. 2013;58(5):845–9.
34. Alberti A, et al. P0. 1 is a useful parameter in setting the level of pressure support ventilation. Intensive Care Med. 1995;21(7):547–53.
35. Mauri T, et al. Control of respiratory drive and effort in extracorporeal membrane oxygenation patients recovering from severe acute respiratory distress syndrome. Anesthesiology. 2016;125(1):159–67.
36. Pletsch-Assuncao R, et al. Accuracy of invasive and noninvasive parameters for diagnosing ventilatory overassistance during pressure support ventilation. Crit Care Med. 2018;46(3):411–7.
37. Iotti GA, et al. Closed-loop control of airway occlusion pressure at 0.1 second (P sub 0.1) applied to pressure-support ventilation: algorithm and application in intubated patients. Crit Care Med. 1996;24(5):771–9.
38. Conti G, et al. Estimation of occlusion pressure during assisted ventilation in patients with intrinsic PEEP. Am J Respir Crit Care Med. 1996;154(4):907–12.
39. Sinderby C, et al. Neural control of mechanical ventilation in respiratory failure. Nat Med. 1999;5(12):1433–6.
40. Kim M, et al. Effects of lung volume and electrode position on the esophageal diaphragmatic EMG. J Appl Physiol. 1978;45(3):392–8.

41. Beloncle F, et al. A diaphragmatic electrical activity-based optimization strategy during pressure support ventilation improves synchronization but does not impact work of breathing. Crit Care. 2017;21(1):1–8.
42. Sinderby C, Liu S, Colombo D, et al. An automated and standardized neural index to quantify patient-ventilator interaction. Crit Care. 2013;17:R239.
43. Di Mussi R, Spadaro S, Mirabella L, et al. Impact of prolonged assisted ventilation on diaphragmatic efficiency: NAVA versus PSV. Crit Care. 2016;20:1.
44. Barwing J, Pedroni C, Olgemöller U, Quintel M, Moerer O. Electrical activity of the diaphragm (EAdi) as a monitoring parameter in difficult weaning from respirator: a pilot study. Crit Care. 2013;17(4):1–11.
45. Piquilloud L, Beloncle F., Richard JC, Mancebo J, Mercat A, Brochard L, Information conveyed by electrical diaphragmatic activity during unstressed, stressed and assisted spontaneous breathing: a physiological study [Internet]. Ann Intensive Care. 2019;9:89.
46. Bellani G, Mauri T, Coppadoro A, et al. Estimation of patient's inspiratory effort from the electrical activity of the diaphragm. Crit Care Med. 2013;41:1483–91.
47. Goligher EC, Laghi F, Detsky ME, et al. Measuring diaphragm thickness with ultrasound in mechanically ventilated patients: feasibility, reproducibility and validity. Intensive Care Med. 2015;41:642–9.
48. Regan EN, Dallachiesa L. How to care for a patient with a tracheostomy. Nursing. 2009;39(8):34–9.
49. Barnett M. A practical guide to the management of a tracheostomy. J Commun Nurs. 2008;22(12):24–6.
50. Truwit JD, Bernard GR. Noninvasive ventilation—don't push too hard. N Engl J Med. 2004;350:2512–5.
51. Bertoni M, Spadaro S, Goligher EC. Monitoring patient respiratory effort during mechanical ventilation: lung and diaphragm-protective ventilation. In: Vincent J-L, editor. Annual update in intensive care and emergency medicine. Cham: Springer International Publishing; 2020. p. 21–35.
52. Roberts C, et al. Non-invasive ventilation in chronic obstructive pulmonary disease: management of acute type 2 respiratory failure. Clin Med. 2008;8(5):517.
53. Carron M, et al. Predictors of failure of noninvasive ventilation in patients with severe community-acquired pneumonia. J Crit Care. 2010;25(3):540.e9–540.e14.
54. Harb HS, et al. Update efficacy of aerosol therapy with noninvasive ventilator approach (non-invasive ventilation and nasal high flow). J Drug Deliv Sci Technol. 2020;59:101922.
55. Faverio P, et al. Noninvasive ventilation weaning in acute hypercapnic respiratory failure due to COPD exacerbation: a real-life observational study. Can Respir J. 2019;2019:3478968.

GPSR Compliance

The European Union's (EU) General Product Safety Regulation (GPSR) is a set of rules that requires consumer products to be safe and our obligations to ensure this.

If you have any concerns about our products, you can contact us on ProductSafety@springernature.com

In case Publisher is established outside the EU, the EU authorized representative is:

Springer Nature Customer Service Center GmbH
Europaplatz 3
69115 Heidelberg, Germany

Batch number: 10732044

Printed by Printforce, the Netherlands